BMAT Worked Solutions: 2003 - 2019

Aroun Kalyana & Rhea Takhar

ISBN: 9798657391138
Email:bmatbook@gmail.com
Independently published

BMAT is a registered trademark of Cambridge Assessment Admissions Testing, which was not involved in the production of, and does not endorse, this book. The authors and publisher are not affiliated with BMAT, Cambridge Assessment Admissions Testing or the University of Cambridge Local Examinations Syndicate (UCLES). The answers, guidance and explanation in this book are purely the opinion of the authors, rather than being an official set of answers or the only way to answer the questions given, and this has neither been seen nor verified by Cambridge Assessment Admissions Testing.

Questions have been reproduced with the permission of Cambridge Assessment Admissions Testing. Please also note that the essays/essay plans were not written by candidates taking the BMAT exam under test conditions and have not been marked nor the commentaries prepared by accredited BMAT examiners.

All the information given in the book is correct as of the time of publishing. The authors do not accept any liability for the data provided in the book, or damages resulting from the use of the data in the book - the authors recommend you check with official BMAT websites to receive the most up to date information. This book contains links to third-party web sites that are not under the control of the authors. The authors are not responsible for the content of any linked site. Inclusion of a link in this book does not imply that the authors endorses or accepts any responsibility for the content of that third-party site.

The information given within the book is simply guidance, and any advice taken from this publication should be taken within this context. As such, the publishers and authors accept no liability for the outcome of applicants' BMAT performance, university applications or other losses. Every precaution has been taken in the preparation of the book - the authors or publishers accept no liability for errors or omissions of any kind. Neither is any liability assumed for damages resulting from the use of information contained herein. If any error has been inadvertently overlooked, the publishers will be happy to make the necessary amendments at the earliest opportunity. Your statutory rights are not affected

Contents Page

Introduction

What is the BMAT?
The BMAT, or BioMedical Admissions Test, is an admissions test that is sat by prospective applicants for entry into certain universities' medicine, dentistry, or biomedical sciences courses. The BMAT is a very important facet of these applications as it provides universities with further data to differentiate their applicants, many of whom already have very high GCSE (or equivalent) scores. It consists of a 2-hour written paper split into 3 sections:

Section 1 (*1 hour for 32 multiple choice questions*): Tests problem solving and critical thinking

Section 2 (*30 minutes for 27 multiple choice questions)*: Tests scientific knowledge typically covered in schools up to the age of 16 - knowledge of Biology, Maths, Chemistry and Physics is required, up to a standard similar to GCSE.

Section 3 (*30 minutes to write an essay, of length no greater than one side)*: This is an essay task which tests the students' ability to organise, collect and develop ideas and communicate them in a concise and effective style.

Therefore, it is essential for students to be well prepared before sitting this examination. The authors', who scored in the top 10% in the 2019 session, recommend that prospective applicants familiarise themselves with the test and its format, learn all the requisite information for Sections 1 and 2, and practice as many papers as possible. Before 2010, past papers followed a slightly different format, and quite a few questions examine content not on current specifications. Additionally, the essay questions before then differ in style to current essay questions, and therefore there is arguably little value gained from attempting those questions.

We recommend that you attempt the 2011-2019 papers first and attempt the previous past papers (2003-2010) if you have extra time and have attempted all the latest papers and the essay questions. Please note that for Section 2, the questions that test knowledge not currently on the BMAT specification are marked clearly on the past papers on the BMAT website and the worked solutions.

The BMAT website offers a wealth of resources which explain the format of the examination in detail, and the specification used. We recommend that you check the website for the latest information.

How do I prepare for the BMAT?
We recommend that you start preparing for the BMAT approximately 1-2 months before the exam. Remember to plan your time effectively as well, as you will also have other commitments in this busy period, such as putting together your UCAS application, and schoolwork amongst other things.

Introduction

By following the flowchart below, you are likely to be well prepared for and successful in your BMAT exam.

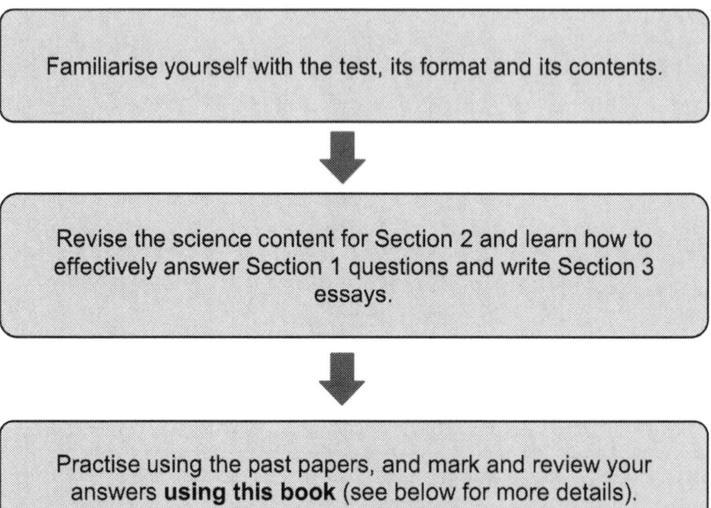

How do I use the BMAT past papers and this book?

All the BMAT past papers can be found free of charge on the BMAT website. Since the actual BMAT examination is a pen and paper examination, we recommend that you print off the papers to best simulate the examination experience. This will help you to build up stamina and enhance your on-the-day exam performance.

- Make sure you sit the exam papers in a quiet room, and remove any distractions, such as phones or computers
- Sit the exam under timed conditions. The BMAT is a time-pressured exam, and therefore it is best to practise all the papers under the same time-pressure
- Remember to mark your papers, and then **review your answers using this book**, so that you identify why you have made the mistake, and how to solve similar questions in the future.
- Keep a record of your scores, so you can see how you are doing and see yourself improving over time [This is always good motivation!] - see page **9** for a table in which you can input your scores.

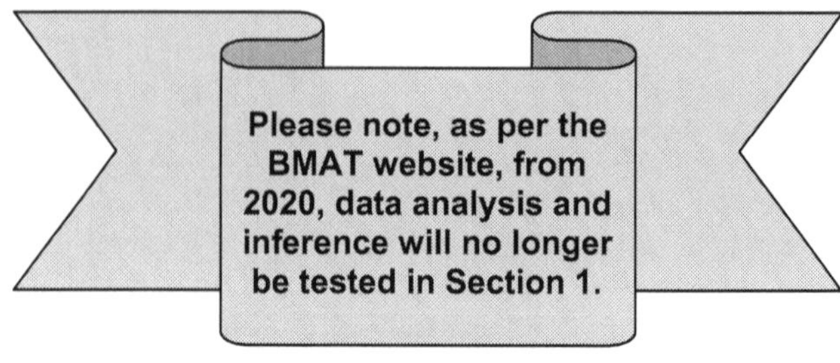

We suggest that you follow this procedure when attempting past papers:

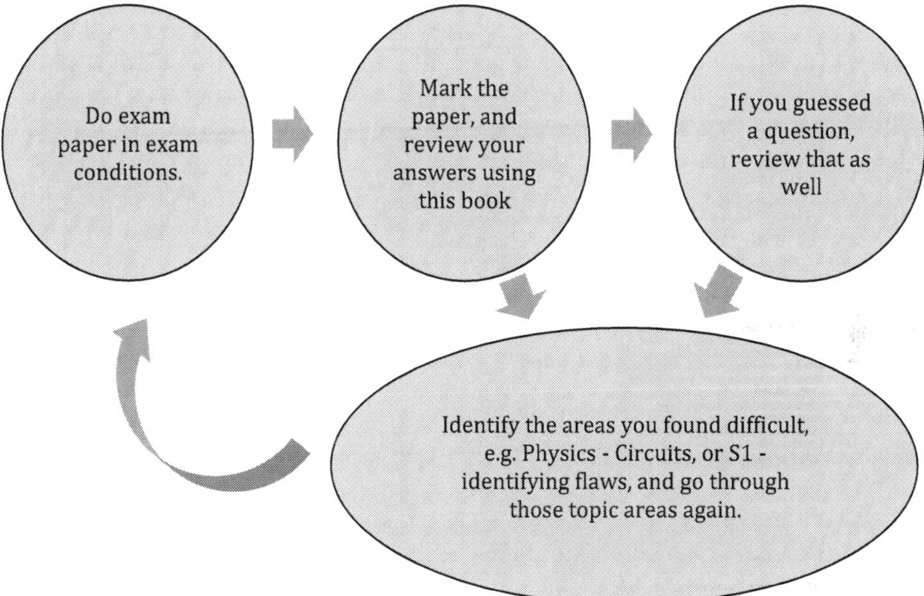

Essay Marking

Often it is difficult to mark your own essays, however, we offer a good value essay marking service. For more information, please email: **bmatbook@gmail.com**

September vs November session

This depends on personal preference and depends on which universities you hope to apply to that require the BMAT. Some universities only accept results from a specific sitting so make sure to check the requirements of each institution you are applying to. Try and spread your workload out, for example, if you are sitting UCAT examinations in the Summer, it may be advisable to sit your BMAT in the November sitting. However, if you are unsure of which universities to apply to, or want to be more tactical in selecting universities for your UCAS form, you may want to do the earlier sitting, as results for this session are usually released before the early UCAS deadline.

Ultimately the decision is a personal one, but regardless of the sitting in which you take your exams, you should thoroughly prepare for the exam.

A note about essay plans in this book

Due to copyright restrictions, we have not been able to reproduce the sub-parts for the questions from 2003-2016. Please use the links provided next to each question to see the individual sub-parts. For your ease, we have left spaces between each section of the essay plan, so that you can see which part of the plan corresponds to each of the 3 sub-parts of the question.

Introduction

Which universities use the BMAT?
At the time of printing, according to the BMAT website, the following universities need students to take the BMAT in either the August/September or October/November session:

University	Course
Brighton & Sussex Medical School	A100 Medicine
Chiang Mai University	Doctor of Medicine
Chulalongkorn University	Doctor of Medicine
Imperial College London	A100 Medicine
Keele University (only overseas for fees applicants)	A100 Medicine
Khon Kaen University	MD02 Medicine/MDX Medicine
King Mongkut's Institute of Technology, Ladkrabang	Medicine
Lancaster University	A100 Medicine & Surgery A100 Medicine & Surgery with Gateway Year
Lee Kong Chian School of Medicine	Medicine
Mahidol University	Medicine, Dentistry
Medical University of Warsaw	DM Doctor of Medicine DMD Doctor of Dental Medicine
Pirogov Russian National Research University	General Medicine Biology
University of Manchester (some international students)	A106 MBChB and A104 MBChB
Navamindradhiraj University	MD Doctor of Medicine
Nazarbayev University	MD
Srinakharinwirot University	A10S Doctor of Medicine
Suranaree University of Technology	MD Doctor of Medicine
Thanmasat University	642901 Doctor of Medicine 6420902 Doctor of Dental Surgery
University College London	A100 Medicine
University of Cambridge	A100 Medicine
University of Leeds	A100 Medicine, A200 Dentistry A101 Gateway Year to Medicine
University of Malaya	Medicine
University of Oxford	A100 Medicine, A101 Graduate Medicine BC98 Biomedical Sciences
Universidad de Navarra	Medicine
University of Pecs	Medicine, Dentistry
University of Rijeka	MD Medicine
University of Zagreb	Doctor of Medicine

Data source: https://www.admissionstesting.org/for-test-takers/bmat/bmat-november/

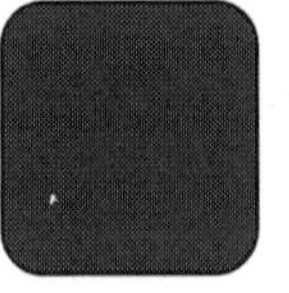

The authors would strongly advise students to double-check the BMAT website and/or the websites of the university for the most up-to-date information.

My Scores

Keeping track of your scores in a table like this will help you track your progress, (hopefully) provide you with some motivation, and importantly allow you to see which areas you need to improve on. We have only included a score grid for papers from 2011 onwards, as these papers are the same style as those you will sit in your examination. Feel free to use this model for the 2003-10 papers if you find this style helpful.

Past Paper	*Completed?*	Mark	Score	Areas I found difficult
Example	✓	*22/35*	*5.1*	*Identifying Assumptions, Circuits [resistors], Ecology [quadrats], Electrolysis [aqueous solutions],*
2011 **Section 1**				
2011 **Section 2**				
2012 **Section 1**				
2012 **Section 2**				
2013 **Section 1**				
2013 **Section 2**				
2014 **Section 1**				
2014 **Section 2**				
2015 **Section 1**				
2015 **Section 2**				
2016 **Section 1**				
2016 **Section 2**				
2017 **Section 1**				

2017 **Section 2**				
2018 **Section 1**				
2018 **Section 2**				
2019 **Section 1**				
Specimen **Section 1**				
Specimen **Section 2**				

Section 3 Year	**q1**		**q2**		**q3**	
	Completed?	**Score**	**Completed?**	**Score**	**Completed?**	**Score**
2011						
2012						
2013						
2014						
2015						
2016						
2017						
2018						
2019						
Specimen						

BMAT 2003

Section 1

Q1	E

It is a good idea to visualise the graph in these sorts of questions. Here, the graph tells you what will happen to the volume of the tank, as its depth (or height if it's easier to picture) increases. The extremities of the graph show that for a small increase in the height, there is a large increase in depth, whereas in the middle section, the depth increases significantly, but the volume only increases slightly, leading to answer option **E**.

Q2	C

The argument in this paragraph is the first line; the author wants ready meal packaging to convey health warnings, because they are '*not good for our long term health*'. Answer option C is the only one that links the reason with the conclusion, and only C strengthens the argument presented. Answer options A, B, D and E are not relevant here, as they do not give reasons for having health warnings on packaging.

Q3	B

General Method: 1 row and 1 column will not have the correct sum, and the value at which they intersect will be the incorrect value. So, add all the values in each row and column and compare with given totals.
Sum Year 7: 30 + 14 + 5 + 101 = 150 (therefore, no value in Y7 is wrong, eliminate A)
Sum Year 8: 33 + 16 + 12 + 89 = 150 (150 ≠ 145, therefore there is something wrong with Year 8)
Sum Cars: 30 + 33 + 16 + 10 = 107 (107 ≠ 102, therefore the wrong value is in this row)
The wrong value is in the car row, and Y8 column, therefore the wrong value is **33 (B)**

Q4	C

The paragraph says that the government is changing university funding from a grant to a loan (a form of debt). We later learn that poorer students are deterred from university because of debt, so we can reasonably infer **C**, that poorer students will be deterred because of the government's decision.

Q5	109

If he has a square grid, he must place a square number of cabbages on the ground. Let us call the number of cabbages he has x, and y the length of the side of the grid.
$x = y^2 + 9$ and $x = (y+1)^2 - 12$
We can equate the two equations together: $y^2 + 9 = (y+1)^2 - 12$
That leaves 20 = 2y, therefore y = 10
Putting that back into the original equation, x= 102 + 9 = **109**

Q6	D

The main conclusion of this paragraph is on lines 3-4: '*It may be undemocratic by favouring some political parties more than others*'. It goes on to say (backing up the above conclusion) that Internet voting would be undemocratic as parties with younger, educated voters would gain more votes (thereby discriminating against some sections of society) = **D**.

2003 Section 1

Q7	A

We need to do the average length of a surgery session/10 = 140/10 = 14 = **A**

Q8	27

(140 x 8.5) [*surgery*] + (408) [*home visits*] = 1598 (we round up to 1600, to make calculation easier)
60 mins in an hour so 1600/60 = 26.6666 which rounds up to **27 hours**

Q9	C

A doctor sees 155 patients a week, so in 50 weeks s/he will have 155 x 50 = 7750 appointments
10,000 [*total population*] / 5,000 [*number of doctors*] = 2,000 so each doctor will have 2,000 patients.
7,750/2,000 = 3.88 = 4 = **C**

Q10	D

We know the number of patients must stay the same, so the overall time doctors spend seeing them must stay the same. Therefore, we can form an equation:
5,000 165 = 4,500 y (we can divide by a factor of 1,000 to get an easier equation)
5 165 = 4.5 y therefore **y = 183 = D**

Q11	A

Compare the difference between the values for each data set (A-D) between 1995 and 2000. For **A**, the difference is the largest (165-140 = 25), therefore we can assume it has contributed the most.

Q12	A

The graph for A shows the data shown in the table - 135 patients a week in 1995 and 155 in 2000.

Q13	B

Let b be the number of people on the bus at the start:
First stop: ⅔b remains, Second stop: 4/9b remain, Third stop: 8/27b remain.
All these people get off at the 4th stop so 8/27b = 8, therefore **b = 18 = A.**

Q14	E

Flaw in the argument: **correlation ≠ causation**
The paragraph assumes with no evidence that there is a link between increasing internet use and increasing obesity and isolation. With no evidence proving a relationship, we can not assume that one causes the other, therefore E is the flaw. The focus of the argument is on disadvantages so A is not correct, B is incorrect since the concluding sentence does not mention only those who spend 8 hours a day, C is not relevant, and D is not relevant as there is no mention of computer games or the TV.

Q15	C

Two pools of six. Let us call the teams in one of the pools A, B, C, D, E and F. Drawing a table will help us visualise:

	A	B	C	D	E	F
A		2	2	2	2	2
B	2		2	2	2	2
C	2	2		2	2	2
D	2	2	2	2	2	2
E	2	2	2	2		2
F	2	2	2	2	2	

Thus, in each pool there are 30 matches, so 60 in total over the two pools (since the other pool will be identical to this one). Each team also plays every other team in the other pool, so 6 x 6 = 36. There is also a final, which is 1 match. Therefore 60+36+1 = 97 = **C**

Q16	C

This is a question testing GCSE maths knowledge. Graphs D and E do not show the line y = 5, therefore they cannot be correct. Only A and C show the line y = 2x, and only C satisfies the inequality, as only in this graph is the value of y greater than 2x.

Q17	B

The paragraph tells us of a negative relationship between number of nematode worms and concentration of fertiliser but does not give a reason to link the two. Since only B refers to the relationship, it is the correct answer. The rest offer explanations for the relationship found, and so cannot be justified by the claim as it does not mention any reason for the relationship.

Q18	5

Make sure you read the whole question before starting. 15 students are taking the BMAT, all of whom take Chemistry. We also know that 3 of these students take all 4 subjects. 13 candidates take Biology, therefore 2 don't and so must be taking Chemistry, Physics and Maths. To maximise the number of boys taking Maths and Physics, we can assume that the 3 who take all 4 are boys, and the 2 who don't take Biology are boys, giving us **5** as our answer.

Q19	D

Julie is therefore 1 hour ahead of Clare, so she will arrive 1 hour before Clare = D. [When Julie's clock reads 11am, Clare's clock will read 10am]

Q20	B

First identify the argument, which is that people should be persuaded to seek medical advice earlier. However, option B says that early consultations '*incurs high costs in doctor's times*', weakening the argument, as it provides a reason why early consultations may not always be beneficial. A, E, D and C are not relevant to the main argument in the text.

2003 Section 1

Q21	7.2

The difference between the two animal's speeds is 50km/h, and we want to work out how long it will take for the cheetah to make up the 100m time difference. Therefore, we work out how long it will take a cheetah to travel 100m, at a speed of 50km/h. Using the formula time = distance/speed, we get 0.1/50 = 0.002 hours, which is 7.2 seconds (multiply hours by 3600 to get seconds)

Q22	E

From the dates given we know the Roman settlement must have existed from at least 88-157AD. Only E supports this, so is the correct answer. C isn't correct, because it could have existed before 88AD (coins could have been made before that haven't been found for example).

Q23	B

Conclusion: '*The habitats of wading birds will therefore inevitably decline if gardening continues to be so popular'.* This statement assumes that gardeners will carry on using peat, and reject alternatives, which is paraphrased by B.

Q24	C

We learn that the Fair E coefficient '*measures the degree of inequality in the distribution of income in a given society'*. The coefficient rises between 1982-2002, and therefore income inequality hasn't decreased, therefore C is correct.

Q25	D

A is incorrect as there is no evidence to say that the rise in inequality is due to fiscal policy.
B is incorrect as it is too vague.
C is incorrect as we don't know what 'better off' specifically refers to; does it mean better nutrition for example?
D is correct as poorer people on Chart 1 have seen a net gain in incomes, but income inequality has increased, and so the richer people must have seen an even bigger increase in income.
E is incorrect as poverty is not mentioned.

Q26	E

Statement 1 could be correct, as the poor haven't increased their incomes as much as they could have, and that is why there is still great income inequality.
Statement 2 is correct for the same reason as D in the previous question (the incomes of the rich have increased more than those of the poor).
Statement 3 could be correct and could explain the increase in income inequality (Fair-E coefficient).

Q27	C

The greater the coefficient, the more unequal a society is. Poland's is 0.2, Ruritania is 0.35, USA is 0.4 and Panama's is 0.6 therefore the order from most equal to least equal is C.

Q28	B

Flaw in the argument: correlation ≠ causation. B explains this.

Q29	E

If the probability of choosing a red sweet is 30%, then the probability of choosing a blue or yellow sweet is 70%. The probability of choosing a blue is then 140/3% and choosing a yellow is 70/3%. So if there were 10 sweets, 3 would be red, 7/3 would be yellow, and 14/3 would be blue. We can't have fractions of sweets, so multiply all by 3, giving a total of 30 [10 x 3]

Q30	C

1 is correct as a maximum of 30% work in the commercial service or both services, means 70% work in only the public health service. 70% > 30% therefore 2 is correct. There is no information about time spent in each service, therefore 3 isn't correct.

Q31	A & C

Put every statement in terms of Anne. A says that Anne is either the same age as or younger than Susan. B says that Anne is older than Susan. C says that Anne is either the same age as or younger than Susan. D says that Anne is older or the same age as Susan. A = C.

Q32	E

Conclusion: '*The government....patterns*'. The evidence for this is that there will be huge consequences for road planning etc, but this assumes that these changes will be long term, and so need to be dealt with, when the scale of the phenomenon is not explicitly mentioned.

Q33	D

1st turn: B > D and C > A. The halfway scores show us that Drumbeat must have been in 3rd position or higher by the first turn, and the last furlong tells us that Bistro must not have been first by the first turn. So CBDA is the starting order, which means that BCAD is the finishing order, which is D.

Q34	C

For 400cm^3 water, 50cm^3 concentrate is needed (water/8 = concentrate). Therefore, C is needed.

Q35	C

At the start up to year 5, deaths > births, so population decreases. After year 5, births > deaths, so population increases. C shows this.

Q36	B

If year 9 is 455AD, then year 72 is 63 years later, so 455+63 = 518AD = B

Q37	C

It says that Gildas was born in the year of the battle of Badon, so knowing his birth date would confirm the date of the battle.

Q38	B

455 + 84 = 539 AD = date according to Welsh Annals
539 - 28 = 511 AD = actual date = B

Q39	506 AD

Maelgwn died in 549AD (455 + 94), and Gildas was 43 at the time of writing the book. If we're looking for the latest date that Gildas was born (and the Battle took place), it would be 549-43 = 506AD.

Q40	C

The last paragraph tells us that the Welsh Annals and dates given by Gildas show that Gildas wrote his book after Maelgwn died, which is only shown in C.

2003 Section 2

Q1	B

Starch starts digestion in the mouth, protein starts digestion in the stomach, and fat starts digestion in the small intestine (duodenum), so B is the answer.

Q2	E

The mass of an atom of uranium is $4 \times 10^{-25} \times 10^{6} = 4 \times 10^{-19}$ milligrams
Then we must multiply by 8 million giving $4 \times 10^{-19} \times 8 \times 10^{6} = 32 \times 10^{-13}$mg = 3.2×10^{-12}mg = **E**

Q3	a – 2, b – 9, c - 6

We use equations in this situation.
3a = 6 so a = 2. 6a = 2c, therefore c = 6, and 2b = 12 + c = 18, so b = 9.

Q4	B

This question tests knowledge not currently on the BMAT specification.
Clockwise moment = anticlockwise moment.
500 x 0.2 = (200 x 0.4) + (200 x x) [note length needs to be in m, not in cm]
20 = (200 x x)
x = 20/200 = 0.1m

Q5	D

At pH 5, methyl orange will be yellow. At pH 5, bromothymol blue will be yellow. At pH 5, phenolphthalein will be colourless. Therefore, yellow will be seen.

Q6	76.8 kJ

We need the following formulae: weight = mass x g and kinetic energy = 1/2 x mass x velocity^2.
Mass = 6000/10 = 600kg. Inputting this into the second equation, we get:
KE = 0.5 x 600 x 16^2 = 76800J = 76.8kJ

Q7	B

Oestrogen stimulates the production of LH, which thus triggers ovulation. Therefore, oestrogen will be highest in B.

Q8	A, C, B, D

This question tests knowledge not currently on the BMAT specification.
Resistors in parallel have lower resistance (because they have the same voltage but a lower current flowing through them) than resistors in series. D will have the highest resistance and A the least therefore. C is more parallel than B, and so the order is A, C, B, D.

Q9	B

First work out the limiting reagent. moles = mass/Mr, so n(hydrogen) = 4.5 and n(nitrogen) = 2. Therefore, we can see that hydrogen is the limiting reagent, as 2 moles of nitrogen need 6 moles of hydrogen to react completely, but we only have 4.5 moles. Therefore, [(4.5 x 2/3) = 3] moles of ammonia are produced. 3 moles of ammonia have a mass of 51g (using mass = moles x Mr)

Q10	B

This is an exponential curve, the general shape of which should be learnt.

Q11	A

Again, these properties need to be learnt. The frequency of the wave does not change during reflection, refraction or diffraction.

Q12	A

In this reaction, two hydrogen atoms are lost, meaning this is an oxidation reaction, as a definition of oxidation is loss of hydrogen.

Q13	D

This question tests knowledge not currently on the BMAT specification.
We create a quadratic inequality as follows: $x^2 - 8 + 2x \geq 0$
We then factorise the LHS: $(x+4)(x-2) \geq 0$
This graph has roots at $x = -4$ and $x = 2$, and since it has a positive x squared term, it is a 'happy' parabola. The inequality asks for the part of the graph above 0, which would be when $x \geq 2$or when $x \leq -4$. Drawing a rough sketch for these questions can help if you are unable to visualise the graph in your head.

Q14(i)	3, 4 & 5

The condition must be recessive as the offspring of 1 and 2 do not have the disease. If the disease was dominant, 4 and 5 would also have to have the condition, as 2 has the condition. Therefore, call G the dominant allele (unaffected) and g the recessive allele (has the condition). Individual 2 is gg, therefore individuals 4 and 5 must have at least one g allele. They must also have one G allele, since otherwise they would have the condition. So 4 and 5 are Gg and are heterozygotes. The only way that 7 can have the disease is if both parents are heterozygous, or if one is recessive. Therefore 3 must also be heterozygous.

Q14(ii)	E

We worked out 3 and 4 are both Gg. Therefore, there is a 25% chance the offspring is GG, a 50% chance the offspring is Gg and a 25% the offspring the individual is gg (has the condition). There is a 50% chance the offspring is female, therefore 0.5 x 0.25 = 0.125 = 12.5%

Q15	4 minutes

Initial count rate = 140 - 20 = 120
After 12 minutes, count rate was 35 - 20 = 15
There were 3 half lives in 12 minutes, so half-life is 4 minutes.

Q16	C

At 70°C, 136g dissolves. Since only 80g was added, all will dissolve. Solubility is measured per 100g of water, yet we are using 200g of water. Therefore, we will need to see at what temperature the solution will become saturated (i.e. when only 40g can dissolve), and this occurs at 46°C. At 20°C, only 27g can dissolve. Therefore, 40-27 = 13. However, we have 200g of water, so 13 x 2 = 26g.

Q17	E

There are many formulas which include voltage. The ones you need to know are voltage = energy/charge, voltage = current resistance, voltage = power/current, voltage = $\sqrt{power\ x\ resistance}$. Only E cannot be made using these equations, therefore E is the answer.

Q18	**1st - jugular vein, 2nd – E, 3rd – B, 4th – C, 5th – A, 6th - D**

Upon leaving the head in the jugular vein, the ADH would flow towards the heart (as veins flow towards the heart). Therefore, after the jugular vein, the first vessel it would flow through is the **vena cava** (E) as that is the major vein flowing to the heart. After flowing through the vena cava, the ADH would flow through the right atrium, right ventricle and then through the **pulmonary artery** (B) to the lungs, where the blood it is in would get oxygenated. It would leave the lungs in the **pulmonary vein** (C), where it would reach the left atrium, and then flow onto the left ventricle. Upon leaving the left ventricle, it would flow through the **aorta** (A), and then would enter the **renal artery** (D), in order to reach the kidney, and the nephron.

Q19	C

This question tests knowledge not currently on the BMAT specification.

First, rearrange the equation given in terms of Energy, giving us: E = f x h.

To work out the frequency (the number of waves that a pass a given a point per second), we need to work out how many multiples of 1×10^{-13} seconds there are in 1 second, which is 1×10^{13}. Therefore, the frequency is $5 \times (1 \times 10^{13}) = 5 \times 10^{13}$ Hz.

$E = f \times h = (5 \times 10^{13}) \times (6.63 \times 10^{-34}) = 33.15 \times 10^{-21} = 3.315 \times 10^{-20} = 3.32 \times 10^{-20}$.

Q20	C

The atom has two shells, and therefore is in period 2. The atom has 4 electrons in its outer shell and therefore must be in group 4.

Q21	E

This question tests knowledge not currently on the BMAT specification.

For this question you need to know that the biceps are involved in flexion (upward movement) and is located on the front of the humerus (on the left of the humerus on the diagram). Similarly, the triceps is involved in extension (the downward movement) and is located on the back of the humerus (on the right on the diagram). Therefore, for the upward movement, the load is furthest on the left (and exerts force downwards), the effort is in the middle (the biceps), and the fulcrum is the elbow (furthest right), which is shown by diagram 3. For the downward movement, the load again is on the left (but this time the effort of the load is upwards), the fulcrum is in the middle (the elbow), and the effort is on the left (the triceps are contracting, and pulling upwards). This is shown by diagram 5.

2003 Section 2

Q22	E

This question tests knowledge not currently on the BMAT specification.
1 and 2 are correct as increasing the speed of rotation of the oil increases the frequency and the amplitude. 3 is incorrect as increasing the speed of rotation does not affect the size of the magnetic field in a generator.

Q23	E

As the atomic number increases, the size of the atom increases, and so does the number of electron shells. This means that the outer/valence electron is further away from the nucleus, so there is a weaker force of attraction between the nucleus and the valence electron, so it is more easily removed. Therefore, the answer is E.

Q24	C

During exhalation, the intercostals relax, the **ribcage moves down and in**, the **diaphragm relaxes and goes dome shaped (more convex)** meaning the **volume of the thorax decreases**. This means the **pressure in the thorax increases**, so air rushes out.

Q25	B

$$\left(\frac{2x^{3/2}y^3}{\sqrt{z}}\right)^2 = \left(\frac{2^2x^3y^6}{z}\right) = \left(\frac{4x^3y^6}{z}\right)$$

Q26	C

After blood passes through Organ X, we can see that there is more CO_2, less salt, less glucose, less oxygen and far less urea. This tells us that Organ X is the kidneys, as it functions to remove wastes from the body. (NB: the reduction in glucose and oxygen is because the kidney respires aerobically). The main difference in the blood before and after it passes Organ Y is that there is a lot more oxygen after passing through the organ than before. Therefore, Y must be the lungs.

Q27	A

We can immediately rule out B and D because drag (air resistance) can never be negative. The parachutist will fall until he/she reaches a terminal velocity. As the parachute opens, the drag will increase sharply, as the parachute provides a lot more air resistance, slowing the parachutist down until they reach a new lower terminal velocity. A is the correct answer because at the newer, lower terminal velocity, the drag force will still be the same, as the weight does not change. Therefore, the drag force will be the same before and after the parachute opens (which is the spike in the graph).

Q28	C

We know that the total positive charges must equal the total negative charges, as the compound is electrically neutral. A is incorrect as it would lead to a final charge of 2- (+2 -3 -1), B is incorrect as it would lead to a final charge of 1- (+6 -6 -1), and D is incorrect as it would lead to a final charge of +3 (+14 – 10 -1). Therefore, only 3 is correct as +10 – 9 – 1 = 0.

Q29	A

For this question, you need to be able to recall the sine rule, and the value for sine 45 ($\frac{1}{\sqrt{2}}$), and sin 60 ($\frac{\sqrt{3}}{2}$),

$\frac{PR}{\sin 45} = \frac{\sqrt{6}}{\sin 60}$, so $PR = \sin 45 \frac{\sqrt{6}}{\sin 60}$, so $PR = \frac{\sqrt{6}}{\sqrt{2}\sin 60}$,

$PR = \frac{2\sqrt{6}}{\sqrt{2}\sqrt{3}} = \frac{2\sqrt{6}}{\sqrt{6}} = 2$

2003 Section 3

To see the marking grid and mark bands that the BMAT examiners will use to mark your essays, please refer to the BMAT website. *To view the full questions, please see:*
https://www.admissionstesting.org/for-test-takers/bmat/preparing-for-bmat/practice-papers/

Explain what you think the author means by the term 'ethical market'.

The 'ethical market' refers to the purchasing and selling of goods (in this case organs) in a moral manner, which prevents the exploitation of people. The article even provides its own definition – 'There *would be only one purchaser, which would buy all organs and distribute according to some fair conception of medical priority. There would be no direct sales, no exploitation of low-income countries and their populations.'*

There are many problems with the legalised sale of organs. For example, even though the article claims that 'exploitation' will not occur, offering money for organs will incentivise lower income groups to sell their organs, as those groups need money the most. This may propagate poverty, as low-income organ donors, are at more risk of illness, and poor health, and can trap themselves and their families in a cycle of poverty.
The legalised sale of organs leads to the issue of removal of the organ. This is a complex, and often expensive, procedure and the organ donor will need extensive pre-operative check-ups and post-operative care. If organs were for sale, donors may wish to make the most profit possible, and thus skimp on such essential care, which could be detrimental to their health, and also amplifies the issue of exploitation of those on low incomes.

However, organ donation also has benefits, as the article points out. Legalising the sale of organs could help solve the current shortage of organs that many countries face. Additionally, many may feel that legalising organ sale is actually in line with the 4 pillars of medical ethics; firstly, as long as patient autonomy is respected, it can in fact be ethical, and as other lives are saved, it can be seen under beneficence.

In conclusion, how ethical legalised organ sale is depends on your own personal viewpoint – just ensure that you back up your point of view. Perhaps what may be key for an 'ethical market' to truly be in place, is if there is sufficient organisation and regulation of the market.

Authors' Tip:

Organ sale and organ donation are very interesting topics, and commonly feature in medical school interview ethics questions (or stations for MMI interviews). We strongly suggest you have a look online for information, and the following websites may be useful starting points:
https://www.ncbi.nlm.nih.gov/pmc/articles/PMC3291132/
https://www.medicalnewstoday.com/articles/282905
https://www.organdonation.nhs.uk/helping-you-to-decide/about-organ-donation/faq/what-is-the-opt-out-system/

2003 Section 3

A little learning is a dangerous thing. (*Alexander Pope*)

The statement means that small amounts of learning/knowledge can be harmful when the person does not know the complete picture, or when the person doesn't know enough. This is because knowing something about a particular topic may give someone misguided confidence that they know what they are talking about, and they may then act upon it, which could lead to potentially dangerous effects. For example, if a patient decided to start a course of treatment themselves, having read very little about their symptoms/condition/treatments on the internet, dangerous side effects could occur. Other examples of when little learning can be dangerous include a pilot wanting to fly a plane loaded with passengers, after just having read about how to fly a plane or having just conducted basic training on a flight simulator. The statement also implies therefore, that not knowing anything about a specific subject area is better than knowing very little, for the fear of the person thinking they are an expert on that subject, based on very little knowledge.

However, sometimes 'a little learning is *not* a dangerous thing'. It may be useful, or indeed essential, to have basic knowledge about certain subject areas, and it may not be entirely realistic to expect people to be in one of two extremes, that of knowing absolutely nothing and that of being an expert.

- First Aid is a common example for this. Being able to perform simple first aid techniques such as bandaging, abdominal thrusts or CPR without knowing the mechanisms behind it is still useful, and would be a helpful skill to know (as opposed to being harmful), as it could potentially save a life.
- Having a basic command of a language when you go abroad can be useful as you will be able to communicate in simple situations, and ask basic questions, such as directions, which may be helpful in certain situations, for example when no one else can speak English.

(The more original the examples, the better your essay will be – make sure any examples you use are concise and relevant to the question!!)

What can determine whether or not little learning is a dangerous thing is the mindset of the learner. If the learner thinks that they are an expert having learnt very little about a subject, and then goes on to act using that basic knowledge in a way that they have not been trained for and with misguided confidence, then potentially that learning will be dangerous. However, if someone learns very little, and understands the limitations of their knowledge, then any task that they perform with that in mind is unlikely to be harmful, as they understand how much of a task is within their scope of understanding. Additionally, the difficulty of a subject area is another factor to be considered. Knowledge about basic, day-to-day tasks, is unlikely to be harmful, but more complex knowledge, like that of flying a plane, or medical surgery needs to be understood fully before the action is undertaken, and in those situations, a little knowledge could be harmful.

It is ridiculous to treat the living body as a mechanism.
The above statement implies that since the living body is so complex, it would be foolish to generalise and regard the human body as simply one large mechanism (or even a series of many mechanisms).

The human body is made up of many different physiological systems, such as the respiratory or the endocrine systems, and many medical schools teach medicine as a 'systems-based' approach. Therefore, many doctors view it useful to take individual parts of the body, and treat them like mechanisms or systems, as this aids in learning, diagnosis and treatment.

However, many people point out the principle of 'emergent properties', where the whole is greater than the sum of its parts. Even though the body may be made up of many different systems, than can be seen as mechanisms, when they come together, through their synergistic interactions, a more complex entity (the living body) is formed, which therefore can't be viewed as a (simple) mechanism. Additionally, the term mechanism implies consistency and uniformity, whereas disease manifests itself in different ways in different people and affects their quality of life in different ways, so a mechanistic approach to the human body may not always be useful. Also, many aspects of the living body, such as the mind, emotion and memory storage may not be able to thought of mechanistically, and as they are constituent parts of the body, some may argue that the body can't be treated as a mechanism.

In conclusion, viewing the body as one single mechanism may not be too helpful due to its complex nature. However, the body can be seen as made up of many different mechanisms, that work together synergistically to create the living human body. It is important to note however, that, a doctor must also view the person holistically, and subjectively on a case by case basis, when coming up with treatment plans, and when trying to treat disease, as simply an objective, mechanistic view would not be sufficient.

2003 Section 3

Our belief in any particular natural law cannot have a safer basis than our unsuccessful critical attempts to refute it. (Karl Popper)

The statement argues that the best way to be sure about any law or theory is by being able to refute/disprove any arguments or conjectures against it. For example, Popper would say that the best way to prove a theory is to see if there are situations where it doesn't hold. Popper here suggests that this may be more useful than actually finding any positive evidence for the theory (since this in turn, may actually be disproven!).

However, some scientific experiments work on the basis of trying to prove a hypothesis, as opposed to refute one. They work on the basis that proof is needed for something to be deemed true or correct, and that falsification alone will not necessarily indicate that this theory is the correct one (just that the others are wrong). For example, Harvey's experiments proved how the body's circulation worked through direct observation and experimentation, as opposed to falsification.

Popper's statement reflects one aspect of the scientific method, the need for continual testing and experimentation, and that in order for a hypothesis to be scientific, it needs to be able to be testable, and in theory falsified. However, many would say that falsification alone cannot describe the scientific method fully, as experimentation to provide evidence for a fact is needed, and falsification alone may not be sufficient proof.

Authors' Tip:

The BMAT website have provided sample answers with commentary to the following questions (https://www.admissionstesting.org/Images/377965-specimen-section-3-sample-responses-with-examiner-comments.pdf). It is helpful to read those answers and commentaries to show you what the examiners want to see in high scoring answers.

BMAT 2004

Section 1

Q1	C

Splitting A with 2 diagonal lines across opposing corners makes 4 triangles. Splitting B with 3 lines going from the midpoint of each side to the adjacent one gives rise to the arrangement. D is made by drawing two vertical lines at the corners of the top of the trapezium and then by drawing a diagonal from the top left to bottom right corner. E can be made by drawing a vertical line down from the top of the arrow to a horizontal line across the square section of the arrow. Finally, a diagonal from the top right corner of the square to the bottom left gives the arrangement. Thus, by elimination C is the answer.

Q2	C

A is not relevant as the argument makes no reference to preference of fatty foods to fruit and vegetables; it merely compares price. B is incorrect because advertisement is not related to the conclusive statement in the passage. C however links directly to the argument because it shows that the whole premise: taxation in order to improve health; is a strong argument; hence why it is correct. D limits the scope to children which is not what the passage does, and E would not strengthen the argument at all; it is entirely unrelated to the conclusion.

Q3	B

To tackle this question, we can approach it systematically. Reading down through the information we can hypothesise that all of the 40 slot-headed screws are 3mm in diameter. This leaves a remainder of 30 that are cross headed and 3mm in diameter. Then, of that 30, we can hypothesise that 5 are 35mm long and 15 are 20mm long, this leaves us with 10 cross-headed, 3mm wide and 50mm long screws.

Q4	A

This is a common type of question: correlation does not equal causation. The answer is A because it hits right at the aforementioned flaw.

Q5	C

This question requires us to set up 2 simultaneous equations: one for Tom and one for Suki regarding their speed. We know speed = distance/time and the equating factor is distance which is 2km. We can call Suki's speed s and Suki's time t.
So, for Tom:
2km = 4s x (t - 0.25 hours). The reason it is 0.25 hours is because Tom cuts off 15 mins of journey time as he leaves later and arrives earlier, and 15 minutes is 0.25 hours.
For Suki:
2km = s x t
Equating and solving simultaneously for the 2 unknowns gives t = 1/3 hour and s = 6km/h
Remember Suki has been walking for 10 mins when Tom leaves so distance = 6km/h x 1/6 hour which gives 1km.

2004 Section 1

Q6	E

A is incorrect as the passage does not assume this, it just states that for those with allergies to animals it isn't appropriate to keep pets; not that they can never have pets.
B is wrong, the passage says, '*everyone who can own a pet, should do so'* and this is the argument in the singular, the passage never refers to the idea of having multiple pets.
C is wrong, the passage states that people '*tend to live longer'* if they keep pets, and that the explanation '*seems to be'* that factors including the '*emotional benefits of affectionate relationships'* do this. But the use of '*seem'* and '*tend'* are conditional, not as absolute as the word '*always'* used in C.
D is wrong as you could have a scenario where one may be allergic to a pet but still appreciate the benefits that the argument has to offer.
E is correct, the argument assumes that everyone should try to live longer because that is the whole point of the reasoning of the passage; to say that having pets tends to correlate with living longer.

Q7	D

Firstly, subtract the cost of the materials Alf bought from what the client paid Bill: £780 - £240 = £540. This means the total profits were £540 between Alf and Bill. The question tells us they split the profits equally meaning Bill and Alf each deserve half of £540 which is £270. However, the question tells us Bill was already paid £780 by the client, and if he only deserves £270 of this, then he owes Alf the remainder; £780 - £270 = £510.

Q8	12.0, 12.5 or 13.0

To do this we can add up the values from the graph (for both men and women together) and this gives us (in millions) approximately 1.2 + 0.1 + 1.4 + 0.3 + 0.8 +1.4 + 0.8 + 1.2 + 0.8 + 5 = 13. These are rounded up values for each bar hence why there are 2 other answers you could have obtained.

Q9	A

We can read from the table that the total number of days spent in hospital for cancer was about 4.3 million and that the total number of episodes of care was 1.4 million for cancer by reading off the graph. If men and women spent equal average times in hospital this means all we need to calculate is the total number of days spent in hospital for cancer/total number of episodes of care in hospital. This comes to 4.3 million days /1.4 million episodes which is about 3.1 days per episode.

Q10	A

We already know that the total episodes of care for cancer is 1.4 million. Thus, lung cancer accounts for 1/7 of 1.4 million coming to 200,000. If the incidence among men is 50% higher for men than women, we know the ratio of episodes men: women is 1.5: 1 or 3:2. This means men count for 3/5 of all episodes; 3/5 of 200,000 is 120,000. It is also worth noting that A is the only answer below 200,000 so you can actually arrive at the answer without needing to do the second stage of calculation.

Q11	A & C

A would directly reduce staying times in hospital for cancer compared to diseases of the circulatory system.
B is wrong because this would in fact counter the effect stated in the question. By increasing the episodes of care for circulatory diseases this actually means that the length of stay per episode is decreased which wouldn't contribute to the difference, it would actually make the two values closer.
C is correct, using similar reasoning to A it means that the length of stay for circulatory diseases is greater than that of cancer treatment.
D is wrong, the number of people who die doesn't have a bearing on the length of time they stay in hospital to receive treatment for their respective diseases during the time that they are alive.

Q12	B & C

John could have answered 6 questions correctly, and 6 with no answer, earning him 6(3) + 6(0) = 18 points. This is the minimum that he could've scored in order to make 18 so we can eliminate A as a result. He could also have scored 7 points correctly, giving him 21 points, and he could have scored 3 incorrectly and not answered 2 to give 18.
However, if John scores 8 points correctly this gives him 24 points. Even if he got the remaining 4 questions incorrect, this would give him 20 points which is not what the question asks for, the question already states that John scores 18 overall. E would give John 9(3) = 27 points, and even if the remaining 3 were incorrect, this would be a total of 24 points which is too many. Hence D and E are wrong as they both give John too many points.

Q13	B

The question wants to know about water as a condition for life as we know it. The passage tells us: '*life as we knew it which began in water, would not exist*' when referring to the importance of the structure of ice. Thus, water ice must be a necessary condition for life so we can eliminate A and D. However, water ice is not sufficient for life itself, so B is correct.

Q14	B

This is a visualisation question requiring you to try and fold up the piece of cardboard in your head. B cannot be formed because of the relationship between the sides with 2 dots and 4 dots. The only way those sides can be adjacent is if the one with 2 dots borders the one with 4 dots with only 1 dot on that side. However, on B both of the 2 dots are closest to the 4-dot side which cannot be.

Q15	D

A is not suggested, just because an argument for animal experimentation is presented, it doesn't mean animal rights are less important than human rights.
B is wrong because the passage gives an example of where animals MAY benefit, but equally animals could experience harm in other ways which aren't mentioned.
C is wrong as there is not clear justification for '*all*' animal experiments as the passage states itself; look out for the strong language here.
D is correct, it matches the conclusion expressed in the last sentence of the passage: '*if the animal population as a whole derives benefit from experiments on only a small minority of animals, those experiments are morally acceptable*'. This is summed up by C.
E is wrong as the conclusion of the passage as explored above already tells us that research can take place, and this includes non-medical research.

Q16	A

In any scenario, if we consider David, we know that he started at 70kg and if he gained weight more than 5kg this places him as heaviest at over 75kg as we know that all of the others lost at least 5kg. This is why all the answers show him as heaviest.
We are told Colin lost more weight than Annie and Barbara and as he was 2rd heaviest to begin with and she was the heaviest this must mean that Colin has to finish lighter than Barbara. Hence A is correct.

Q17	A

The conclusion of the passage is in the first sentence; that '*the worst of what ensued'* is that '*it isn't yet history'*. This is summarised by A; as the worst aspect of the spill is that its consequences aren't over.
C can't be asserted from the information in the passage. Although B, D and E may be true, they don't reflect the main conclusion of the passage.

Q18	C

The surface area of the 1cm^3 cube (10mm x 10mm x 10mm = 1000mm^3) in cm is 1cm x 1cm x 6 faces = 6cm^2
The surface area of the 0.0001mm^3 cube in cm^2 is 0.01cm x 0.01cm x 6 = 0.0006cm^2
The number of 0.0001mm^3 cubes in the 1cm^3 cube is 1000/0.0001 =. 1,000,000. So the total surface area of all of the smaller cubes is 1,000,000 x 0.0006cm^2 = 600cm^2
So the increase is 600cm^2 - 6cm^2 = 594cm^2

Q19	D

A, B and C can immediately be considered red flags given their use of strong language like '*will'* and '*cannot'* because this shows they are absolutes. E is wrong because the passage makes reference to the lack of an active lifestyle in younger people, not that exercise itself has a lesser effect in younger people than older people. Hence D is correct.

Q20	D

The information at the beginning of the passage tells us that the maximum daily salt intake is 6g and reading down the "all" column for the men, we can see that 15% of all men had 6g or less (note this is a cumulative percentage). So, if there are 567 men in total and 15% of them have 6g or under of salt, 15% of 567 = 85.05 hence D is correct.

Q21	7.6

We can find the median by interpolation for women using the information in the question, it is the amount taken by 50% or less of those women in the survey. 50% sits between 31% and 66% in the column for all women; and these percentages are for 6g and 9g respectively.

31%	50%	66%
6g	x	9g

Hence: x-6/9-6 = 50-31/66-31
This simplifies to: x-6/3 = 19/35
Therefore x = 57/35 + 6 = 7.6

Q22	A

As the table shows cumulative percentages for men; we know that:
3g or less: 4%
6g or less:15% - 4% = 9%
9g or less: 39% - 15% = 24%
12g or less: 60% - 39% = 21%
15g or less: 79% - 60% = 19%
18g or less: 91% - 79% = 12%
The only graph that matches this information is A.

Q23	B

A doesn't affect anything, whether the results were presented cumulatively or not the percentage per age group wouldn't change.
B is correct; if there was a larger number of a particular age group then they would be biased in the sense that they would be over-represented.
C is wrong; by this logic all would be still in proportion to the true values of the study.
D is wrong, this doesn't actually matter as the figures given are proportionate to the age range.
E is wrong; if the data is used to estimate data for 19-64-year olds, then no data is needed from people under 19 or over 64.

Q24	10

20 patients were booked but 2 didn't attend, so of the 18 patients:
1 takes 12 minutes.
17 take the normal 5 minutes = 85 minutes.
Aside from this there is an urgent phone call taking 8 minutes.
There is also an emergency appointment taking 5 minutes.
All surgery was completed by 11am so the 20 minutes free don't need to be used.
The total time taken is therefore: 12 + 85 + 8 + 5 = 110 minutes.
The surgery session is 2 hours long = 120 minutes. Thus, the doctor must have been 10 minutes late.

Q25	B

A is not assumed, the last line of the passage says: '*if gardening continues to be so popular*' which clearly shows it may stop being popular.
B is correct; the passage states that '*gardeners are being encouraged to use alternatives to peat*' but in order for '*the habits of wading birds*' to '*inevitably decline*' this must mean that gardeners would ignore encouragement to use peat alternatives.
C is wrong, environmentalists are not even mentioned in the passage.
D is wrong, cost is not mentioned as a factor in the passage.
E is wrong, it doesn't matter about other animals because the habitats of wading birds are the only thing this passage is concerned with.

2004 Section 1

Q26	A

Start by mapping out the times when each lighthouse is off (when time 0 is the when they became visible at the same moment as in the question):
When Lighthouse 1 turns off: 3; 14; 25, 36, 47, 58, 69, The interval is 11 seconds as it is the time the light is on plus the full time the light is off.
When Lighthouse 2 turns off: 2, 11, 20, 29, 38, 47, 56, The interval is 9 seconds as again it is the time the light is on plus the time the light is off.
As we can see 47 is common to both, but now we have to subtract 15 because that is how long ago, they first became visible at the same moment. 47-15 = 32

Q27	B

Work out by what factor the volume and surface area would increase with the changes stated in the question:
The volume would go from $\pi r^2 h$ to $\pi(2r)^2(2h) = 8\pi r^2 h$ so increases by a factor of 8.
The surface area would go from $\pi r^2 + 2\pi rh$ to $\pi(2r)^2 + 2\pi(2r)(2h) = 4\pi r^2 + 8\pi rh$ which is an increase by a factor of 4.
So, the mass of metal would be 4 lots of the original (800g) = 3200g
The mass of water would be 8 lots of the original (15.6kg-800g = 14.8) = 118.4g.
N.B remember to realise that 15.6kg is the total mass; hence why finding the water mass involves subtracting the mass of the cylinder itself. The total mass comes to 121.6kg.

Q28	C

If 30% work at least some of the time in the commercial sector, this includes those working in both the commercial and the public health sectors. Thus, 70% must only work in the public health service. Hence statement 1 is correct.
Thus, statement 2 is correct as 70% > 30%
Statement 3 cannot be deduced because we are only told what proportion of people work in the 2 sectors; not how much of their individual time they spend in each aspect of their work.

Q29	E

We can work out the mass of sodium chloride in 200ml of 30g/l solution (it is 200ml as we know that 50ml was accidentally spilt): mass = volume x concentration so mass = 0.2l x 30g/l = 6g
The mass in 50ml of 20g/l is 0.05l x 20g/l = 1g
So, the total mass is 7g in 250ml. Concentration = mass/volume = 7g/0.25l = 28g/l

Q30	B

We can immediately eliminate A and D because they are the wrong patterned graph; the cyclist is going faster and therefore will have a lead over the runner for the first leg. We can then eliminate E because it shows a plotting at 2km, but we know the plots will be at 1km, 2.5km, 3km and 4km to coincide with the different sections as shown in the question.
I have included a table for fullness for how to solve the last stage:

Time taken (minutes)	Flat	Mud	Uphill	Downhill
Runner	10	22.5	10	7.5
Runner cumulative	10	32.5	42.5	50
Cyclist	2	30	15	1.5
Cyclist cumulative	2	32	47	48.5

We can clearly see that at the end the cyclist has a lead of 1.5 minutes (as 50 minutes – 48.5 minutes = 1.5 from their cumulative end values). B is the only graph to match this pattern.

Q31	A & C

Take each statement and formulate an inequality:
Anne is not older than Susan: A≤S
Susan is younger than Anne: S<A
Susan is at least as old as Anne: A≤S
Anne is not younger than Susan: S≤A
We can quickly see that A and C are the same.

Q32	14%

Percentage decrease = change/original x 100
Therefore, in this instance = 700/4900 x 100 = 14%

Q33	B

A is not correct; the passage states earlier in paragraph 3 that whiplash is recorded as '*strains and sprains*' so it wouldn't matter what proportion of recorded '*strains and sprains*' were from whiplash.
B is correct, taking the line '*in 1987, 75 per cent of BI claims were for sprains and strains, and 45 per cent for "all other injuries"*'. Adding this up comes to 120% overall, which is concerning, but if there is an overlap of strains and sprains with other injuries this would account for the proportions as they are in the passage.

Q34	22

We know that from 1980 to 1993 the number of BI claims per 100 insured vehicles rose 33% to 29.3. This means that the number of claims per 100 in 1980 was 29.3/1.33
To help the ease of calculation; we know that 1.33 is approximate to 4/3 so 29.3 divided by 4/3 is actually 29.3 x ¾ = approximately 22

Q35	B & C

The trend is that BI claims that involved a property damage claim rose 64%.
A does not explain this; even if whiplash wasn't considered a "*bona fide*" condition this would mean that the number of BI claims would actually decrease so this isn't right.
B is correct, if lawyers have a no-win-no-fee policy this means that more people would want to pursue a property damage claim as even if they were unsuccessful, they wouldn't be losing out.
C is correct; if you had a strain or sprain then pursuing damages could be difficult with difficult qualification on severity but if the car has been damaged then one would pursue a property damage claim; as well as a BI for the strain or sprain; hence the increase in likelihood of both.

2004 Section 2

Q1	B

Recall from biology that blood returns to the heart from the lungs via the pulmonary vein (2) then enters the left atrium (3) followed by the left ventricle (4). From there it leaves the heart via the aorta (1) and goes to the body. When it returns to the heart it does so via the vena cava (7) and then enters the right atrium (6) and right ventricle (5) before leaving the heart to go to the lungs by the pulmonary vein (8).

Q2	B

Recall that the area of a triangle is given by ½ base x height. Thus, it can be written as:

$$\frac{4+\sqrt{2}}{2} \times (2-\sqrt{2}) = \frac{8-2\sqrt{2}-2}{2} = \frac{6-2\sqrt{2}}{2} = 3-\sqrt{2}$$

Q3	q = 3, r = 12, s = 3, t = 6

You may find writing equations based on their number each side of the given equation for each species to be useful with these sorts of questions to avoid trial and error.
Copper: q = s
Hydrogen: r = 12 (this is 1 solved)
Nitrogen: r = 2s + t
Oxygen: 3r = 6s + 6 + 2t
If we substitute r = 12 in for Nitrogen and Oxygen we get:
Nitrogen: 12 = 2s + t
Oxygen: 36 = 6s +2t +6 so 30 = 6s + 2t
We can then solve these two simultaneously to obtain values for t and s; and to do so we can double the nitrogen equation so the t's will be eliminated.
Nitrogen: 24 = 4s + 2t
Oxygen: 30 = 6s +2t
Subtract Nitrogen from oxygen giving:
6 = 2s so s = 3 (This is the second solved)
We know q = s from earlier so q = 3 as well. (This is the third solved)
We can substitute values for r and s into the initial nitrogen equation to solve for t:
t= r – 2s = 12 – 2(3) = 6 (This is the fourth solved)

Q4	E

This question tests knowledge not currently on the BMAT specification
This question tests knowledge on moments; so, using the equation:
Moment = force x perpendicular distance to the pivot
N.B. you must convert to metres.
Moment = 60N x (0.16m + 0.04m) = 12Nm
We know that clockwise moments = anticlockwise moments
So, moments about the piston = 12Nm = force x perpendicular distance to pivot
= force x 0.04m
Thus force = 12Nm/0.04m = 300N

Q5	0.32A

This question tests knowledge not currently on the BMAT specification
The charge per ion is 1.6×10^{-19} and there are 2×10^{18} ions travelling between the electrodes in 1 second so the overall charge per second (which is equal to current as Q=It so I = Q/t) is $2 \times 10^{18} \times 1.6 \times 10^{-19} = 3.2 \times 10^{-1} = 0.32$A

Q6	E

When expiring, the pressure (Z) needs to increase by decreasing the volume so the diaphragm (Y) will relax to resume its dome shape to decrease the volume. The external intercostal muscles (X) will also relax so the ribcage moves down and in to decrease the volume. E matches this.

Q7	i) E, ii) B, iii) A, iv) C

i) this substance would have a high melting and boiling point given its giant molecular structure as lots of energy would be needed to break the strong covalent bonds. It could, like graphite, conduct electricity when solid, or could not conduct electricity at all like silicon dioxide. giant molecular structures don't tend to conduct when molten. The only row that matches this is E.
ii) Metals have high melting and boiling points as well as good conductivity when solid and molten due to their delocalised electrons that are free to move and carry a charge throughout the structure. The only row that matches this is B.
iii) Ionic compounds have high melting and boiling points as lots of energy is needed to overcome the strong electrostatic forces between ions. They cannot conduct substances when solid, only when molten so A is the answer.
iv) A liquid at room temperature and pressure is going to be a simple molecule meaning it will have a low melting and boiling point, as well as poor conductance due to not having any delocalised electrons. This is C.

Q8	E

You can answer this by working out the empirical formula of the compound:
Approximately 80% is Tungsten, meaning the remaining 20% is oxygen.

	Tungsten	Oxygen
Percentage	80	20
Ar	184	16
Percentage/Ar	0.43	1.25
Ratio of Percentage/Ar in whole numbers	1	3

So as W:O is 1:3 the formula is WO_3

Q9	7.2m

We know that KE = ½ mv^2 and that v = 12m/s so substituting this in gives KE = ½ m (144) = 72(mass). We are also told that all of the KE is converted to GPE (recall GPE = mgh) so this means 72m = mgh where g = 10N/kg so 72m = 10mh
We can divide both sides by m and divide the LHS by to obtain h; giving 7.2m

Q10	A & B

This question tests knowledge not currently on the BMAT specification
A:$cos(\alpha)$ = obtuse and in the second quadrant therefore negative for cos.
$cos(\theta)$ = acute and in the first quadrant therefore is positive for cos.
Therefore, it follows that $cos(\alpha) = -cos(\theta)$
The value remains the same because $\alpha + \theta = 180$
B:$sin(\beta)$ = reflex and in the fourth quadrant therefore is negative for sin
$sin(\theta)$= acute and in the 1st quadrant therefore is positive for sin
As β+θ =360 this statement is true.
C: $\gamma = \theta$
As these angles are the same (as they are alternate angles) C is not true because $tan(\gamma) = tan(\theta)$
D:$\theta + \alpha = 180$and $sin(180) = 0$ not 1 so D is false.

Q11	B

This question tests knowledge not currently on the BMAT specification
We can see that the pyruvic acid has gained 3 hydrogens and we know that this is the definition of reduction hence B is correct.

Q12	D

	X_R	X_R
X_r	$X_r X_R$	$X_r X_R$
Y	$Y X_R$	$Y X_R$

We can see from this Punnet square that any son of the grandfather will not carry the recessive alleles, only the daughters will. This means that 4 and 5 would be carriers so we can eliminate E and F. 5 has no children so cannot pass on any alleles, but 4 has 2 children. If we know that 4 has a recessive allele, then despite the genotype of 3 the male offspring still has a chance of carrying a recessive allele. Thus, D is the answer.

Q13	D

This question tests knowledge not currently on the BMAT specification

$$x^2 \geq 8 - 2x$$
$$x^2 + 2x - 8 \geq 0$$

Factorise this quadratic:

$$(x+4)(x-2) \geq 0$$

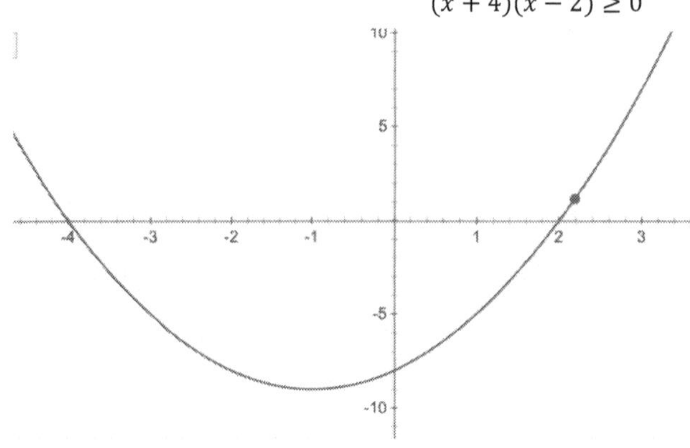

Remember that in order to come up with the final inequalities you need to quickly sketch a graph of the quadratic to see the roots: Here we can see that the proportion of the quadratic where y≥ 0 is when $x \leq -4$ and $x \geq 2$

Q14	D

This is a question about diffusion; smaller molecules can diffuse faster than bigger molecules hence why the ammonia travels faster to the other side of the tube and the product is formed closer to the HCl end. A cannot be deduced because more atoms does not necessarily mean a larger molecular mass. The boiling point does not come into this, they are both gaseous at room, temperature as they are simple molecules. C would result in a band closer to ammonia because the diffusion gradient would be lessened, ammonia's concentration would have to be higher for a ring to form closer to the HCl. Reactivity is not relevant here.

Q15	i) false, ii) false, iii) true, iv) false, v) false

(i) when the switch closes, we know that V_1 and the bulb are connected in parallel meaning the voltage remains the same across each of them. So (I) is false.
(ii) the reading on the ammeter will not increase, it will stay the same. As we have just seen voltage will remain the same, and the resistance is the same also because no components have been changed. Hence as V=IR, I will also remain the same.
(iii) When S_2 is closed the reading on A_2 will increase because a secondary branch is now available to the current, which will take the path of least resistance, hence the overall resistance has decreased due to this alternative path. If V remains the same and R decreases, this means I will increase due to V=IR.
(iv) The above reasoning also explains why when S_2 is closed the A_3 reading will increase, the other path that becomes available lowers resistance thus increasing current, hence why this statement is false.
(v) Because S_3 is closed this means there is a shorter circuit that the current can take (hence there is a short circuit) meaning that the current will now only flow round the top portion of the circuit (as this has negligible resistance) and not travel to any components; hence why the reading on A_2 will actually decrease.

Q16	B

Out of the 3 people, there are 3 combinations for how only 1 of them can suffer from a long-term illness: SNN, NSN, NNS (where N = not suffering which has a probability of 3/4, S = suffering which has a probability of 1/4)
So, the probability for each one of these combinations is ¼ x ¾ x ¾ = 9/64
This means the probability for all of these combinations is 3 x 9/64 = 27/64

Q17	D

At terminal velocity weight = air resistance. Weight = mg = 90kg x 10N/kg = 900N (note g is given in the question as 10N/kg)

Q18	D

You can draw out a simple primary amine such as methylamine and count up the number of each atom. You will see that there is 1 Carbon, 5 Hydrogen atoms and 1 Nitrogen atom. The answer choices only have options for H as 2n + something, so we know that 2n is 2 in this case (as n=number of carbon atoms). Hence, 2(1) + something = 5 hydrogens, so the additional part must be +3. So, the general formula is $C_nH_{2n+3}N$

2004 Section 2

Q19	A, D & E

Sex cells are haploid cells containing half the amount of DNA in a normal body cell. A, B, D and E are the ones containing a haploid amount of DNA, but B isn't actually possible normally because egg cells always contain an X chromosome; hence why only A, D and E are normal.

Q20	C

The equation for electrical power is P = IV. Taking each answer option in turn we can see whether each expression can show this.
A – we know that Q = It so I = Q/t. Substituting this into P = IV gives P = QV/t
B – P = IV and as V = IR we can substitute V into the 1st equation getting P = I(I)R = I^2R
C – this is not possible. If we try and substitute I = Q/t into P = I^2R we get P = Q^2R/t^2 which is not the answer choice with the terms given
D – this is straightforward; it just is the equation P = VI
E – V = IR and rearranging for I gives I = V/R. Substituting this into P=IV gives P = V^2 / R

Q21	D

This question tests knowledge not currently on the BMAT specification
The hepatic portal vein carries blood between 2 organs, the liver and the gastrointestinal tract (among others) whereas the others only carry blood to 1 organ. Because of this, only the hepatic portal vein will have a set of capillaries at either end.

Q22	F

We know that from P to Q the atomic mass doesn't change but the atomic number has gained 1, showing the emission of a beta particle, as when the electron is emitted a neutron is transformed into a proton raising the atomic number by 1.
From Q to R the atomic number decreases by 2 showing the emission of an alpha particle. We can therefore eliminate A, B, C and D from the answers.
The value of X is A-4 as we can see that from Q to R an alpha particle is emitted, and this would lead to a decrease in the mass number by 4. Hence the answer is F.

Q23	E

This question tests knowledge not currently on the BMAT specification
The information in the question tells us that oxygen from air displaces water; and that carbon monoxide displaces oxygen showing that order of increasing bond strength is:
Water < oxygen < carbon monoxide

Q24	C

This question tests knowledge not currently on the BMAT specification
P relaxes and R contracts (this is an antagonistic pair of muscles). Q contracts (you can tell on the diagram that it has become shorter and fatter). Similarly, from the shape of T you can see that it too has become shorter and fatter indicating it has contracted. This means S must have relaxed as these are also an antagonistic pair of muscles.

Q25	D

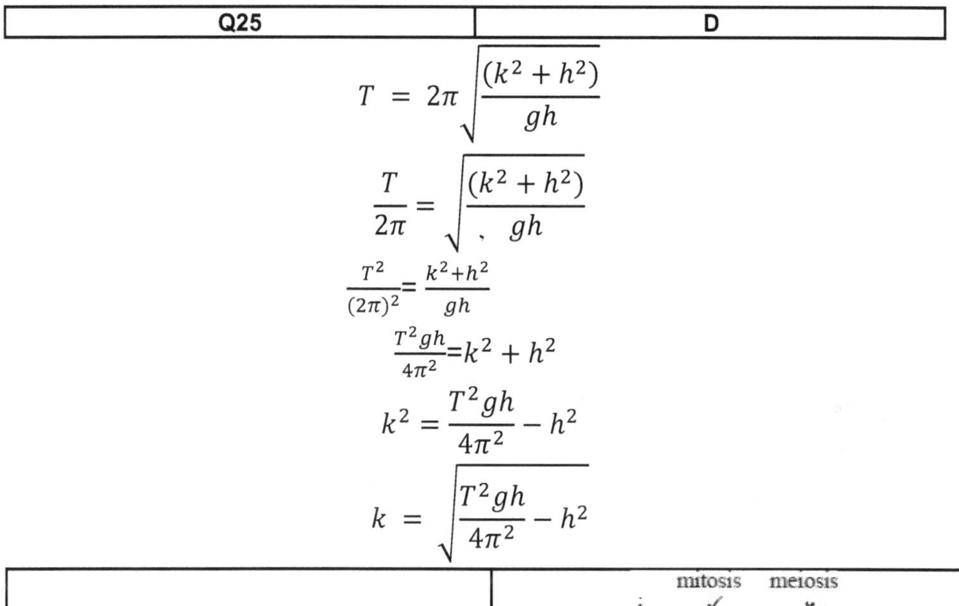

$$T = 2\pi\sqrt{\frac{(k^2+h^2)}{gh}}$$

$$\frac{T}{2\pi} = \sqrt{\frac{(k^2+h^2)}{gh}}$$

$$\frac{T^2}{(2\pi)^2} = \frac{k^2+h^2}{gh}$$

$$\frac{T^2 gh}{4\pi^2} = k^2 + h^2$$

$$k^2 = \frac{T^2 gh}{4\pi^2} - h^2$$

$$k = \sqrt{\frac{T^2 gh}{4\pi^2} - h^2}$$

Q26		mitosis	meiosis
	i	✓	✗
	ii	✓	✓
	iii	✗	✓
	iv	✗	✓
	v	✓	✓

This question tests knowledge not currently on the BMAT specification

4 or 5 correct for 1 mark

(i) mitosis creates daughter nuclei that are identical to the parent nucleus

(ii)in mitosis and meiosis all chromosomes are replicated in the process (mitosis 1)

(iii) meiosis leads to the formation of gametes

(iv) haploid nuclei contain half the amount of DNA in a normal body cell hence are gametes, so only mitosis produces these

(v) both processes produce cells with distinct chromosomes

Q27	C

We know that the factorised form of the equation will be:

$(x+a)(x+b) = 0$, where both a and b are the roots of the equation.

The question tells us that: $a+b = 7$ and $ab = 9$

Solving this simultaneously by rearranging the first equation for a gives:$a = 7-b$

So $(7-b)(b) = 9$

$$7b - b^2 = 9$$

So $b^2 - 7b + 9 = 0$

N.B. doing the same for b will give the same form of equation.

Alternatively, it may be helpful to remember that quadratics can also be written in the following form:

$$x^2 - (sum\ of\ roots)x + (product\ of\ roots)$$

2004 Section 3

To see the marking grid and mark bands that the BMAT examiners will use to mark your essays, please refer to the BMAT website. *To view the full questions, please see:*
https://www.admissionstesting.org/for-test-takers/bmat/preparing-for-bmat/practice-papers/

Individual freedom and the rule of law are mutually incompatible.

This statement suggests that we cannot simultaneously live lawful lives and retain our freedom.

Individual freedom generally constitutes the ability to do as one pleases, taking whatever course of action one wishes. It is clear that this is not what we have in the UK, we cannot act in a way that is harmful to others if it contravenes the law; this could be argued to be an infringement of freedom. We cannot go wherever we please freely, we are limited by the law as to what we can and cannot do.

On the other hand, you may wish to mention how individual freedom does not equal absolute freedom as this isn't constructive or fair to others. There is no way that we could allow absolute freedom for the individual in society because it would be an antinomian chaos which many would argue to be unethical and unproductive for humanity. In addition, just because the rule of law exists this is not to say that we cannot break the law as we are all too aware law-breaking is commonplace. Freedom has not been infringed; freedom has been exercised but will be punished for violating the law.

You could mention pioneers of individual freedom such as John Stuart Mill, who believed freedom from state interference was really important, unless our actions cause harm to others.

You may wish to question further what individual freedom really means, and whether we could even comprehend such a concept without a rule of law. What is freedom unless you have some parameters by which to define it?

It is worth trying to bring a sense of balance and perspective back to the question as well. The statement says the two are "mutually incompatible" but you may wish to refer to your own life experiences to judge for yourself whether you think you have had individual freedom and what your feelings are about that. Do you think they have been mutually incompatible in your life; or does that depend upon how you define individual freedom? For example, I am well aware that I haven't experienced absolute individual freedom, but that actually makes me quite happy; I have always had a set of rules to guide my behaviour and I have also experienced freedom of my actions within the rule of law.

There is more to healing than the application of scientific knowledge.

This gets at the arguably wider role of healing than through science; such healing could include emotional therapy or homeopathy.

Arguably, there is much more to healing than simply the application of scientific knowledge: healing is often associated with something emotional or spiritual, when one reaches a place of balance and happiness. Take for example, a hypothetical patient who had cancer in their mouth leading to extensive surgery to remove tumours leaving him cancer free but with scarring and reduced aesthetics of the face. Although scientific knowledge has "healed" the man; he is not healed mentally or emotionally. Potentially therapy could do this for him, or the homeopathic effects of a treatment.

Relating this back to medicine, there is a strong argument to diverge away from the "paternalistic" style of some doctors to simply tell patients what to do as opposed to engaging with their patients socially and emotionally to come to a more patient-centred and balanced form of care.

However, there is a problem with relying on healing methods that aren't validated through the application of scientific knowledge. For example, take our hypothetical patient from earlier; imagine he didn't have any surgery and just took a homeopathic treatment hoping it would "heal" him. This led to his detriment and ended up worse off. You may wish to show here just how important evidence-based medicine is and that the empirical nature of scientific knowledge allows us to apply it as a form of healing because it is reliable, peer-reviewed and repeatable.

So maybe you could conclude that a balance of these aspects of treatment is important, with a focus on scientific knowledge.

Authors' Tip:

The nature of medicine and the debate between allopathic and homeopathic/alternative medicine is an interesting topic, and with homeopathy/alternative medicine relatively common nowadays, it may be useful for you to read up about it. For more information, please see the NHS page on homeopathy, which can be accessed using the link below:
https://www.nhs.uk/conditions/homeopathy/

2004 Section 3

Our genes evolved for a Stone Age lifestyle. Therefore, we must adopt Stone Age habits if we are to be healthy.

This statement argues that the function of our genetic constitution should be fulfilled in the way that it was designed for; this being survival in the Stone Age.

You may wish to argue against this statement on the grounds that it seems like a fallacy of composition (you could possibly reference David Hume here) to say that we must behave the way we are designed. This seems reductive, simplistic and not necessarily true. Logically, for example, we are capable as a species of creating computers and advanced technologies. Humans from the Stone Age would not behave with these kinds of higher cognitive functions; they wouldn't be regarded as Stone Age habits, yet it would seem absurd to us to not fulfil the potential of the human mind despite the fact that our genetic make-up seems to push towards a Stone Age type human.

Alternatively, you may think that some Stone Age habits include ideas such as the "Selfish Gene" that Richard Dawkins is a proponent of; in that we are designed genetically to try and benefit ourselves and the people around us that we care about; and this could be equated to primeval Stone Age habits.

In today's society, there is an arguable need to refer back to Stone Age habits with regards to being self-sufficient, less gluttonous, and more fit. Humans in the Stone Age were responsible for hunting for themselves, finding their own food and going long periods of time without food; contrastingly in our society we suffer from obesity and inactivity hence why a return to these habits could be welcome.

You may conclude that while the statement has well-founded sentiments, we ought not adopt all Stone Age habits and make a return to their way of life, but rather adopt a few where we see fit, and where they would essentially benefit our lives and society.

Authors' Tip:

'*The Selfish Gene'* by Richard Dawkins is a good book to read in preparation for medical interviews, especially at more scientific institutions, such as the London universities (KCL, UCL and Imperial) and Oxbridge.

BMAT 2005

Section 1

Q1	C

This can be done by simply counting up the number of each type of square. There are 9 black large squares, 9 medium white squares and 20 small grey squares. This ratio of large: medium: small is 9:9:20 which can be approximated to 1:1:2

Q2	D

The argument's conclusion is that schools should revert to traditional school days, as adult life is competitive. Therefore, the assumption (something that links the reasoning given with the conclusion to make the argument cohere) is that it should be school sports (as opposed to other aspects of school life) that should prepare children for adult life, which is option D. A is not relevant to the argument, B is not needed to accept the conclusion, and C weakens the conclusion, as opposed to being an assumption.

Q3	B

A bird has two legs, and a sheep four. Let us call the number of birds, b, and the number of sheep, s. In this way we are able to form two simultaneous equations, and subsequently solve them.

$b + s = 13$ (Julia)

$2b + 4s = 36$ (Tim)

Doubling Julia's (2J) gives $2b + 2s = 26$. Doing $T - 2J \rightarrow 2s = 10$, so **s = 5 = B**

Q4	A

We need to find an answer that best explains why if the universe is expanding, galaxies can still collide, which is answer A. B is too specific to be correct (just because we have one example doesn't mean we can generalise to <u>all</u> galaxies). C doesn't link the two statements, D doesn't provide an explanation, merely an analogy/observation, which isn't relevant, and E doesn't provide an explanation which links the two statements.

Q5	30 to 49

This question requires an ability to read and scan the tables quickly. The question tells us that between 1991 and 1995 the cancer death rate between ages 30-54 was higher in females, therefore we only need to look through ages 30-54, as outside that range, male deaths would be higher between 1991-95. Go through the age categories from 30-54 and compare whether for a particular age range there are more female deaths than male (you also will need to compare time period as well). We see that between the ages of 30-49, across all time ranges, the female cancer death rate exceeded the male one.

Q6	B

First, identify the conclusion, which in this case is the last line; '*since our consumption of natural pesticides……our health is at greater risk from natural pesticides than from synthetic ones*'. Therefore, to weaken the argument, we need to show we are at less risk from natural pesticides, which is what B says. A and C strengthen the argument, and D is not relevant.

Q7	£10,500

£350,000 falls in the 3% tax bracket, so the stamp duty will be 0.03 x £350,000 = £10,500

Q8	C

As stamp duty is a percentage of the property price, as opposed to a fixed amount. There should be diagonal lines on the graph, so D is incorrect. There must be large increases in stamp duty payable near the boundaries, so there should be near vertical lines, so B is incorrect. The stamp duty percentage increases for each price range, and so the diagonal lines should get steeper each time, as opposed to having the same gradient each time, so A is incorrect, and C is the correct answer.

Q9	B

On the first £120,000 we pay no tax.
On the next £130,000 we pay 1% so £1300 tax.
On the final £50,000 we pay 3% so £1500 tax.
So £1300 + £1500 = £2800

Q10	£3,300

Let's work out the tax on £260,000. For this price, tax is 3%, so £7800 tax
Now let's work out the tax that he pays by cheating the taxman. He pays 1% on his £250,000 (as the question tells us to round to the nearest £100, it is far easier to use £250,000 than £249,999). So, tax is £2500. Remember he also pays an extra £2000 for this agreement, so total paid is £2500 + £2000 = £4500. So, £7800 - £4500 = £3,300

Q11	A

If all students who study Spanish also study French, then the circle for Spanish must be inside the circle for French. Therefore, the circle on the right represents those who study German. Therefore, the shaded area represents those who study German and French, but not Spanish.

Q12	E

E is the correct answer as if the argument is correct in saying that '*even children under 15 are known to use it*', and '*those who start smoking before the age of 15 have a much higher risk of becoming schizophrenic in later life*', it would mean we would have to wait and see if the rates of schizophrenia in the population increases in the future, in order to weaken the conclusion that '*since the incidence of schizophrenia in the population has remained stable whilst the use of cannabis has been increasing, it cannot be true that smoking cannabis causes schizophrenia*'. A is in favour of the argument, B isn't relevant to the conclusion as schizophrenia is not cancer, C is not relevant here as it isn't specific enough, and D is not relevant to our conclusion.

Q13	B

Call the incident light y. 0.8y would pass through the first pane of glass. Therefore, 0.8 x 0.8y = 0.64y would pass through the second pane of glass. However, this is not the only light that will pass through. Some of the light that passes through the first pane of glass, will get reflected by the second pane of glass, and then get reflected back by the first pane of glass and pass through the second pane of glass = 0.8y x 0.15 x 0.15 x 0.8 = 0.0144.
So, 0.64 + 0.0144 = 0.6544 ~ 65%. (Note, that reflection between the two layers will occur indefinitely, but the light transmitted will be minutely small for each subsequent reflection)

Q14	E

The conclusion is that '*nuclear power...will have to continue to be used in 2050'*.
1 is correct because the argument assumes that as nuclear power will have to continue to be used in 2050, the government's economic growth goal has to be met, which is an assumption/weakness.
2 is incorrect because that is not relevant to the argument which links energy consumption with the need to carry on using nuclear power by 2050.
3 is correct because the passage only mentions present rate of development of renewable sources, and at this present rate the renewables will be unable to meet the shortfall in supply. This is a weakness, as the passage assumes that no increased development in these energy sources will occur.

Q15	D

Let us call the price at which the corner shop buys 4 packets 4x. Let us call the normal price of 3 packets 3y. So 3y/4x = 1.2 as we learn that she makes 20% profit. Rearranging, we get y = 1.6x. So normally the profit is 4y/4x = 4(1.6x)/4x = 6.4x/4x = 1.6 so 60% profit is made.

Q16	D

When the dipstick measures 0.15m, there are 400l of oil in the tank. After the delivery, there will be 900l (400l + 500l) of oil in the tank, so looking on the graph, the dipstick will read 0.6m

Q17	E

The passage makes the point that the '*natural beauty of the countryside*' is forest, and that had human activities, such as crop agriculture or the grazing of livestock, not occurred the countryside would still be forest, and therefore it is not wind farms alone that are destroying the countryside, but also other factors. E, thus, best completes the passage. A is not relevant as the passage talks about the countryside, B is an assumption not supported by the passage, and C and D are irrelevant to the argument at hand.

Q18	C

The conclusion of the passage is that '*we should not tolerate such aggressive behaviour in a civilised society Any player acting in this way should be...banned from the club's next three games*'. For the banning of players to have any effect, the argument must assume that banning players would reduce the incidence of aggressive behaviour, which is C.

Q19	3200 (allow 3100)

The division annual rate (start) is 37,838. Dividing that by 12 will give us a monthly rate of 3153, which rounds up to 3200.

Q20	F

F is the correct answer as all three factors are '*confounding factors*' as they are all reasons why the decrease in crime may not be attributed to improvements in CCTV alone.

Q21	9%

% change = (new amount – original amount)/original amount x 100,
So, in the target area = 131-161/161 x 100 = -30/161 x 100 = ~-18.6%
In the division, (6442-7164)/7164 x 100 = -722/7164 x 100 = ~-10%. The difference between them is roughly 9%.

Q22	22%

Discounting vehicle crime gives us a start annual rate of (1526 – 279) = 1247, and an end annual rate of (1098 – 126) = 972. Therefore, the percentage change, discounting vehicle crime, is (972 – 1247)/1247 x 100 = -275/1247 x 100 = 22% (doing -275/1250 is an easier calculation yielding the same answer)

Q23	E

1 is correct as providing data for crime in the buffer area will allow you to see whether crime has simply been displaced to surrounding areas.
2 is incorrect as it isn't relevant, as the question asks about the effects on crime in the buffer area.
3 is correct as data in the buffer area helps us build a better picture of whether crime is falling just in the buffer area, or in the whole division.

Q24	A & C

A is correct because there are no students who had scores between 0-25% meaning the easy questions were answered correctly by all, including the weakest candidates. C is also correct because there are many students who scored between 90-100%, meaning that many students were able to correctly answer the hard questions, and not just the most able.

Q25	C

For this question, it is easier to work through the answer options until you encounter the correct answer (which in this case would be a missing line, which represents being able to travel directly between two points). A is incorrect, as to get from X to C you have to go through I. B is incorrect, as to get to I from A you have to go through C. D is incorrect as to get to G from F you have to go through E. E is incorrect as to get to X from J you have to go through I. C is the only correct answer.

Q26	A

The passage tells us that the medullary bone is only found in females, therefore any specimen with a medullary bone must be female and can never be a male. Therefore, the absence of such a bone is a **necessary condition** for male sex determination. However, it is not a **sufficient condition**, as it is possible for a female specimen to have an absent medullary bone, as the passage states that the '*medullary bone remains undetectable during brooding and until the next ovulation*', as '*shell formation depletes the bone*'.

Q27	B

1 is correct as 70% of the inhabitants are not in the 17-34 age range. Therefore, if all of the non 17-34 residents took the car, then there would still be 5% of the inhabitants remaining who took the car. Therefore, that 5% must have to be within the 17-34 age range, which is 1/6 of the age range (30% of the population are 17-34).
2 is correct because if all the people who took public transport were 16 & under, then that would only be 15% of the total population. Since the population of people 16 & under is 30%, then no more than half can possibly take public transport
3 is incorrect because it is entirely possible for all those who walk/cycle to be over 60, as only 10% walk/cycle, whereas 15% of the population are over 60.

Q28	B

At first look, you may think that the next number will be 1, because 14 – (3 + 5 + 5) = 1, but this is not possible as 1 is an odd number, and the question says that the machine never generates more than 5 odd numbers. Similarly, by this logic, 3 would also be incorrect. Now look at the number sequence, and find 4 numbers which add up to 14, the first set being 4 4 2 4. Therefore, the next four is 1 5 6 2, and the next is 4 2 5 3. That leaves us with 5 5 x y, where x and y are the next two digits. As 5 + 5 + x + y = 14. Therefore, x can't be 4, as because if it was, then y would have to be 0, which isn't possible, therefore B = 2 is . Therefore, the correct answer is B = 2.

Q29	F

First identify the conclusion of the argument, which in this case is the last line, '*so global travel helps to immunise the population*'.
1 is correct as according to the passage, frequent global travellers gain immunity to infectious disease, but if the majority of British residents aren't frequent travellers, then the majority of Britain wouldn't be immune.
2 is also correct, as just because you are immune to a number of infectious diseases, does not necessarily mean that you are immune to bird flu.
3 is also correct because human nutrition depends on other factors other than the strength of the economy, and therefore just because the economy is strong it does not mean that childhood nutrition is at a sufficient level that children have developed immunity.

Q30	**D**

There are 4 situations one needs to consider, with each situation being when one of the cars is the best. If the first car is the best, then the chance of buying the best car is 0. If the second car is the best, then the chance of buying the best car is 1. If the third car is the best, then the chance of buying the best car is ½ (as he could also have picked 2, as long as 2 was better than car 1). If the fourth car is the best, then the chance of buying the best car is 1/3 (as he could also have picked cars 2 or 3). Therefore, the sum of the probabilities is 0 + 1 + ½ + 1/3 = 11/6. However, as there are 4 possible situations that could all equally occur, the probability of choosing the best car is ¼ x (11/6) = (11/24) = D
Alternatively, if probability isn't your strong point, you may want to write out all the potential combinations (for example, if the 1st car was the best, the 2nd was the second best, the 3rd was the third best and the 4th was the worst, we would write it as 1234). By doing this way, you will see that there are 24 combinations, 11 of which lead the buyer to buying the best car.

Q31	A

1 is correct because the passage provides both advantages and disadvantages to taking aspirin, and then goes on to say that it should only be taken by those who meet certain medical conditions (when a patient is found to have a 3% or higher chance of a first heart attack or stroke within five years).
2 is incorrect because the statement is too general, the text only states that 80% of men should take it over 50, it doesn't mention anything about women, and also acknowledges that 20% of the male population over 50 wouldn't need to take it.
3 is incorrect, as there is no comparison of different risks with age presented in the paragraph. All the text says is that 50% of the male population will have reached threshold by 40, and that 80% will have reached it by 50 – do not confuse these stats with what statement 3 talks about.

Q32	**D**

From the rules given in the question, we can work out that the number is:
(2 x 5 x 5 x 5) + (3 x 5) + 1 = 266 = D

Q33	**B**

1/3 x 247 million is roughly 82 million = number of people who visited alternative therapists
425 million visits were made, so 425/82 = ~5 = B

Q34	**C**

A is not correct because the passage says that conventional doctors also care about the overall well-being of patients, just that it comes at a '*premium*'
B is incorrect because of the different modalities between the statement and the passage. The passage claims that there is a '*lack of central definition of alternative therapies'* so some may aim to treat diseases.
C is correct because the passage says this, '*the time it takes to get to know their patients is…at a premium…. this is the void that alternative medicine appears to be feeling'*
D is incorrect, as just because alternative health practitioners may believe this, there is no evidence in the text to say that conventional doctors do not.
E is incorrect because the text does not mention that alternative therapies have no side effects.

Q35	D

The main point paragraph 3 makes is that doctors and conventional medicine have changed, and now doctors don't have enough time for all patients ('*premium*'), and so many have turned to alternative medicine, which is what D says. A is not implied by the text as invasive procedures aren't mentioned, B is not true as although doctors acknowledge that it is getting harder to combine the art of healing with the science of medicine, that doesn't mean that doctors support alternative therapies. C is also incorrect as the text does not talk about pharmaceutical companies, nor their influence or interests.

2005 Section 2

Q1	A

This question tests knowledge not currently on the BMAT specification.
The tidal volume is the volume of air that a person inhales during a normal breath. B is the total lung capacity, C is the inspiratory reserve volume, D is the expiratory reserve volume, and E is the inspiratory capacity.

Q2	B

The answer is B, as a burning splint makes a squeaky pop sound in hydrogen, is put out in carbon dioxide and a glowing splint relights in oxygen. A is incorrect as none are unsaturated compounds, C is incorrect as only carbon dioxide causes an effect in limewater, and D and E are incorrect as all three are gases, and so do not have pHs.

Q3	D

This question tests knowledge not currently on the BMAT specification.
Summing the atomic numbers (54 + 38 = 92), shows us that there is no change in protons, therefore A and C are incorrect. Summing the mass numbers (139 + 95 = 234), we see that the uranium has a mass number 4 higher than the sum of its products, therefore 4 neutrons must have been given off.

Q4	C

We know that current always flows through the path of least resistance. Therefore, we need to lower the resistance of two resistors in such a way that the current will flow from one of the lower resistance resistors, through the ammeter, and through the other lower resistance resistor. This would only work if we changed both p and s, or both r and q. Therefore, C is correct.

Q5	D

This question tests knowledge not currently on the BMAT specification.
Emphysema occurs when the alveoli become damaged, and so their SA is reduced. D is the only answer mentioning the alveoli, so is correct.

Q6	C

First rearrange the equation in terms of y: $y = \sqrt{\frac{z}{x}}$

Substitute the values given in the question:

$$y = \sqrt{\frac{1.2 \times 10^{13}}{3.0 \times 10^{-6}}}$$

Simplify, using the laws of indices,

$$y = \sqrt{0.4 \times 10^{19}} = \sqrt{4 \times 10^{18}} = 2 \times 10^{9}$$

Q7	A

As one molecule of glucose breaks down to form two molecules of pyruvic acid, the reaction must be a decomposition reaction. As hydrogen is lost, the reaction must be an oxidation reaction (H_{12} breaks down into 2 H_4 molecules, so 4 H is lost), so A is correct.

Q8	A

Since B and D have short lashes, while both her parents and her sibling C have long lashes, the allele for long lashes must be dominant. Therefore, both A and her husband must be heterozygotes. A must be heterozygous for lash length, because otherwise it would not be possible for her to have children, some of whom have long lashes, and some of whom don't, given that her husband has long lashes. C and E could be either homozygous dominant, or heterozygous, while B and D must be homozygous recessive.

Q9	C

If B is increased by 40%, we can set up the following proportionality statement:

$$A \propto \frac{1}{(1.4B)^2}$$

Therefore,

$A \propto \frac{1}{1.96B^2}$ which is $A \propto \frac{100}{196B^2}$ which is $A \propto \frac{25}{49B^2}$

As the answers given are all quite close, we need to be careful here. A is now 25/49 of its old value, which is just slightly over 50% of the old value. Therefore, the decrease must be slightly under 50%, which is answer option C.

Q10	39 cm

This question tests knowledge not currently on the BMAT specification.

This question is slightly more difficult than regular GCSE moments questions, as we have to take into account the weight and effects of the uniform beam. The centre of mass of the beam is in the middle, and so is 15cm to the left of the pivot.

clockwise moments = anticlockwise moments

$10 \times 800 = 200x + (15 \times 10)$ [Note the 15 x 10 comes from the weight of the bar]

$8000 = 200x + 150$

$7850 = 200x$

$x = \frac{7850}{200} = 39.25cm = 39cm$

Note: even though the SI units for distance is m, we can work in cm here because all the distances are in cm, and the question wants the answer in cm.

Q11	D

Sodium carbonate decahydrate is $Na_2CO_3 \cdot 10H_2O$, as 'deca' means 10.

The total Mr is (2 x 23) + 12 + (3 x 16) + (10 x [16 + 2]) = **46 + 12 + 48 + 180** = 286

The Mr of the decahydrate is 10 x [16+2] = **180**

Therefore the % by mass is $\frac{180 \times 100}{46+12+38+180}$ (or more conventionally written, $\frac{180}{286} \times 100$)

Q12	B

This question tests knowledge not currently on the BMAT specification.

This requires recall of the knowledge of what happens to the ciliary muscles and suspensory ligaments, and the subsequent effects on the lens during accommodation. When seeing far objects, the ciliary muscles relax, the suspensory ligaments tighten, and the lens becomes less convex.

2005 Section 2

Q13	A

$$y = \left(\frac{x^2 + 2ax}{b}\right)^{1/2}$$
$$y^2 = \frac{x^2 + 2ax}{b}$$
$$by^2 = x^2 + 2ax$$

This next step is relatively complex, you need to recognise that we can complete the square on $x^2 + 2ax$. Completing the square gives us $by^2 = (x + a)^2 - a^2$

$$by^2 + a^2 = (x + a)^2$$
$$(by^2 + a^2)^{1/2} = x + a$$
$$\mathbf{x = (by^2 + a^2)^{1/2} - a}$$

Q14	B

Time = Distance / speed
Time = (0.1m + 0.1m)/500 = 0.2/500 = 0.0004seconds = 0.4ms

Q15	D

For an exothermic reaction, the ∑bonds made must be greater than the ∑bonds broken, since ΔH is negative (and ΔH = ∑bonds broken - ∑bonds made).
Therefore $x + 3y < 6z$ which is $6z > x + 3y$ = D

Q16	i) D, ii) C, iii) G

This question tests knowledge not currently on the BMAT specification.
i) A tendon joins muscle to bone, which can only be D
ii) A ligament joins bone to bone, which can only be C
iii) For a muscle to be antagonist, it must work in an opposite direction to the other muscle in its pair and is usually located on the other side of a bone. Therefore, G is the answer.

Q17	A

First expand the brackets, and we get

$$(\sqrt{5} - \sqrt{2})(\sqrt{5} - \sqrt{2})(\sqrt{5} + \sqrt{2})(\sqrt{5} + \sqrt{2})$$

Notice that if we write this differently, we get two pairs of 'difference of two squares' making simplification far easier

$(\sqrt{5} - \sqrt{2})(\sqrt{5} + \sqrt{2})(\sqrt{5} - \sqrt{2})(\sqrt{5} + \sqrt{2}) = (5 - 2)(5 - 2) = 3^2 = 9$ = A

Q18	B

Let us assume that the rock was made wholly out of U-235, as that will give us the maximum possible age. The ratio is 1-part uranium to seven parts lead, so there are 8 parts in total.
At time 0: (0 years): 8 parts uranium, 0 parts lead
After 1 half-life: (7.1×10^8 years): 4 parts uranium, 4 parts lead
After 2 half-lives: (1.42×10^9 years) : 2 parts uranium, 6 parts lead
After 3 half-lives: (2.13×10^9 years): 1-part uranium, 7 parts lead.
At this point, the ratio is correct therefore the maximum possible age of the rock is B.

Q19	B

Moles of NaOH needed to neutralise acid = cv = 2 x 0.05 = 0.1 moles
Therefore, 0.05 moles of acid were used, as there is a 2:1 ratio.
mass = (moles x Mr), so Mr = (mass/moles) = 4.5/0.05 = 90 = B

Q20	C

The movement of a substance which requires oxygen is **active transport**, which is the movement of a substance against its concentration gradient (from an area of low concentration to an area of high concentration). Looking through the answer options, C must be the correct answer as the concentration of magnesium ions is lower in Cell L than in cell K.

Q21	A

As triangle ABC is equilateral, AC and BC must also be xcm.
Dealing with the semicircle, xcm is the length of the diameter. The area of a semicircle is $\frac{\pi r^2}{2}$, so the area of the semicircle is $\frac{\pi\left(\frac{x}{2}\right)^2}{2} = \frac{\pi x^2}{8}$

To work out the area of the triangle ABC, we need to split the triangle in half.

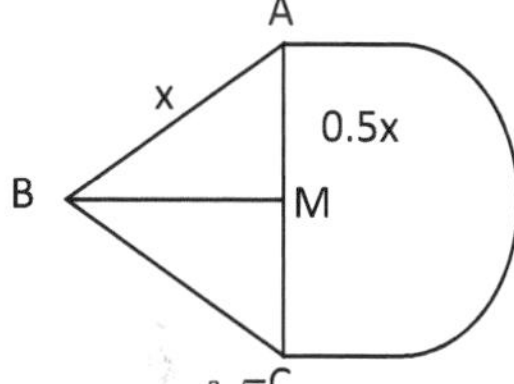

AM = ½ x, and we can work out BM by Pythagoras.

$BM = \sqrt{x^2 - \frac{1}{4}x^2} = \sqrt{\frac{3}{4}x^2} = \frac{x\sqrt{3}}{2}$

The area of the triangle ABM is $0.5 \times 0.5x \times \frac{x\sqrt{3}}{2} = \frac{0.25x^2\sqrt{3}}{2} = = \frac{x^2\sqrt{3}}{8}$

We double this to get the area of ABC (as it is made up of ABM + ACM) = $\frac{x^3\sqrt{3}}{4}$

So the total area is: $\frac{x^2\sqrt{3}}{4} + \frac{\pi x^2}{8} = \frac{2x^2\sqrt{3} + \pi x^2}{8} = \frac{x^2(2\sqrt{3}+\pi)}{8} = A$

Q22	D

g on that planet would be 2.5ms^{-2}, as g on Earth is 10ms^{-2}.
Therefore, on that planet, GPE = mgh = 1 x 2.5 x 20 = 50J

GPE = KE, and KE = ½ mv^2, so $v = \sqrt{2E/m}$

$v = \sqrt{100/1} = \sqrt{100} = 10.0 = D$

Q23	B

In order to avoid algebra, it may be quicker to calculate the relative mass of carbon in each of the four compounds given (A-D). Each compound has 4 carbon atoms (total mass of 12 x 4 = 48), therefore we are looking for the compound that has total mass 60 (as 48 must be 80% of the total compound).

In A, $\%\, mass\ of\ carbon = \frac{48}{48+9+2} = \frac{48}{59} = incorrect$

In B, $\%\, mass\ of\ carbon = \frac{48}{48+8+4} = \frac{48}{60} = CORRECT$

In C, $\%\, mass\ of\ carbon = \frac{48}{48+7+6} = \frac{48}{61} = incorrect$

In D, $\%\, mass\ of\ carbon = \frac{48}{48+6+8} = \frac{48}{62} = incorrect$

2005 Section 2

Q24	A

The right atrium contains deoxygenated blood, while the left atrium has oxygenated blood. If there was a passage between them, the left atrium would contain deoxygenated blood, meaning therefore, that the left ventricle and subsequently the aorta would contain deoxygenated blood = A. (Note, if blood flowed from left to right atria, this wouldn't be problematic, as blood from the right atrium goes to the lungs to get oxygenated anyway).

Q25	B

Force = pressure x area, with pressure in Pa and area in m^2
2.0 cm^2 is 0.0002 m^2
152mmHg is 1/5 of 760mmHg, therefore 152mmHg is 20kPa = 20,000Pa
So, F = 20,000 x 0.0002 = 4N.

Q26	D

This question tests knowledge not currently on the BMAT specification.
The most reactive element would be the hardest to displace from its oxide; Na is the most reactive out of those elements, so D is correct.

Q27	0.8

For these questions, it is essential that we draw a diagram.

BD is a diameter of the circle, as D is opposite B, so BD is 20cm. The angle CBA is 90° as the angle in a semicircle is 90°. The point at which the two diameters (AC & BD) is the origin. Therefore, OD = OC = OA = OB = 10cm.

We have a right-angle triangle ABC, so we can use Pythagoras to find lengths.

$BA^2 + BC^2 = AC^2$ so $144 + BC^2 = 400$.
$BC^2 = 256$, so BC = 16.

Using the sine rule, $\sin BAC = 16 \times \frac{\sin 90}{20}$
sine 90 = 1, so sin BAC = $\frac{16}{20} = 0.8$

As angles in the same segment are equal, BAC = BDC, so sin BAC = sin BDC, so sin BDC = 0.8

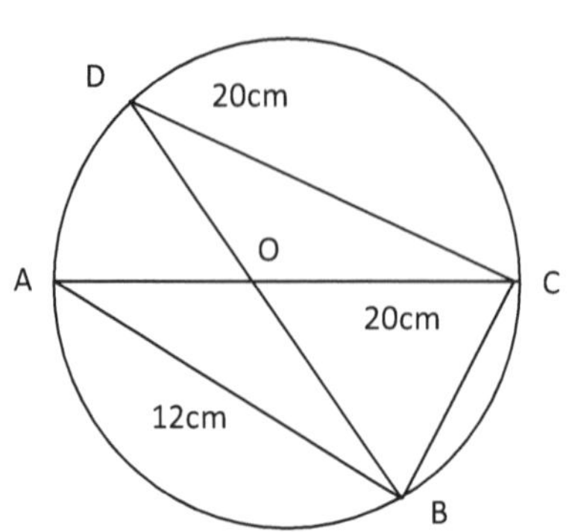

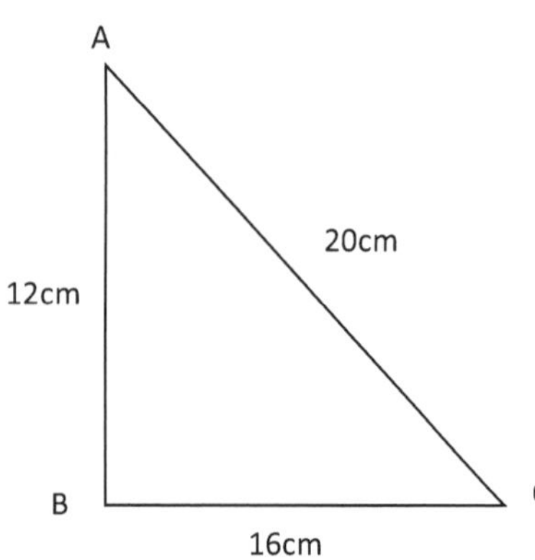

2005 Section 3

To see the marking grid and mark bands that the BMAT examiners will use to mark your essays, please refer to the BMAT website. *To view the full questions, see:*
https://www.admissionstesting.org/for-test-takers/bmat/preparing-for-bmat/practice-papers/

Question 1 was written to widen access to the exam paper, as in the past, students hoping to study Veterinary Medicine would also have to take the BMAT. VetMed students no longer take the BMAT, and so in its current iteration (2017 onwards), there are none of these questions, so the authors have not included worked essays for these and recommend that you only attempt these after having attempted all the previous ones.

Science should leave off making pronouncements: the river of knowledge has too often turned back on itself. *Sir James Jeans (1877-1946)*

The statement addresses the ability of scientific knowledge to be completely valid/true, and here 'pronouncements can refer to any (accurate/reliable) scientific statement of truth, such as laws, theories or statements about results/experiments that have been undertaken. The statement tries to convince the reader that science should avoid these pronouncements, as too often they have been proven to be false.

There are many examples of biomedical pronouncements that have subsequently turned out to be false, you only need to turn to history to find some. In the 2nd century AD, Galen came out with the pronouncement that the body was composed of 4 humours, and that an imbalance in any of these led to character traits, such as aggression, and disease. We now know that this is untrue, and Galen's theories have been disproved by many scientists, such as Harvey. In more recent times, the Andrew Wakefield scandal is another example of a pronouncement that turned out to be false. Wakefield claimed that there was a link between the MMR vaccine and autism, and 'proved' his results by falsifying data and gravely abusing autistic children through unethical procedures. Further experiments were later performed, and there was found to be no link between MMR vaccine and autism, leading to Wakefield's article being removed from the Lancet (where it was published), and the original co-authors removing their names/support for the article. Wakefield's results led to fear among parents in the subsequent years regarding vaccinating children, and has led to a rise in the number of unvaccinated children, reducing the herd immunity of populations (and potentially endangering children's lives), and this event is evidence for the danger of making pronouncements.

However, scientists should still make pronouncements, as it is through these that science can ultimately progress and advance. If no one pronounced anything, and everything was uncertain, then development would surely be impeded. Additionally, certain life-saving drugs have been developed based on pronouncements, for example based on pronouncements about the structure and function of cells – without these, those treatments wouldn't have been developed. By making pronouncements, scientific discoveries can be shared internationally, and other experts can assess their lines of thinking/experiments/methods through peer review, increasing the reliability (and accuracy) of experimental findings.

Perhaps what is necessary is for people to realise that scientific pronouncements (while the majority are correct), carry a degree of uncertainty as they are limited by current knowledge, technology, and expertise. Scientific pronouncements, at their core, must be able to falsified, and there is always the chance of them being disproved in the future, but that does not mean that they shouldn't be made.

With limited resources and increasing demand, doctors will not in the future be concerned about how to cure, so much as whether to cure.

The statement means that in the future, where there will be greater demand from a growing population, varying lifestyles and a more ageing population structure, and fewer available resources (due to resource depletion, climate change, overpopulation etc), medical professionals will be more focused on whether someone should receive treatment/cure, as opposed on curing the patient. This will be due to the demand for medical treatment/care outstripping supply. Therefore, the overall focus may shift from finding cures to certain diseases to maximising the remaining resources and treating the most people possible.

Limited resources and increasing demand can be caused by growing populations (overpopulation), food/water insecurity, problems caused by climate change and resource depletion. Other factors include a more ageing population structure, with populations having more complex medical needs (the older a person gets, the more medical conditions a person, on average, will develop). Because of these factors, it could be possible that we may have to prioritise certain patients for treatments over others, which could result in the death of others (who could have been cured if resources were available) – this has a host of moral and ethical problems and decisions.

It is the duty of a government to provide for all the needs of all its citizens, and it should adapt to the changing global situation. The NHS core principles describe the function of the NHS as being a system which provides <u>comprehensive care to all.</u> Therefore, for the NHS to carry on abiding by its principles and acting as a public healthcare system, it means that the government should ensure that resources for medical care should always match demand.

However, another of the NHS' principles is to providing the best value for the taxpayers money, and this may mean that certain treatments for very rare conditions may not be cost effective to offer on the NHS, due to its limited monetary resources. Therefore, while ensuring there are sufficient resources to meet all the demand may be the theoretical solution, it may not always be practically possible, and compromises may have to be made.

Authors' Tip

Deciding which treatments to offer is a complicated process, and in the UK, this falls under the remit of the National Institute for Health and Care Excellence (NICE). Common medical school interview questions involve asking students to consider which treatments out of a group of 4 should be offered, and there are many factors to consider – a utilitarian perspective may be the most useful, and we suggest you read up on QALYs (*Quality Adjusted Life Years*)

BMAT 2006

Section 1

Q1	C

	Seabirds	People
Ratio today	80	1
% change	-60%	+25%
Ratio 20 years ago	200	0.8

If seabirds used to be 100%, then decreased by 60% that means 40% equates to 80.
Therefore, 100% equates to 80/0.4 = 200
If people used to be 100%, then increased by 25% that means 125% equates to 1.
So, 100% = 1/1.25 = 0.8.
Putting 200:0.8 in terms of a ratio of seabirds to 1 person we need to do 200/0.8 = 250 hence the ratio is 250:1

Q2	E

A is incorrect, the last line clearly says that freedom of speech needs to '*have limits put upon it*' to sustain democracy which has the feature of tolerance. This means they can coexist but in a limited way.
B is wrong, the passage does not reference the law at all as a method of limitation.
C is wrong, although both are key features of democracy that is not the conclusion of the passage; the conclusion is that freedom of speech has to be limited.
D is wrong, we do not know that tolerance is more important than freedom of speech, we are just told that if freedom of speech is allowed then tolerance is lost. There is no reason why the two could not be equally important.
E is correct, this sums up the last line well that freedom of speech has to be limited.

Q3	B

This is a tough visualisation question; you may find it easier to leave this question to the end and then cut out the shapes and try and fit them on each shape to see which ones are possible. It may also be worth looking at the angles on the 4 smaller tables and working out which shapes are very much possible; and what is not; for instance we can eliminate 4 on the basis that it would need 4 of the same type of smaller table; but we only have 2 of each type. Similarly, 2 would need 2 of 1 type at each end but that leaves a rhombus in the middle that cannot be formed of either type of table.

Q4	C

The statement's conclusion is that '*political journalists are not doing their job properly*' and that is because they have excluded '*all other important political issues*'. The first line also states that '*the media have an important role to play...since a democracy requires that voters are well informed about political issues*'. This assumes that it is the job of political journalists to do this informing, as C states.

Q5	62 seconds

Train 1 (the first train mentioned) has to travel the entire length of the tunnel plus its own length of 80m = 695m.
Train 2 has to travel 40m to the tunnel, the entire length of the tunnel (615m) and its own length of 120m = 775m.
Clearly train 2 has to travel further and being as they both travel at the same speed, the time taken or both trains to have completely emerged from the tunnel is the time taken for the slowest train (train 2) to get through the tunnel.
So, train 2 has to travel 775m at 45kh/h. We can convert the speed to m/s as our answer needs to be in seconds. So 45000m/3600s = 12.5m/s.
Time = distance/speed = 775m/12.5m/s = 62 seconds.

Q6	C

A cannot be asserted; we do not know that the influence is more in 1 direction than the other.
B cannot be asserted; they could be well aware for all we know.
C is correct, we know they clearly publish articles about dangers of anorexia and the use excessively thin models to promote the latest fashions.
D is wrong, '*the public*' is not the subject of the passage; young women are and this may not be true, the public could be interested in a different body type to the ones in these articles.
E is wrong, although it could be correct, it cannot be drawn as a conclusion from the passage.

Q7	B

Reading along to the 'total' column and row we can see that White pupils attain 55.1% (5 grades A* to C) and Asian students gain 58.7%. This is a difference of 3.6% which rounds to 4%.

Q8	E

Reading down the '*other than English as a first language'* column to "total" and looking at the greatest figure in the KS 2-4 VA measure we can see that (excluding the white group) Chinese pupils have the greatest figure here at 1036.0.

Q9	D

A is not best supported by the data, reading the total column for boys and girls respectively for KS 2-4 VA measure we can see boys have a score of 977.5 and girls of 997.3 and a 0.2 difference is not massive.
B is not supported; looking at the column for '*other than English as a first language*' to the total row and the total x total row we can see that for white people 6485/486,887 speak a different first language to English. For mixed people it is 1210/12,085, for Asians it is 30,349/35,252 (which is clearly the largest of the whole lot), for Black people it is 7053/20391, and for chines it is 1785/2316 and for *'other'* it is 3336/4928. Hence it is Asians, not Chinese who support the data shown.
C is incorrect, if we take the difference in % with 5A* to C, we can see that white pupils have a difference of 57.3-48.0 = 9.3%. However, for mixed pupils. The difference is 59.4-50.9 = 8.5% which is clearly a smaller difference.
D is correct; reading across the 'total' row comparing % with 5A* to C between '*English with a first language*' and '*Other than English as a first language*' we can see that only the mixed pupils perform better, with 55.0% with English as a second language compared with 54.7% with English as their first language.

Q10	D

A - This is a possible explanation for the difference.
B – This is also a possible explanation, if boys mature later then they may experience less improvement during the time that they are less mature
C - This is also plausible, if boys are not focussed on improvement in academic pursuits because they are more interested in non-academic pursuits this accounts for the lack of improvement
D – This is not a possible explanation, the question says '*for all ethnic groups'* so it doesn't matter how large the gap in improvement between boys and girls is for the Asian group because the difference in improvement is across all ethnic groups not just Asians.

Q11	E

1 – this helps to explain the results, we can see that the less time one has spent smoking, generally the more words they can recall. Recollection is similar to learning and remembering and 1 does support this notion.
2 – this also helps to explain the results, knowing that cannabis affects the brain long-term does help to explain the results, as we are dealing with 2 groups who have been smoking for a number of years
3 – this could also help explain the results; although it isn't down to the cannabis itself but rather a different factor: IQ levels.

Q12	A

The cost of each of the 3 boxes normally is \$1.50. 60% of this is paid to the supplier: 60% of \$1.50 = 90c
The cost of 3 boxes for the price of 2 is 2(\$1.50) = \$3 so the cost of each box is \$1.00. 60% of this is paid to the supplier (make sure to read the question that the supermarket's gross margin remains the same at 40% meaning the proportion paid to the supplier stays at 60%).
60% of \$1.00 = 60c.
So, we can tell that the supplier has to reduce the price of the cereal from 90c to 60c, which is a reduction of 30c.

2006 Section 1

Q13	68p

Working from lowest stamp upwards we can see that:
The 23p stamp can be paid for by the 23p denomination
The 32p stamp can be paid for by the 32p denomination
The 37p stamp can be paid for by the 37p denomination
The 49p stamp can be paid for by the 49p denomination
The 50p stamp can be paid for by the 50p denomination
The 32p stamp can be paid for by the 32p denomination
The 62p stamp can be paid for by the 42p denomination and the 20p denomination
The 68p stamp cannot be paid for by only 2 stamps alone; it requires at least 3.

Q14	C

A – this doesn't apply because we are not talking about the application of a method, we are talking about the method as a whole
B – this is not a weakness because it is essentially what the first line of the passage states and later goes on to contradict
C – this is the answer. The fact that scientists who study fingerprinting all agree that it is completely reliable (which is an opinion) does not mean the method is reliable, as we know that no one knows whether the technique is reliable.
D – this is not a weakness because it does not undermine the experts' opinion as they don't cite length of time as to why they think fingerprinting is reliable.

Q15	C

When attempting these questions, it is useful to first try and pinpoint the towns for which 2 sets of information are provided, as this narrows down possibilities.
Taking Ruilick, we know that Wellbank is due east of it, and Aultviach is due north of it ('*due*' meaning directly in this sense). The only town for which this is the case is E hence E is Ruilick. We then know that A is Aultviach and F is Wellbank.
Taking Aultviach, we know that Clashandarran is south and east of it, this could be B, C, D or G; but we also know that Rheindown is due south of Clashandarran and the only location with a town directly south of it is B; hence B is Clashandarran and D is Rheindown.
We are then told that Beauly is south and west of Windyhill. Being as the only options for towns left are C and G, this means that Beauly must be G and C must be Windyhill.

Q16	B

1 – this is not an assumption; we are told that '*many countries in the developed world have set targets*' but this doesn't mean less developed countries haven't; we are just told it is '*considered unrealistic to expect such restraint*' by them. Eliminate A and C.
2 – this is not an assumption, in fact the passage end by asking such a question, not answering it in this way. Eliminate D and E.
3 – this is not an assumption; non-improving levels of prosperity doesn't mean that countries necessarily have to choose between acting to reduce global warming problems or alleviating current levels of poverty in developing countries
4 – this is assumed, the question of choosing between the two situations in the last line assumes that the improvement of the economy can only come at the production of greenhouse countries that will contribute to global warming problems.

Q17	B

Start with the initial amount and work backwards (the fact that we know she had exact change for the bubble gum means that all the money was spent): £125 and subtract the cost of buying each of the kids (10 in total) a 25p packet of bubble gum each. £125 - 10(£0.25) = £122.50
If 2 chose to go on Apocalypse; they also went on the Carousel which amounts to 2 x (£9 + £3.50 = £25. Subtracting this from £122.50 = £97.50 left over for the other 8 kids.
The ride options are either Armageddon + Dodgems = £7.50 + £5 = £12.50. Let x kids do this.
Or Armageddon + Helter Skelter = £7.50 + £4.50 = £12. Let y kids do this.
We can form some simultaneous equations now and solve:
X + y = 8
£12.50x + £12y = £97.50
We can multiply the first equation by 12 and eliminate y: 12x + 12y = 96
Then we can subtract this from the second equation:
£12.50x + £12y = £97.50
12x + 12y = 96
£0.50x = £1.50, and so x = 3

Q18	C

The argument made is that people shouldn't complain about the use of pesticides because farmers need to use them to maximise yields (as supermarkets are so competitive on pricing) in order to avoid making a loss. This assumes that the use of pesticides is the only way to avoid making a loss.
For the record, A is not a flaw as it is use in general, not the manner of use that is bothersome. B is wrong because the argument doesn't contradict itself, it highlights both of these points presenting them as reasoning as to why pesticides need to be used. D is irrelevant to the conclusion as it isn't to do with avoidance of a loss with regards to supermarkets. E is not a flaw because the argument already says that the damage to humans is only alleged.

Q19	E

From the 8th to the 15th Ayesha has missed 6 scheduled sessions (as she takes Saturday's off) meaning she has to make up 18 days to get back to fitness. However, 14 days after she returns, Ayesha has a sore shoulder on the 15th causing her to miss an additional 4 sessions on the following 4 days. At this point, Ayesha has actually made up for 4 of the missed sessions (12 days) making her 2 sessions (6 days) behind her peak fitness. (N.B we exclude counting on Saturdays' because they are not scheduled days).
So, if she was 2 sessions behind, and now due to injury is an additional 4 sessions behind, this comes to a total of 6 sessions which means she needs to make up 18 days excluding Saturdays. We know she will restart training on Thursday 4th May (after her shoulder has healed) and 18 days later (plus 2 days for the 2 Saturdays she won't swim on) comes to 24th May.

Q20	B

In 2004 there were approximately 31250 GPs (reading off the top graph) and of them, 12500 were female. 12500/312500 = 12.5/31.25. This is clearly less than 50% so we can eliminate C, D and E, and it is also clearly greater than 12% so B is the only reasonable answer.

2006 Section 1

Q21	C

Check the key, approximately 49% of female GPs in 2004 were part time. We already know from Q20 that there were 12500 female GPs and about half of this Is 6250 which approximates to C.

Q22	D

In 1994, about 12% of 27500 GPs were part time (3500) and this means 88% were full time (24000). If part timers do 50% of normal hours, this is the same as regarding half the number of part timers and adding them to the number of full timers, i.e. 3500/2 + 24000 = 25750.

In 2004, about 25% of 31250 GPs were part time (7800) and this means 75% were full time (23500). If part timers do 50% of normal hours, this is the same as regarding half the number of part timers and adding them to the number of full timers, i.e. 7800/2 + 23500 = 27400

Hence, the number of hours has risen from 25750 to 27400 which is a rise of approximately 10%.

Q23	B

The average of the individual guesses is:

(40 + 37 + 26 + 19 + 9 + 4)/6 = 135/6 = 22.5

If we know 4 is closer than 40 to the true weight, we know that the middle value between these numbers can be done by doing: 40-4/2 = 36/2 = 18. 18 + 4 = 22. Hence, if Suzie's value is closer than Wally's we know that the answer has to be lower than 22 so we can eliminate C, D and E.

We are left with A and B, 20 and 21 each. We are told that the average, 22.5 is closer than any other guesses, but Mary guessed 19. 19 is closer to 20 than 22.5 so A can't be right. B however, is 21 which is closer to 22.5 than 19 so is correct.

Q24	C

The passage states that for an epidemic the virus needs to be able to be transmitted easily, but that the current virus of H5N1 cannot be transmitted easily between people, but that if it behaves like a mutated influenza virus it could become more easily transmissible, making an epidemic more likely. This is what C says.

A is unrelated to the conclusion, and D is wrong because the virus could mutate making it transmissible. C is wrong because it suggests that an epidemic would become likely with mutation which is not the case as mutation could actually result in no change to the ease of transmission of the virus.

Q25	B

Take an easy time limit, like 1 hour. We know that the hour hand will cover an area of 1/12 x pi x $(6.3)^2$ which is approximately 3.3pi.

The minute hand will cover its entire area which is pi x $(8.4)^2$ = 70.56 pi

We can see the ratio will therefore be: 70.56 : 3.3 meaning we can clearly eliminate C, D and E because looking at the numbers this doesn't fit. We can also eliminate A as 3.3 x 16 = 52.8 which is far less than the 70.56 we need. Hence B is the answer.

Q26	D

1 – this is correct, if worldwide demand for electricity had grown and the argument had been followed through, this would mean that more electricity would be demanded from fossil fuel generators and the new green technologies may not be able to supply the electricity sufficiently given that experts have only made a prediction as to their capabilities, and this is not fool proof.
2 – this is also dangerous, if the rate of electricity supply by green technology cannot keep up with growing demand then there are not enough supplies of electricity which is unsafe.
3 – this is not showing why the conclusion could be unsafe, the argument is about the danger of a shortage of supply of electricity not about how waste can be stored.

Q27	5 hours

The route is x km on the flat, y km climbing to the summit, y km downhill and x km flat again (as the question says their route is reversed).
2x + 2y = 20km according to the question.
We also know that the time taken = distance/speed which in this case = x/4 + y/3 + y/6 + x/4 = 6x + 8y + 4y + 6x/24 = 12x + 12y/24 = 0.5(x+y) hours
But we can rearrange our first equation giving: 2(x+y) = 20 so x+y = 10
Hence, 0.5(x+y) = 5 hours.

Q28	B

The trend of the graph is that as population increases in 2005 the population in 2006 will also increase, up to a certain population, after which any increase in 2005 results in a decrease in population in 2006.
A does not explain the trend, it would support a straight line of y = x not this curve.
B is correct, the high mortality due to starvation when the population gets to a certain point causes the reduction in population in the following year.
C is wrong, this still doesn't explain the decrease in population after a certain point.
D definitely doesn't match the pattern; this pattern is supposed to hold throughout the survey not just the middle years.
E does not match the above pattern.

Q29	D

1 may be concluded, it says '*may*' in it which is a good sign as this is not strong language. It also makes sense that if in humans less of the dangerous substance is made than in animals that it may be less dangerous to humans.
2 – this is the opposite of what the passage says, the passage says cooking above 120 degrees is dangerous as it produces acrylamide.
3 - the passage tells us that cooking potatoes this way makes them absorb more fat and that eating more fat is bad for one's health.

Q30	A

If we first count how many 1cm cubes are along each edge (including the 3cm cubes split into 3 x 1cm cubes) we get 8. Hence, in the entire cube there would be 8 x 8 x 8 = 512 1cm cubes.
We are told that under the outer layer are just 2cm cubes with a volume of 2 x 2 x 2 = 8cm^3.
So, we need to subtract the volume of all the 1cm cubes (each with a volume of 1cm^3) and the 3 cm cubes (each with a volume of 3 x 3 x 3 = 27cm^3).
We can count 8 x 3cm cubes which will have a volume of 8 x 27cm^3 = 216cm^3
We can also count 20 inner 1cm cubes per face (so 120cm^3 total) and 24 outer 1cm cubes so 144cm^3).
512 – 216 – 144 = 152cm^3 which we know is made up of 2cm cubes only. So, we divide this volume by the volume of a 2cm cube:
152/8 = 19 which is A

Q31	B

This is relatively straightforward: the last paragraph reads: '*the three, who recently looked down on Google'* which implies that they now no longer do so as they now want to '*form alliances'*. Hence B is correct.
A is not necessarily true, Google may not be achieving what Microsoft achieved in computer systems, we just know that Microsoft doesn't want anyone to do so. This doesn't imply reliably that Google are doing so.
C is not reliably inferred, the big three '*wonder'* if an alliance will stop Google, not that it is the only way of doing so.
D is wrong, just because jockeying produces rich entertainment and opportunities for consumers, this is not to say that an alliance would detrimentally affect consumers.

Q32	B

If an 80% boost (180% or 1.8 times 2005 revenue) was the equivalent of more than £1.2 billion, then sales at the end of 2005 would be 1.2billion/1.8 which is approximately 2/3 billion or £666,666. Out of the statements, we already know A is false, it has to be at least the value stated, hence B is correct. C is wrong, this could be too low a cap, as could D. This is because we are not told how much more revenue was made.

Q33	C

A – The text does not allude to Google's triumph.
B – being a '*knight in shining armour'* is subjective and implies Google is saving the others, when really it is a competitor.
C – This can be reasonably inferred; an alliance would weaken Google's monopoly which is a danger
D – This is not implied by the text at all.
E – we do not know that Microsoft is afraid, we just know that it does not want anyone '*repeating on the internet what it achieved'* but this is not necessarily fear.

Q34	C

1 would certainly indicate that Google is making the pace by striking a corporate link that otherwise could have benefited Microsoft, this is what the 3rd paragraph suggests: that such a link was '*snatched...from under the nose of Microsoft*'.
2 certainly indicates that Google itself is making the pace as the end of the 3rd paragraph suggests: they have revenue that '*represents a lot of advertising*'.
3 is not a reason for Google to be making the pace, it is too general.

Q35	A

A – this is true: '*jockeying offers rich entertainment and opportunities for consumers*'
B - '*have to*' is strong language that is wrong here because the act of companies merging is suggested once they encroach upon one another but is not suggested to be the only course of action in such a scenario.
C - '*cannot*' is again strong language and the author does not express this absolute sentiment.
D – This is wrong, the last paragraph tells us they wonder if they can form an alliance which indicates they may merge, not that they will never merge.
E – This is wrong, just because the passage is focussed on the threat Google poses doesn't mean it is the only threat to Microsoft. We know that all of the companies compete with one another.

2006 Section 2

Q1	E

We know that insulin supports the conversion of glucose to glycogen to reduce blood glucose concentration. Hence, if insulin is lower than normal this means there is low blood glucose as most of the former blood glucose has been converted to glycogen. This means we want regions of the graph where glycogen will be converted to glucose to oppose this to try and increase the blood glucose concentration. Hence, this will be the regions of the graph where there are falling levels of glycogen: these are 3 and 5.

Q2	C

A and B are explained by T's simple molecular structure as they are relatively low. Molecules with simple molecular structure also tend to have low conductivity in solution because they have no ions or electrons free to move and carry a charge throughout the structure, so D is not the answer either.
C is the answer because the solubility in water isn't really explained by the bonding and structure of the molecule.

Q3	F

There are 32×10^{20} atoms of X and over 8 years 2 half-lives will have taken place, meaning that the number of X nuclides remaining will be $\frac{1}{2} \times \frac{1}{2} \times 32 \times 10^{20} = 8 \times 10^{20}$. This means that 24×10^{20} of Y have been produced (as X decayed into Y). The question tells us that initially there were 4×10^{20} Y nuclides meaning that the total sum of Y nuclides 8 years later would be $24 \times 10^{20} + 4 \times 10^{20} = 28 \times 10^{20}$.

Q4	B

To keep water in the body, we want ADH to be secreted because that will increase water reabsorption in the kidney. Hence, we can eliminate A, D and E. This will make urine more concentrated. In the nephron more water will be reabsorbed to fulfil this. The only factor that discriminates between the right and wrong answers now is the blood concentration. If we want to increase water reabsorption, the blood concentration needed to be high in the first place so we can eliminate C and F and come to B.

Q5	C

We know that alkali metals and halogens are the most reactive. The former is because they have 1 outer electron that is very easy to lose and the latter is that they have 1 electron to gain (because they have 7 outer electrons already) in order to have a full outer shell.
Hence, we can eliminate B, E and F because they don't have 1 or 7 outer electrons.
But the question asks for a non-metal so we can eliminate D for being an alkali metal.
Out of A and C, C is the correct answer because it has the fewest subshells meaning that it is more electronegative; it has a stronger power to attract electrons than A as it has a smaller atomic radius and less shielding of inner subshells of electrons.

Q6	A

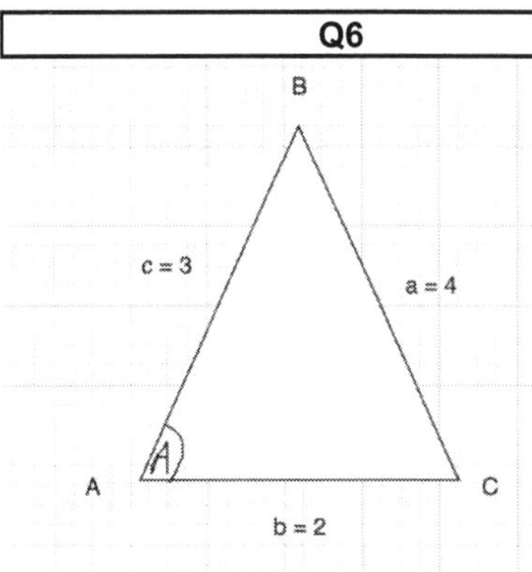

This question tests knowledge not currently on the BMAT specification.

Step 1: rearrange the given expression for cosA

$$\frac{a^2 - b^2 - c^2}{-2bc} = cosA$$

Step 2: substitute our numbers in from the diagram and solve:

$$\frac{4^2 - 2^2 - 3^2}{-2(2)(3)} = \frac{16 - 4 - 9}{-12} = \frac{3}{-12} = \frac{-1}{4}$$

Q7	A

1 – this is wrong, microwaves are part of the EM spectrum so are transverse
2 - this is true; microwaves can travel at the speed of light in air
3 - ultrasound waves are used in pre-natal scanning
4 – infrared waves are used in thermal imaging
5 – microwaves are EM waves so can travel through a vacuum

Q8	C

We are told that the lower quartile is 115, meaning the probability of having a heart rate of less than 115 is ¼. We are told that the upper quartile is 165, meaning the probability of heaving a heart rate less than 165 is ¾, hence the probability of having a heart rate greater than 165 is ¼.
There are 2 scenarios by which the question could be fulfilled. Either, all 4 of the members are going to have heart rate of over 165; or 3 will have a heart rate of over 165 and 1 will have a heart rate of less than 165.
In the first scenario the equation is:
$(¼)^4$ x 4 = 1/256 as the probability of being over 165 is ¼ and this has to happen 4 times and be multiplied by 4 for each of the people.
In the second scenario the equation is:
$(¼)^3$ x (¾) x 4 = 12/256 as 3 people have the probability of being over 165 and this happens 3 times, but 1 person has a probability of being under 165. In total we have to multiply by 4 for each of the people.
Adding the two probabilities gives our answer:
12/256 + 1/256 = 13/256

Q9	B

1- adding a catalyst doesn't speed up the rate of reaction, it just speeds up the time taken to reach equilibrium
2 – adding more ammonia will cause the reaction to move forwards to reduce the ammonia concentration; this will increase the yield of the salt.
3- by increasing the pressure, the equilibrium will shift to the side with fewer gaseous moles which is the RHS so the yield will increase
4 – the reaction I exothermic in the forwards direction so by increasing the temperature, the equilibrium will shift to try and decrease the temperature by moving in the endothermic direction, which is the backwards reaction. This will decrease the yield.

Q10	D

If two heterozygous plants are crossed, we have the following Punnet square:

	R	r
R	RR	Rr
r	Rr	rr

The question tells us that recessive alleles prevent seedling development, so these plants will never develop into mature ones. This means out of the remaining genotypes 2/3 are heterozygous as we have two Rr and 1 RR left. 2/3 is approximately 67%.

Q11	C

The question tells us that the force is transmitted hydraulically, and we know that pressure across fluids is the same, so if the pressure applied at X is $3N/cm^2$ then the pressure transmitted to Y is the same.

Q12	E

$$r = 1 - \frac{6\Sigma d^2}{n(n^2-1)}$$

$$r - 1 = \frac{6\Sigma d^2}{n(n^2-1)}$$

$$(r-1)n(n^2-1) = 6\Sigma d^2$$

$$\Sigma d^2 = \frac{(r-1)n(n^2-1)}{6}$$

$$\Sigma d^2 = \frac{(r-1)(n^3-n)}{6}$$

Q13	B

It is worth thinking that the only product that isn't gaseous is K_2CO_3 as at 200^0C water is water vapour and CO_2 is a gas also. Hence, the loss in mass will be the difference between our starting mass of $KHCO_3$ and our ending mass of K_2CO_3.
The first thing to do is to work out the moles of $KHCO_3$. We can work out the Mr:
39+1+12+3x16 = 100
Thus, the moles = mass/Mr = 50g/100 = 0.5 moles. This means the moles of K_2CO_3 is half of this as they are in a 2:1 ratio, so 0.25 moles of K_2CO_3 are produced.
The Mr of K_2CO_3 is 2x39+12+3x16 = 138
Hence the mass of K_2CO_3 is moles x Mr = 0.25 x 138 = 34.5g
So, the loss in mass is 50g – 34.5g = 15.5g

Q14	x = 3, y = 1

You may consider rearranging the second equation for y and substituting it into the first equation. (You could rearrange for x and do the same and you will come to the same answer ultimately).
So, if 2x-y = 5 then y = 2x-5
Substituting this into our first equation gives:
$4x^2 + (2x-5)^2 + 10(2x - 5) = 47$
$4x^2 + 4x^2 - 20x + 25 + 20x - 50 = 47$
$8x^2 - 72 = 0$
$8(x^2 - 9) = 0$ so x = +/- 3 but the question asks for the positive solution so x = 3
If x = 3, we can substitute this into the equation y = 2x - 5 to find y:
Y = 2(3) - 5 = 1 hence x = 3, y = 1.

Q15	E

The place with the highest concentration of glucose is 2, this is because the carbohydrate rich meal has just been consumed and the glucose has been hydrolysed in the stomach and intestines. Hence, we can eliminate A, B, D and F.
The place with the highest concentration of urea is 3 because the liver is the site of deamination. Hence, we can eliminate C and come to E as our answer.
For the record, the place with the lowest concentration of oxygen is 3 also because blood has travelled through several organs to get there and is the closest to the vena cava which we know has the lowest oxygen concentration.

Q16	2 m/s^2

The object of mass 20kg will have a weight of 200N. So, the resultant force acting on the object is 240N upwards – 200N of weight downwards = 40N upwards.
We know F = ma, so a = F/m = 40N/20kg = 2ms^{-2}

Q17	E

1 – this is incorrect, the nucleus would have a relative mass of 40 if the mass number is 40 (as this is the sum of the mass of the protons and neutrons, and electron mass is negligible).
2 – this is incorrect; the electron configuration is 2, 8, 8, 2, hence it is in Group 2 not group 8.
3 – this is incorrect; we now it is in Group 2, and these metals form 2+ ions when they lose their 2 outer electrons.
4 – this is correct as we have already established from its electron configuration.
5 – this is incorrect; we know that as it is in Group 2 it is a metal.

Q18	C

We can see that 21% of inhaled air is oxygen, and 16% of exhaled air is oxygen meaning 5% of the air with oxygen is absorbed.
If 500cm^3 is breathed 14 times a minute this equates to 7dm^3 inhaled a minute. The question asks about absorption in 4 minutes though so 7dm^3 x 4 = 28dm^3 inhaled.
So, 5% of 28dm^3 = 1.4dm^3.

Q19	C

This question tests knowledge not currently on the BMAT specification.
We know that in low light levels the pupils will dilate so that more light can enter the eye. This means we can eliminate A and D.
The radial muscles contract and the circular muscles relax hence C is correct.

Q20	E

The upper branch is in series, so has a higher resistance than the lower branch which is in parallel. We know this because in series total resistance is just summing the resistance of each component, but in parallel it is summing the reciprocal of the resistance across each component.

If we use V = IR, we can see that if V stays the same across both branches, but R is higher in the upper branch, this branch will have lower current whereas the lower branch has a smaller R so a larger current.

Now R_3 has the smallest current going across it because it is branched again. If V = IR, and R stays the same and I is the lowest, this means V_3 will be the lowest. Hence, we can eliminate A, B, C, and D.

Comparing V_1 to V_2 we can see that there is the same amount of current going across V_1 and V_2 but the resistance preceding V_1 is greater than that of V_2 (referring to the 1st paragraph's logic) so using V=IR, V_1 will be smaller than V_2.

Hence, the final order of increasing potential difference is:

V_3, V_1, V_2

Q21	9

$$\left(\frac{32^{1/5}+9^0}{81^{3/4}}\right)^{-1}$$

$32^{1/5} = 2$ as $2^5 = 32$

$$9^0 = 1$$

$81^{3/4} = ((81)^{1/4})^3 = 3^3 (as\ the\ 81^{1/4}\ is\ 3) = 27$

Substituting these into the original equation gives:

$(\frac{2+1}{27})^{-1} = (3/27)^{-1} = 27/3 = 9$

Q22	D

A – this is incorrect; the activation energy is V+W not X

B – although Z may have more energy than U, X is not the route taken with a catalyst, Y is because it is a lower energy pathway which is the pathway a catalyst takes. Also, W is not the activation energy, again it is V + W. Hence this is wrong.

C – Y is the route taken when a catalyst is present, V is the heat of reaction, but the reaction is endothermic not exothermic so this aspect of the statement is wrong.

D – this is fully correct, X is the route taken without a catalyst as it has a higher activation energy, V + W is the activation energy and V does have a positive sign as the reaction is endothermic.

Q23	C

Wave speed = frequency x lambda
Frequency of red light = c/lambda (N.B frequency of light does not change, that's why we can ignore the fact that the speed changes, because the wavelength will change so as to keep frequency the same). So, we can eliminate A, B, E and F.
Recall that the speed and direction of light changes during refraction and can be summed up by this acronym: FAST: Faster - Away / Slower - Towards. We can see from the diagram that the blue light is closer or more 'towards' the normal than the red light meaning it is slower than red light. Hence, we can eliminate D leaving C.
(Alternatively, you could use the fact that blue light has a higher wavelength than red light and follow through by using the fact that frequency remains the same, so a higher wavelength means a lower speed).

Q24	E

1 – this is correct; you can recall this from your notes
2 – this is incorrect; oxygen debts are formed from anaerobic respiration
3 – this is incorrect; aerobic respiration also produces water which is a waste product
4 – this is true, reduced aerobic respiration will transfer less energy meaning less active uptake of mineral ions can occur
5 – this is incorrect; the little oxygen that is present is aerobically respired; the 2 types of respiration happen in conjunction
6 – this is true, aerobic respiration only forms lactic acid

Q25	B

This question tests knowledge not currently on the BMAT specification.
Instead of spending lots of time on this question trying to balance sides it is much faster to realise that 4 protons are converted into Helium (which has 2 protons and 2 neutrons). Hence, 2 of our original protons must have been converted to 2 neutrons which is shown by B.

Q26	A

$$a = \frac{k}{b^2}$$

Substitute the values for a and b into the rearranged expression for k:

$$k = b^2 a$$

$$k = 4^2 \times 9 = 16 \times 9 = 144$$

Now rearrange the expression for b:

$$b = \sqrt{\frac{k}{a}} = \sqrt{\frac{144}{4}} = \sqrt{36} = +/-6$$

Take the positive answer which is 6.

Q27	5 seconds

We are told charge density = charge/surface area and that on the large sphere it is $0.25C/m^2$
We can rearrange this to find out the charge = surface area x density
$= 0.04m^2 \times 0.25C/m^2 = 0.01C$
We are told that the large sphere is charged at a rate of 2mA and so we can use Q = It to work out t (the time interval).
t= Q/I = 0.01C/2mA = 0.01C/0.002A = 5 seconds

2006 Section 3

To see the marking grid and mark bands that the BMAT examiners will use to mark your essays, please refer to the BMAT website. *To view the full questions, please see:* https://www.admissionstesting.org/for-test-takers/bmat/preparing-for-bmat/practice-papers/

Our zeal to make things work better will not be our anthem: it will be our epitaph. *(*Bryan Appleyard*)*

This statement gets at the fact that advances in modern technology are not ultimately going to be beneficial for us; they will lead to our demise (an epitaph being words to the memory of a dead person).

The statement has been made when thinking of the dangers of advancing modern technology to a point where it is detrimental to society. One example of this is the advancement of Artificial Intelligence, whereby machines can be programmed to make decisions independent of human input. This is particularly dangerous when one considers the concept of defence and nuclear weapons, if a machine controls this the humanitarian element of control is essentially lost. This is worrying as the human methods of democracy and decision making could be overridden by a machine leading to avoidable death and destruction.

Another example of detriment from the advance of modern technology includes the loss of jobs due to the mechanisation of several industries. Jobs involving hand-made items, or the distinct human touch could be redundant if a machine is able to perform the same operation more cheaply and efficiently. This is arguably the loss of creativity and “humanity”.

Having said this, there is no doubt that the rise of technology and its accessibility in more homes than ever before gives a platform and a measure of equity to the access of information to more people than ever before. It is extremely common for most adults (and teenagers these days) to have a smartphone that contains a computer and access to the internet at all times. This means information is at your fingertips which leads to innovation, learning and advancement.

In addition, although we discussed how advancement can be dangerous for some industries, it is equally and perhaps more so integral to it. From aviation to retail to computer science and medicine technology gives us tools to explore further like never before. Taking medicine as an example, the ability to use gene therapy as a means of providing the most tailored treatment possible pushes the boundaries of technology today; and medical advancements in surgery and prostheses using robotics and 3D printers is changing and saving lives.

Try to think about aspects of your life that are impacted by the dangers and the benefits of technology; writing about personal experience gives clarity and originality in your work.

Higher education and great numbers – that is a contradiction in terms. *(Nietzsche)*

This statement puts forth the notion that higher education should only be undertaken by a relatively small number of people as this is what one would expect from the term "higher education". One would assume that as one passes up the ranks of levels of education, each one more advanced than the previous, that the number of people at each stage would also decrease; similar to a pyramid hierarchy based off of meritocracy.

Higher education is commonly associated with developing yourself into a speciality of sorts, where previously you may have taken fewer subjects, you may now narrow your scope down or refine the level of study to one higher with more nuanced points; and with greater engagement with academic literature.

What you understand by "higher education" could be interpreted as university as is a common association. However, you may wish to argue that higher education includes apprenticeships, college students or others pursuing education beyond the compulsory years within the UK.

You may argue that qualitatively higher education is different from other forms of education, in that the ratio of teaching staff to students is significantly larger, meaning more teachers per pupil, leading to more individualised and stimulating teaching. You could discuss the focus on being independent and accountable for your own learning, and also having a greater responsibility with regards to what you can do within your own learning. Take Chemistry, for example: if one studied Chemistry at university they would find much more responsibility placed on them to use higher technology, more precise equipment in practical work than they had ever used before at school.

When arguing that it is indeed possible to deliver higher education to a large proportion of the population you may wish to consider the role of technology and the internet as a platform by which many people can sign up to take online courses; the MOOCs or Massive Open Online Courses offered by some universities come to mind. These courses can include a variety of styles of learning (including visual and auditory) and include videos, text, animations and podcasts as a multi-media approach to the supply of information. They can also be pitched at a variety of different levels, maximising participation as those of several different levels of education could take part.

For those reading this shortly after the lockdown due to the COVID-19 pandemic you may wish to consider how university lectures are currently being delivered and you could use this as evidence of how higher education can be delivered to a larger proportion of the population.

2006 Section 3

The main benefit of 'patient consent' is that it relieves doctors of blame for bad decisions.

The argument underlying the statement is that by consenting to a treatment, a patient takes responsibility for that decision; not the doctor (even if it ends up being a bad decision).

The benefits of patient consent generally include the fact that the patient is now informed, they have a good understanding of what the treatment will entail, they have been alerted as to the pros and cons of the treatment as well as what role they will need to take in their own care. On top of this, they have been given the reasoning behind why this treatment option was chosen as opposed to another or no treatment at all. It also reduces litigation of doctors given that on the whole, the supply of more information ensures the patient is willing to undergo treatment.

Information given during the consent process allows patients to retain autonomy, one of the four pillars or medical ethics. It is also detailed by GMC documents (for example you could look at the GMC ethical guidance for doctors if you wanted to do further reading). In order for the patient to be able to give consent, they are tested for competence and the needs for consent are detailed here: https://www.nhs.uk/conditions/consent-to-treatment/

An example of where patient consent would be meaningful is if they could voluntarily give their consent without coercion, having been fully informed. To do this they also need to have capacity which involves being able to understand information given to you, retain it, make a decision regarding the information and communicate it back. Consent can be given verbally, as written consent, or non-verbally (e.g. holding out your arm for a blood test). So a situation such as a patient giving consent for surgery involves them being tested for capacity, being told about all of the risks and benefits of the procedure as well as the alternatives (or no treatment at all) and making a decision based on this information. In this instance, consent would be meaningful.

Consent would not be meaningful if the patient was told to sign a document allegedly giving consent without being informed of the risks or benefits of the treatment, and/or without being tested for capacity.

Clinical decisions ought to be made on a best-interests basis; that is whether the treatment or lack of treatment given is in the best interest of the patient. This involves using clinical expertise, using evidence-based medicine as far as possible, and the needs and wishes of the patient themselves. An example of where this could be deemed to go wrong is if a patient may be quite happy to take a drug that hasn't got a sound evidence basis where the doctor has had a lapse of clinical judgement but this is not acting in the best interests of the patient. Having all 3 ensures fullness and the best clinical outcome. You can read more about this at the following link: https://www.ncbi.nlm.nih.gov/pmc/articles/PMC3477329/.

However, it is worth noting that at the end of the day, if a patient does not want a treatment that will benefit them, there's nothing doctors can do about it: 'Ultimately, if a patient is deemed to have capacity, the patient's autonomy/wishes reign supreme, and this should be respected in the clinical decision-making process'.

BMAT 2007

Section 1

Q1	B

After the first year of growth, the tree will be 1m.
After two years of growth it will be 1m + [0.1 x (30-1)] = 1m + (2.9m) = 3.9m
After three years of growth it will be 3.9m + [0.1 x (30-3.9)] = 3.9m + 2.61m = 6.51m = 6.5m.

Q2	C

The passage argues that other events in history have caused similarly dangerous and devastating effects (air raids on Hamburg and Tokyo for example, and '*conventional bombing*') to WMDs, and therefore the fact that they are '*uniquely dangerous*' is easily disproved. A is incorrect because the passage doesn't discuss the morality of WMDs, B incorrect as the passage doesn't deny that they are devastating, just that they aren't the only serious threat. D is incorrect for similar reasons.

Q3	C

The easiest way to solve this question is to add an extra column to the table, titled 'increase' to be able to see how much each person increased by (as a proportion of the total increase).

Representative	Increase
Asquith	60,000
Burton	40,000
Coleridge	50,000
Darwin	100,000
Elgar	50,000
Total Increase	300,000

The table shows us that Elgar and Coleridge had the same increase, which was a 1/6 of the total increase. We also know that Darwin had an increase double that of Elgar and Coleridge, which was a 1/3 of the total. Therefore, we need to find a pie chart which matches these facts, which is C.

Q4	A

The conclusion of this passage is '*To reduce this loss of young life, the driving test should require a much higher level of mastery of driving skills*' and it says that drivers wouldn't be allowed until they had more driving experience.
1 is correct as it weakens the argument, as the passage doesn't acknowledge that there are many young drivers who are highly skilled who are involved in serious accidents, and therefore the level of skill may not be the problem.
2 is incorrect as it does not refer to the skill of the driver, which is the crux of the argument
3 is incorrect because it supports the argument, as opposed to weakening it.

2007 Section 1

Q5	B

Looking at the table we can immediately rule out maternity, as its occupancy is roughly 60% whereas, learning disabilities (the row above it), has a much higher occupancy (which can be seen as 4,134 is very close to 4,899). The remaining rows may not easily be worked out by eye, so at this point it is good to calculate the remaining, using approximations to make calculations quicker.
Acute: 93/110 = ~85%
Geriatric: 24/27 = ~89%
Mental illness: 28/32 = 87.5%
Learning disabilities: 4/5 = 80%
Therefore, B (geriatric) has the highest occupancy.

Q6	B

The argument states that more young people should take up boxing as every time a boxing club has been set up in a high-crime area, there has been a reduction in violent crime. Here the flaw/weakness in the argument can be seen as correlation does not equal causation, and there could be other leisure activities that reduce the crime rate more than boxing. Therefore, B is correct. A & C are not relevant to the conclusion while D actually strengthens the argument.

Q7	E

There are only two ways that the bulbs can be ordered, so that the colours alternate.
The 1st permutation: YRYRYR
The 2nd permutation: RYRYRY
Both will have the same probability of occurring, so let us work out the probability of the 1st permutation occurring
The probability of the first flower being yellow, is ½, and subsequently, the probability that the next flower will be red is 3/5. The probability the following flower in the sequence will be yellow is 2/4, the probability of the next being red is 2/3, the probability of the next being yellow is ½, and the probability that the final one is yellow will be 1.
So, multiplying the probabilities (the 'AND' rule), we get
$\frac{1}{2} \times \frac{3}{5} \times \frac{2}{4} \times \frac{2}{3} \times \frac{1}{2} \times 1 = \frac{12}{240} = \frac{1}{20}$
As there are two permutations, the total probability is $\frac{1}{20} + \frac{1}{20} = \frac{1}{10}$

Q8	C

The author presents the idea that many people think that if they can't explain something, then it must be paranormal. He then goes onto to argue against this idea presenting evidence of '*fire-walking*'; therefore, C is the correct answer. A and B are too definitive for the scope of the passage (as the passage neither rules out paranormal experiences, nor states that everything can be explained, rather it says that for the majority of what may be thought as paranormal events, an explanation can be found). D is incorrect as the passage states that they do occur, just that they are thought of as paranormal or mystical.

Q9	E

For this 2kg, its ber is [30 x 2 + 70] = 130. The cat has sepsis, so its mer will be 1.6 x 130 = 208kcal. Therefore, it will need 7 x 2.08 = 14.56g of protein = E.

Q10	C

This cat's ber is [70 x $1^{0.75}$] = 70 Its mer is 70 x 1.3 = 91kcal. Therefore, its maintenance protein requirement is 0.91 x 7 ~ 6.34g.
CCFR has 1 kcal/ml, so will need 91ml for the cat to receive its mer of 91kcal. However, 91ml of CCFR has 91 x 0.06 = 5.46g of protein. Therefore, the cat is receiving [6.34 – 5.46] = 0.88g, so it's receiving 0.9g too little of protein = C (we have rounded 0.88 to get 0.9)

Q11	C

For this question, we need to work out what the ratio of protein to calories in each of the feed formulae in the answer options is, and then match it with the requirement of a cat with renal failure which is 4g of protein per 100kcal.
FCH has 1.4g/1.3kcal, which as we can see is too high (as in 130kcal, there will be 140g)
CCFR has 0.06g/1kcal which is 6g/100kcal which is too high
ES has 0.04g/1kcal which is 4g/100kcal – this is the correct answer
OHN has 0.05g/1.1kcal which is roughly 4.5g/100kcal – this is too high
EMF has 0.08g/2.1 kcal which is roughly 4g/105 kcal – this is too low.

Q12	C

100kcal worth of CCFR feed (the correct one) will have 6g of protein (this is the amount we need), so the ratio is 6:100.
CCF has 0.09g of protein, for each kilocalorie and ES has 0.04g of protein per kilocalorie so we can set up an algebraic equation, where F is the volume of ES feed added.
0.09 x 100ml + 0.04F = 0.06 (100 + F) [Note, the 100 + F is the total final volume]
9 + 0.04F = 6 + 0.06F
3 = 0.02F, so F = 150ml.

Q13	C

We can see that in the 16-24 category, just less than 10% had drunk on x days or more.
Using trial and improvement, we can work out the value of x.
When x = 3, the % is 10 + 7 + 4 + 2 + 3 = 26% which is too high
When x = 4, the % is 7 + 4 + 2 + 3 = 16% which is too high
When x = 5, the % is 4 + 2 + 3 = 9% which is just less than 10%. Therefore, x = 5 is correct

Q14	A

The argument's main point is that dogs were more active/anxious than usual, because they could hear sounds from rocks scraping or breaking underground before an impending earthquake. Therefore, the dog's hearing is the important thing. A is correct, as if dogs who couldn't hear weren't more anxious, it shows that the argument is correct in thinking that it was the sounds that the dogs were hearing that made them more anxious. B is not relevant to the argument, C doesn't affect the strength/weakness of the argument, and D weakens the argument, as it says that sounds aren't produced before an earthquake.

Q15	C

Paul received 116 votes, and thus Elaine must have received 58 votes. The number of votes for Paul and Elaine make up 2/3 of the total votes, so 116 + 58 = 2/3 of x, where x is the total number of votes. Therefore 174 = 2/3x, so x = 261 votes. Therefore, Ann received 87 votes. Thus, Paul won the election by a margin of 29 votes (116 – 87)

2007 Section 1

Q16	A

The problem with the above argument is that it says that just because a phenomenon has occurred for a group of people, it will occur for every individual, which is summarised in D. B is incorrect as the argument does not bring into account lifestyle, C is incorrect as the conclusion '*So it's clear that someone who is awarded a PhD in Sweden will live longer than they would have done if they had not studied for a higher degree*' only refers to Sweden, and doesn't assume that this trend occurs in other countries. D is incorrect as there is a flaw in reasoning; those with PhDs are the healthiest people is not the same as only the healthiest people are awarded PhDs, and the article only assumes the former.

Q17	B

The above argument's conclusion is that '*today's smokers find it harder to give up than did their predecessors, since smokers are now inhaling more nicotine*'.
1 is incorrect as it doesn't refer to the amount of nicotine
2 is correct as if people smoked fewer higher nicotine content cigarettes, then the overall amount of nicotine inhaled would stay the same
3 is incorrect as it isn't relevant to the conclusion and doesn't affect the amount inhaled.

Q18	B

He is able to buy 50 paving slabs for £140. Each paving slab is 0.7m x 0.7m and so has an area of $0.49m^2$. Therefore, the total area that Bob can slab is 50 x 0.49 = $24.5m^2$.
This slabbed area is twice as long as it is wide, so the width is w, and the length will be 2w.
Therefore, 2w x w = 24.5, so $2w^2 = 24.5$
$w^2 = 12.25$, so w = 3.5m.
Therefore, the width of the flower bed is 5m – 3.5m = 1.5m = B

Q19	B

The faster driver's average lap time is 66 seconds, whereas the slower driver's is 70 seconds. When the faster car laps the slower one, it means that it will have done one more lap than the slower one, so we can create the following equation, where x is the number of laps
66x = 70(x-1), so 66x = 70x – 70, so 70 = 4x, so x = 17.5
So the faster car will lap the slower one after 17.5 laps
17.5 x 66 = 1155 seconds, which is 19 minutes and 15 seconds = B

Q20	D

% of men screened positive = [(number of true positive + number of false positive)/1000] x 100.[(21 + 85)/1000] x 100 = 106/1000 x 100 = **10.6%**

Q21	C

Those who were found to have cancer were:

- 26% of those who had abnormal PSA levels, so 26% of 10%, which is 0.26 x 0.1 = 0.026 = 2.6%
- 0.8% of those with normal PSA levels, so 0.8% of 90%, which is 0.008 x 0.9 = 0.0072 = 0.72%

So, 2.6% + 0.72% = 3.32% = C

Q22	A

False positives in the PSA test: 74% of 10% = 0.74 x 0.1 = 0.074 = 7.4%
False positives in the DRE test: 85/1000 = 8.5%
Therefore, there are fewer false positives in PSA than DRE, so P is correct
False negatives in the PSA test: 0.8% of 90% = 0.72%
False negatives in the DRE test: 16/1000 = 1.6%
Therefore, there are fewer false negatives in PSA than DRE, so Q is correct

Q23	B

The chance of getting a false positive on the PSA test is 7.4% (0.074). The chance of getting a false positive on the DRE test is 8.5% (0.085)
0.074 x 0.085 = 0.00629. 0.00629 x 1000 = 6.29 ~ 6 = B.

Q24	D

The passage states that the internet doesn't allow the physical movement of goods across the world, and therefore it is not needed for globalisation, only that the internet makes the exchange of ideas easier. Therefore, the internet is neither a necessary nor sufficient condition.

Q25	B

334,000 + 54,000 square km of farmland would produce 35 billion gallons of ethanol per year. Therefore, each square km of farmland produces (35,000,000,000/388,000) ~90,000 gallons of ethanol. 54,000 x 90,000 = 4,860,000,000 = 4.9 billion = B.

Q26	C

Using the data given in the question, we need to work out how many possible combinations there are. We can see that there are 4 combinations.
Window **8A, 8B**, Pete, Aisle, Maurice, Noola, Olive
Window Olive, Noola, Maurice, Aisle, Pete, **8E, 8D**
Window **8A,** Maurice, Noola, Aisle, Pete, **8E**, Olive
Window Olive**, 8B**, Pete, Aisle, Noola, Maurice, **8D**
Only two out of the four combinations have two vacant seats together, so the probability of that occurring is ½ = C.

Q27	C

6/50 chickens had rings on the second day when they were rounded up, and 50 have rings in total. Therefore, we can set up and equation, where x is the total number of chicken.

$$\frac{6}{50} = \frac{50}{x}$$

$$x = 50 \times \frac{50}{6} \sim 417 = C$$

Q28	A

The passage concludes that sleeping with the light on during infancy causes increased rates of myopia/nearsightedness in children, as there is a correlation between the two variables. The flaw in the argument is that correlation does not always equal causation – A is correct as it provides another reason which may explain this relationship, as it suggests that myopia is more likely to present in children who have myopic parents (through inheritance). B and C do not give other reasons why the correlation may have occurred, whereas D actually strengthens the argument, providing more evidence for the correlation.

Q29	C

The conclusion is that the purchasing of diamonds is morally unjustifiable because the human cost for the war-torn countries that they may have come from is too high. The first sentence tells us that this '*human cost*' is due to the money from diamond sales going to finance military rebellion of groups opposing legitimate governments. C is therefore correct, as it provides a contradiction to this, saying that diamond sales benefit the 'recognised governments' of the countries, weakening the argument.
A is incorrect as it doesn't weaken the argument that diamonds have too high a cost, B is irrelevant to the conclusion as it doesn't mention diamonds, while D doesn't talk about diamonds and their relation to wars/governments, so isn't correct.

Q30	E

This is a visualisation question – if you find these questions difficult, the authors recommend you cut out the shapes during your practice to see how the nets transform int 3D shapes. Only nets Q and S will fold into cubes (when folded the two triangles will fit together to form a square).

Q31	B

1. MHR = 217 – (0.85 x 60) = 217 – 51 = 166bpm
2. Add 4 beats for 55+ year old elite athletes = 166 + 4 = 170bpm
3. Subtract 14 beats for swimming training = 170 – 14 = 156bpm = B

Q32	D

A is not correct as we do not know the absolute values for the wages, only the relative wage increases compared to someone who left school at 15.
B is not correct for the same reason as A.
C is not correct because women who leave education when they are 22 earn less than those who left when they were 21.
D is correct for the same reason as C.
E is not correct as it is not possible to tell this from the graph, which shows us only the proportional wage increase relative to those who left education at 15.

Q33	C

Correlation ≠ causation are common BMAT questions, and this is one of them. The authors assume that the increase is caused by the education, when there may be other factors causing this relationship – C explains this and is so correct. A is incorrect, as the authors have already said that these figures are averages, B is not correct as cannot be inferred from the data, D is not assumed by the text and can be used to weaken the authors' arguments and E is not assumed as the data provided is just wages relative to the wages of those earned by someone who left at age 15 (and not relative to the wages of a 15 year old!).

Q34	B

The question asks us to find a cause for why trade union members have lower financial returns on their degrees, and B gives us a reason. A is not relevant to the relationship as the number of people who sign up to a trade union doesn't affect the relationship between membership and financial return from a degree, C wouldn't be an explanatory reason for the relationship as it refers to those who have degrees, D isn't relevant and E is wrong for the same reasons as A.

Q35	D

Older people who left education earlier but earned more is contrary to our trend; if this was not true our general trend and best fit lines would be stronger and have a higher gradient, therefore the effect of these older people on the graph is that it has caused the gradient to be lower, as our trend has been weakened.

2007 Section 2

Q1	B

The table shows us that there is no protein in the fluid. Therefore, the fluid must have been taken from a part of the kidney after the glomerulus/Bowman's capsule, as ultrafiltration must have already occurred, so we can rule A out. We also see that the fluid is 99% water, which means that the fluid must be in a part of the kidney before the Loop of Henle and collecting ducts, so B (the proximal convoluted tubule) is correct. We can also tell that B is correct as there is still some glucose left.

Q2	B

If element x is in period 2, it means that it has two electron shells, the first of which must be full. Element y has six more protons that element x, therefore must be in either period 2 or period 3 (so A is incorrect), and therefore will have two or three electron shells, the first of which must be full. Therefore, B is correct as both will have full first shells. C is incorrect, as this is not true if x is in groups 3-8, and D is incorrect as the increase in nucleon (mass) number is not always the same as the increase in atomic number (# of protons).

Q3	α = 220, β = 40

Placing a sheet of paper between the source and the detector means only beta particles will be detected (as alpha has a very small penetrating power and will be absorbed by paper). Therefore, the beta particles count rate was 60 – 20 = 40 bpm (we minus 20 to account for background radiation). The total count rate (removing background radiation) was 260bpm, as 280 – 20 = 260. To get the count rate caused by alpha, we do 260 – 40 = 220bpm (the 40 is caused by beta particles).

Q4	A

Let us create an equation for the new value of A, using what the question has told us:

$$A = \frac{(1.5x + 1.5y)^2 \times 0.8z}{2P} Q$$

$$A = \frac{2.25(x + y)^2 \times 0.8z}{2P} Q$$

We can ignore the variables, as we are only looking at the percentage change in A.

$$A = \frac{2.25 \times 0.8}{2} = \frac{1.8}{2} = 0.9$$

Therefore, the new A is 90% of the old A, so its value has decreased by 10%.

Q5	E

Exhalation: intercostals relax, ribcage moves down and in, diaphragm relaxes and goes dome shaped, volume of thorax decreases, pressure in the thorax increases and the air rushes out. Therefore 1 and 3 are correct.

Q6	A

$$t = 2\pi\sqrt{\frac{2lR^2\left(W + \frac{w}{3}\right)}{n\pi r^4 g}}$$

$$\left(\frac{t}{2\pi}\right)^2 = \frac{2lR^2(W + {}^{w}/_{3})}{n\pi r^4 g}$$

$\frac{t^2}{4\pi^2} \times n\pi r^4 g = 2lR^2(W + {}^{w}/_{3})$ which is $\frac{nt^2r^4g}{4\pi} = 2lR^2(W + {}^{w}/_{3})$

$$\frac{nt^2r^4g}{8\pi lR^2} = W + \frac{w}{3}$$

$$W = \frac{nr^4gt^2}{8\pi lR^2} - \frac{w}{3} = A$$

Q7	300

For this question, we need to use this formula: $\frac{n_s}{n_P} = \frac{v_s}{v_p}$ and V = P/I to work out the output voltage/voltage on the secondary coil. The output voltage = 500W/10A = 50V.
So: $\frac{n_s}{1500} = \frac{150}{250}$, therefore $n_s = 1500 \times \frac{50}{250} = \mathbf{300}$

Q8	B

This question is surprisingly simple once you realise that you have to use oxidation states. The O_4 has an oxidation state of -8, and since the molecule of iron oxide is electrically neutral, the sum of the oxidation states of the 3 iron atoms must be +8. The only way to achieve this is by having 2 Fe atoms with an oxidation of +3, and 1 Fe atom with an oxidation state of +2 per molecule. Therefore, 1/3 of the iron ions are Fe^{2+}.

Q9	B

When the heart is pumping blood to the lungs, blood flows out of the right ventricle, through the pulmonary artery. At the same time, blood is pumped out of the left ventricle to the rest of the body through the aorta. Therefore, both atrioventricular valves will be closed (this prevents backflow of blood into the atria), and both semilunar valves will be open, to allow blood to flow from the ventricles into the major arteries (left ventricle leads into aorta, and right into pulmonary artery).

2007 Section 2

Q10	D

The precipitate is PbI_2; to get the greatest height of the precipitate, you need to have the greatest number of moles of lead iodide, and therefore the greatest number of moles of the limiting reactant. The mole ratio of potassium iodide to lead nitrate is 2:1, so in order to work out which reactant is limiting, we divide n(KI) by 2, and then see whether the number of moles of lead nitrate or potassium iodide is the smallest. The smallest value will tell us the limiting reactant, and this value will be the number of moles of lead iodide. To work out the number of moles, we use the formula n = cv.

	$n(Pb(NO_3)_2)$	[n(KI)]/2	Which chemical is limiting?	$n(PbI_2)$*
A	0.005 x 2 = 0.01	(0.01 x 2 = 0.02)/2 = 0.01	N/A (all the chemicals will be used up)	0.01
B	0.0025 x 5 = 0.0125	(0.0025 x 5 = 0.0125)/2 = 0.00625	KI	0.00625
C	0.0075 x 3 = 0.0225	(0.005 x 5 = 0.025)/2 = 0.0125	KI	0.0125
D	0.005 x 4 = 0.02	(0.0075 x 5 = 0.0375)/2 = 0.01875	KI	0.01875

* $n(PbI_2)$ is equal to the $n(Pb(NO_3)_2)$ if lead nitrate is the limiting reactant, or equal to half the number of moles of KI if KI is the limiting reactant, as there is a 2:1 ratio between KI and PbI_2.

The greatest number of moles of lead iodide occurs in D, so D is the correct answer.

Q11	E

1 is correct as this is possible during a change of state (think of the flat parts of a cooling curve). 2 is correct as heat can pass through a vacuum in the form of radiation. 3 is correct because steam is in a higher energy state (gas) than boiling water, and so has more energy. 4 is correct – a convection current is set up when a container of water is heated or cooled.

Q12	E

This question tests knowledge that is not currently on the BMAT specification.

The mean (Q_2) of this data set is 850 steps, and the upper quartile (Q_3) is 1000 steps. ¼ of the data set lies between the upper quartile and the mean, so there is a ¼ probability of a member having taken between 850 and 1000 steps.

Since we want to know the probability of 3 of these members having taken between 850 and 1000 steps, we do ¼ x ¼ x ¼ = 1/64 = E.

Q13	C

This question tests knowledge that is not currently on the BMAT specification.

The calf muscles contracting provides the effort, the load is the downward force exerted by the foot and the fulcrum are the toes. Therefore, the load is between the fulcrum and the effort.

Q14	A

The most exothermic reaction will be the one between the most reactive group 1 element and the most reactive group 7 element. Out of the group 1 elements in the answer options, caesium is the most reactive, and fluorine is the most reactive group 7 element, so A is the correct answer.

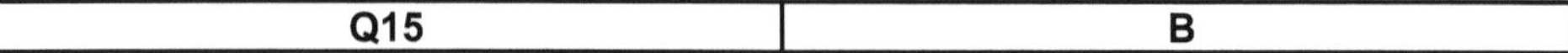

Q15	B

This question tests knowledge that is not currently on the BMAT specification.
The shorter the wavelength of light, the more refraction that occurs – therefore the violet light will get refracted the most as it has the shortest wavelength. Therefore, A, C and E are incorrect. Both rays of light will follow similar refractory paths, so D is incorrect, and since the light enters/is incident in the top half of the air bubble, it will refract out of the top half of the air bubble, so B is correct.

Q16	C

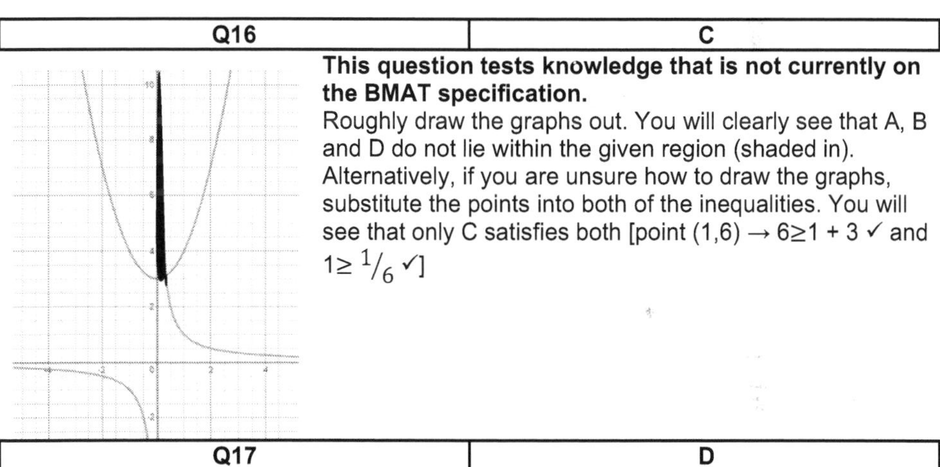

This question tests knowledge that is not currently on the BMAT specification.
Roughly draw the graphs out. You will clearly see that A, B and D do not lie within the given region (shaded in). Alternatively, if you are unsure how to draw the graphs, substitute the points into both of the inequalities. You will see that only C satisfies both [point (1,6) → $6 \geq 1 + 3$ ✓ and $1 \geq {}^{1}/_{6}$ ✓]

Q17	D

Only the males in this family tree get NPS, so we can infer that it is sex-linked, with the allele for NPS carried on the X chromosome. Call the allele for NPS X^N and the normal allele (the one that doesn't cause NPS) X^n. Looking at the family tree, we can see that 8 and 9's father (the black square) must have a genotype of X^NY, and therefore X and Y must be both X^NX^n (heterozygous), as they don't have the condition. They would have received a X^N from their father, and a X^n from their mother. Therefore, since 8 and 9 must be heterozygotes, we are left with answer options D or E.

This means that we have to see whether 4 or 5 must also be a heterozygote. 1 must have the genotype X^nY since he doesn't have the condition, and 2 must be X^NX^n since her son has the condition, and therefore must have received the X^N from her. (Note: 2 is a heterozygote, but B is not the correct answer since as seen in the previous paragraph 6 can be X^nX^n or X^NX^n). We are unable to deduce the genotype of 5 as she can be either X^nX^n or X^NX^n. 4 must be a heterozygote however, as just like her mother, she doesn't have NPS and she is married to a man who doesn't have NPS (X^nY), yet has a son who has NPS, so she must be the one to pass on the X^N allele.

2007 Section 2

Q18	D

The number of moles of H_2O in 6g of ice is mass/Mr = 6/18 = 0.3333 moles of H_2O
1 mole = $24dm^3$ at RTP, so 0.3333 moles of H_2O is $8dm^3$ = $8000cm^3$.

Q19	700N

This question tests knowledge that is not currently on the BMAT specification.
Clockwise moments = anticlockwise moments.
The weight of the bar will be a clockwise moment, as the weight will be exerted from the midpoint of the bar, which is 1.5m right of the pivot. Call the weight of the bar, w.
4.5 x 100 + 1.5b = 1.5 x 1000
450 + 1.5b = 1500
1.5b = 1050
b = 700N

Q20	A

The longest side is the hypotenuse, or c, thinking in terms of Pythagoras' rule. If we call the remaining side a, then we have the following formula, which we can solve for a.

$$a^2 + \left(3 + 2\sqrt{5}\right)^2 = \left(6 + \sqrt{5}\right)^2$$
$$a^2 + 29 + 12\sqrt{5} = 41 + 12\sqrt{5}$$
$$a^2 = 12 \; a = \sqrt{12} = 2\sqrt{3} = A$$

Q21	E

Platelets are involved in clotting, so a low platelet count would mean low levels of clotting. White blood cells are needed for defence against disease, so a large number of abnormal WBCs would mean low disease resistance. Red Blood Cells transport oxygen and aren't affected so oxygen transport is unaffected/stays at normal levels.

Q22	D

1 is correct (you will need to be able to recall the formulae of common compounds).
2 is incorrect, ammonia solution is alkaline, so will have a pH greater than 7.
3 is correct as ammonia has a simple molecular structure.
4 is incorrect as it is alkaline, so it will turn damp red litmus paper blue.
5 is incorrect as it is a gas at room temperature.
6 is correct as both nitrogen and hydrogen are non-metals, so bonding is covalent.

Q23	E

For the purposes of this question, an artery can be viewed as a cylinder, with length x mm, cross-sectional area A, and volume Ax.
The volume of blood flowing through the artery per second is the same as the volume of the artery divided by time it takes one RBC to pass through the length, so
$V = \frac{Ax}{T}$, therefore $A = \frac{VT}{x}$. However, A here, has units (ml/second x seconds)/mm which is ml/mm whereas we want A in mm^2. A ml is $1000mm^3$, so we must multiply $\frac{VT}{x}$ by 1000 to get A in mm^2.

Q24	A

The volume of the cylinder is $\pi r^2 l$. The volume of a sphere is $4/3\pi r^3$, so the volume of a hemisphere is $2/3\pi r^3$. Therefore, total volume is $\pi r^2 l + 2/3\pi r^3$ which is $\pi r^2(l + 2/3r)$ which is $\pi r^2(3l + 2r) = \pi r^2(2r + 3l)$ = A.

Q25	A

The top of the fractionating column is the coolest, and where the fraction with the lowest boiling point condenses and runs off. Therefore, C and D are incorrect. The answer is A, as the temperature in the flask will be the average of both boiling points. This is because the flask will need to be hot enough to evaporate the hexane, but not the heptane.

Q26	C

For this question, a clear understanding of the roles of the ovarian hormones in the menstrual cycle is needed. Oestrogen is needed to thicken the lining of the uterus, and a high concentration of progesterone maintains the lining of the uterus – thus a fall in progesterone concentration leads to the breakdown of the uterine lining.

Q27	D

1 is correct as beta emissions results in the atomic number increasing by 1, as a beta particle is a neutron which turns into a proton and a high energy electron, the latter which is ejected from the nucleus.
2 is correct because beta radiation is absorbed by the skin.
3 is incorrect as the radiation will attack all cells; it is not cell specific.

2007 Section 3

To see the marking grid and mark bands that the BMAT examiners will use to mark your essays, please refer to the BMAT website. *To view the full questions, see:* https://www.admissionstesting.org/for-test-takers/bmat/preparing-for-bmat/practice-papers/

The technology of medicine has outrun its sociology. [*Henry E. Sigerist (1891-1957)*]

This statement means that the levels of innovation that we have reached in terms of technology allows us to do many more medical interventions/treatments/procedures, but this technological innovation has occurred at a faster rate than the rate at which societal opinions/views have changed and progressed.

For example, many medical technologies are available at present, but are currently not implemented in society regularly today, as society rejects them on the basis of the treatment not being in line with society's ethical standards, or being against the cultural, religious or personal beliefs of those within the society. For example, embryonic stem cells have been seen as a way to cure diseases such as type I diabetes, where non-functioning islet cells are replaced with those capable of producing insulin. However, a large part of society objects against this treatment, as an embryo has to be destroyed to access these stem cells, and many people view an embryo as a 'potential life'.

Additionally, new medical technologies are, on the whole, very expensive, and so only limited to the very rich – since the whole population does not have access to these treatments, it can be interpreted that the technology of medicine is outrunning its sociology. As Sigerist himself says, under a private medical system, where the number of physicians is '*determined by need but by the per-capita spendable income of the population, large sections of the population have no medical care at all or certainly not enough'* we can see how his statement holds some truth.

A way of addressing this problem would be with education – society can be educated on how modern technologies can still fit in with their code of ethics/religious beliefs. For example, many religious believers use certain parts of their holy texts to justify advances in technology related to gene technology; for example, even though it may be seen as playing 'God', as long as it betters the (quality of) life of the person receiving the treatment, genetic engineering/gene editing can be seen as part of the religious duty of kindness/caring for others.

Public health systems, such as the NHS, could be a way of addressing the problem Sigerist describes, as they ensure that everyone has access to (the majority of) current treatments, regardless of their ability to pay, thereby reducing the inequality in healthcare.

Alternatively, researchers or scientists could try and alter their technologies to fit in with the views of society, so that they can be more readily accepted and used. For example, researchers are currently looking at using and reprogramming adult stem cells (ASCs) [*induced pluripotent stem cells*] for treatments, as opposed to using embryonic stem cells, as there are fewer ethical issues involved with ASCs as no embryo/person is killed.

Authors' Tip

The ethics of stem cell use is still a hot topic today, and ever more research is being carried out in this field of research, as it is becoming a more viable option to treat debilitating diseases such as Stargardts Macular Dystrophy, and more common conditions like diabetes or leukaemia. Stem cells and their ethics of use may come up at interviews. For more information on the types of stem cells, their use in research and the ethics involved, have a read of this article: https://bbsrc.ukri.org/documents/1007-stem-cell-resourse-edition3-pdf/

Our unprecedented survival has produced a revolution in longevity which is shaking the foundations of societies around the world and profoundly altering our attitudes to life and death [*Tom Kirkwood, BBC Reith Lectures, 2001*]

The statement means that the increases in life expectancy worldwide due to improvements in medicine and nutrition are profoundly affecting many institutions which make up societies, such as healthcare systems and social care networks, as well as changing societies' opinions on life and death.

The world has seen great reductions in death rates, but in many countries a decline in birth rates haven't followed (those who take A Level/IB Geography/Sociology will know about the Demographic Transition Model), meaning that this increase in longevity has resulted in overpopulation, which is putting great stress on the world's finite resources, such as fossil fuels. Food and water insecurity is also growing (partly due to climate change, which can be seen as caused partly by overpopulation).

Additionally, a more ageing population has placed far more stress on healthcare systems worldwide, as the elderly population tend to have more medical conditions (more comorbidities), and thus more complex health needs. An ageing population also puts more stress on the younger population, who end up getting taxed more.

Improvements in healthcare mean that we fear death and disease less, as there is a greater chance that we will be cured should we contract any disease or injure ourselves, which has meant that people participate in more risky activities that put their lives at risk.

In contrast, people may view that a revolutions in longevity aren't 'shaking the foundations of societies around the world' as not all countries are experiencing this, for example war-torn countries, and those in the developing world, and that this revolution is merely making societies adapt to different challenges in the future. Additionally, many opinions on death have remained unchanged, as many people are unsure what happens after death, and there still remains a great deal respect for the dead, and the way deaths are handled.

The way we are governed, our biological and social need, and our relationships with others, have on the whole, remained unchanged, so perhaps an increase in longevity is simply a natural progression that comes with technological innovation, and hasn't really 'shaken' society to a great extent.

2007 Section 3

Irrationally held truths may be more harmful than reasoned errors.
[Thomas Henry Huxley]

The statement addresses truths in science, and means that truths that you hold with no/little background/reasoning are more dangerous than statements that you believe to be true but are false, which you have reached after much reasoning/deliberation. Huxley warns here about the dangers of believing in statements, which although may be factually correct, have been backed up with very little evidence/justification and have not been put through the rigours of the scientific method.

The wording of the statement is rather ambiguous, and there are really 2 options for what irrationally held truths are:

- a factually true statement that has not been backed up by sufficient evidence or justification and cannot be or has not been justified/proven using conventional methods, such as the scientific method.
- truths in the sense that they are 'true' to the individual, so they may hold at truth that unicorns exist.

We will run with the first definition for this essay plan, but the other definition is also equally valid. For example, in the past, people based medical treatment on superstition, and although superstition/supernatural events as the cause of disease has now been disproved, some of their treatments were successful. Following such truths would be harmful, because the treatments would not have worked on everyone, and could have been dangerous to others.

However, if someone makes a 'reasoned error' – that is a mistruth/false statement that has been backed up with logic or reason, the person is more likely to reach a reasoned truth when they review their method and see their errors/have it peer reviewed or critiqued.

However, sometimes 'irrational truths' are actually helpful, and used today in conventional medicine. For example, in the treatment of some mental health conditions, **electroconvulsive therapy (ECT)** (*sending electrical currents in the brain to trigger small seizures, relieving the symptoms of some mental health problems)* is used, There is currently little understanding/reasoning behind how it functions, but since the treatment works in some cases, it is still used today. If people rejected irrational truths completely, such treatments may not be available, affecting the quality of life of sufferers.

However, reasoned errors can be more harmful than irrationally held truths in certain circumstances.

- In some situations, the answer is the most important part, and not the method, for example:
    - in drug calculations, making a reasoned error could have potentially life-threatening effects if someone is given an incorrect dose, regardless of whether their method was the correct one – in this case, getting the correct answer by an irrational/illogical/incorrect method would be better.
    - making a mathematical (reasoned) error in architecture, can have extremely damaging consequences, as the integrity of the building and its foundation could be easily compromised.
- They can be worse because people will be unlikely to change their scientific appraisal method; so people will be teaching the “right way” of reasoning to their pupils, which is actually wrong, and leads to an error; unless someone else points out it is wrong. So, for a short period of time, people think they are correct and have reasoned well (because humans around them arbitering this process agree) however, the mistake is still unknown.

What is important is that people have a logical reasoning behind these methods, so that if they have made an error, they are able to review their chain of reasoning to identify where they have gone wrong. However, it may be difficult to convince someone who thinks they have a logical method that their method is in fact not correct. Additionally, it may be difficult to convince those who hold ‘irrational truths’ that their reasoning is in fact irrational.

BMAT 2008

Section 1

Q1	D

If some Malgons are Zanders and all Zanders are Tvints this means some Malgons are Tvints. You may find it easier to quickly construct a Venn Diagram to see that the Zanders are a subset of Tvints.

Q2	C

C paraphrases the conclusion. The conclusion of traditional evolutionary theory is that '*animals are never altruistic*' and that even if they show examples of '*reciprocal altruism*' such as with the birds, they have '*clear paybacks*' so are not selfless but '*will benefit*' them.
A – we cannot draw this as a conclusion from the information.
B – It isn't said that this theory is discredited.
D – this may be true but doesn't relate directly to the passage's comments about traditional evolutionary theory which states that that animals are never altruistic.

Q3	B

Totalling all of the screws of each diameter and length gives 250. Out of these, there are 38 that are suitable (20 4mm in diameter and 35mm long and 18 4mm in diameter and 40mm long). 38/250 as a percentage is 15.2% which is 15% to the nearest 1%.

Q4	A

The argument is essentially saying that it isn't sufficient to try and justify animal testing by saying that their '*use has been involved in the major discovery of drugs*'. Hence, the last line sets us up to ask an important question: whether they are '*crucial in proving the necessary weight of evidence on effectiveness and safety of drugs*' not whether animals have been used in major drug discoveries. This is A.

Q5	E

We know that the grey die is the conventional die because 3 clearly opposes 4 (and these total 7 as one would expect).
So now looking at the white die if we try and orient the two positions so that the 6 is the same position, we see that 4 opposes 5, and 3 also opposes 1. This leaves 6 and 2, so these have to be opposite one another.

Q6	D

1 – this is true; the headline is made with regards to thinks of a digital nature yet the survey was only about social networking which is only a small portion of digital applications; so older men could still be using them just as much; just different ones.
2 – this is true; a single survey cannot show a divide growing, that would require at least 2 surveys to observe changes over a period of time.
3 – we do not know whether or not the survey was unrepresentative.

Q7	D

We know that the total area is $20m^2$ and there are 2 lots of 0.4m x 0.4m squares (2 x 0.16 = $0.32m^2$) there are 6 lots of the 0.4m x 0.6m rectangles (6 x 0.4 x 0.6 = $1.44m^2$) and there are 6 lots of the 0.6m x 0.6m squares (6 x 0.6 x 0.6 = $2.16m^2$). Hence the total area of the patio that is black is 0.32 + 1.44 + 2.16 = $3.92m^2$
Hence, 3.92/20 x 100 = 3.92 x 5 = 19.6%

Q8	39%

At the top of the table we need to compare the relative risk values for left-handed and non-left-handed women respectively. The left-handed women have a risk of 1.39 and the non-left-handed women have a risk of 1; hence the percentage increase = 1.39-1/1 x 100 = 39%

Q9	B

The information in the question tells us that 426 women in the group had breast cancer. The total number of person-years can be calculated by adding the figures for person-years for left-handed women and non-left-handed women at the top of the table: 153422 + 19119 = 172541. We are asked to calculate per 1000 person-years, so we need to divide this figure by 1000 then solve. 426/172.541 = 2.47 to 2 dp which rounds to 2.5

Q10	A

For those women with a BMI of over 25, we can see that there are 144 non-left-handed women and 20 left-handed women totalling 164 women overall. The total number of person-year for these women = 57458 + 7787 = 65245. So, per 1000 person-years this will be 65.245.
164/65.245 = 2.5 to 1 dp

Q11	D

A – this is incorrect; normalising to 1 for right-handed (non-left-handed women) women just means that all the figures are comparable, there is no effect on the apparent increase, because the figures don't show a decrease. For instance, the ratio of risk of right-handed to left-handed women could be 1:0.75 but it just so happens that there is always a higher risk for left-handed women; not that the method of data presentation is skewing the results.
B – we can see that actually non-left-handed women (right-handed women) had more children than left-handed women so this actually supports the idea that having kids reduces the risk of breast cancer, not the other way round.
C – if they are unlikely to change the hand with which they write then this is essentially inconsequential, why would that change the proportion of women who wrote with their left hand; and therefore had a higher risk of breast cancer?
D – This is correct. There is a causal reason as to why the number of left-handed women will have a higher susceptibility to breast cancer and it explains the increased risk to this group.
E – This would not explain the apparent increase. Because the incidence is divided by the number of women in each group, this makes the two figures comparable as the calculation represents a proportion.

2008 Section 1

Q12	A

We need to calculate a 25% decrease of £1560, which is equal to 75% of £1560 = £1170. Of this, we know that only adults are charged (as indicated by the question) so we can multiply this sum by 1.4 (1.4 representing 140%, a 40% increase on the takings at the last match). 1.4 x £1170 = £1638.

Q13	E

1 - although the increase in activity by pressure groups were correlated with more people thinking flying was more of a problem than cars, this does not mean the former caused the latter, as the statement suggests.
2 – this statement must be true, '*the number of people who think that flying is the bigger contribution*' tells us that clearly there are people who think this, and we already know that this is wrong as '*cars still make a greater contribution to climate change*' than planes.
3 – this statement sums up the last line: '*47% thought that air travel should be limited, but only 15% were willing to fly less often*'. Clearly, that means 32% believed air travel should be limited but weren't willing to fly less often.

Q14	A

Steve Cram clearly has the slowest time but if you look up the table for dates prior to 16th July 1985, of people who ran quicker times, you will see that Saïd Aouita must have held a new world record. After that, the next quickest runner at a later date was Noureddine Morceli; followed by Hicham El Guerrouj. This means 3 runners have set new world records.

Q15	D

A – overproduction or underproduction of a protein does not necessarily lead to a negative effect on health, imagine if the quantity of protein was irrelevant to the body.
B – this is not true, an 89% increase in one protein and a 32% decrease in another is not necessarily negligible hence this cannot reliably be concluded.
C – this is not necessarily true, just because the survey was conducted to simulate a one-hour long phone call, this does not give us any evidence to suggest phone calls longer than this are detrimental.
D – this is correct. The human body clearly has a reaction of sorts, as 2 protein levels are altered.

Q16	D

We need a graph that reflects the change in volume, initially the volume will increase rapidly a the cross-sectional area of the tank from the top downwards increases; hence the volume will increase at a greater rate than the measurement on the dipstick leaving us with C, D or E as these show this initial pattern.
Then, as the cross-sectional area becomes constant in the cylindrical region of the tank, the rate of increase of volume and the measurement on the dipstick will be directly proportional on the line y = x so we can eliminate C and E for not showing this. Hence the answer is D. For fullness, going to the bottom of the tank, the cross-sectional area decreases, meaning the graph will plateau at a vertical asymptote.

Q17	A

1 – this is plausible, if artists can reach a broader population with the same message then it follows that it is more likely that more people will hear about and implement the advice.
2 – this is not a good challenge. Whether or not the artists are affected and begin to change their own lifestyle, that does not get over the issue the author raised, which is why it is they who have been chosen to watch the concert.
3 – again, the effect on the artist is not the focus of the author, the author's point is that the artists were chosen to do the concert given their lifestyles.

Q18	A

We can start by working out the bounds of each droplet of the chemical (the question tells us the value has been rounded to the nearest 0.01cm^3) meaning the range is actually between 0.015 - 0.025cm^3 . The same can be done with the water, it is between 5cm^3 - 15cm^3. If the solution "must not" be greater than 1% that means we need to consider every scenario and ensure that this is not the case within the given bounds. The way to do this is to imagine we have the most concentrated solution possible, i.e. the largest droplet size and the smallest water volume. Hence, the largest number of 0.025cm^3 droplets in 5cm^3 water to ensure that the concentration does not exceed 1%. So, 1% of 5cm^3 is 0.05cm^3 and 0.05/0.025 = 2 droplets.

Q19	79

'Those who took on more intense exercise – the equivalent of running half an hour a day - extended their lives on average by 3.6 years' so the average life span would increase from 75 to 78.6 which rounds to 79 (the question asks for the nearest year).

Q20	C

The increase in life expectancy due to walking 30 minutes a day – 1.4 years
The increase in life expectancy due to running for 30 minutes a day – 3.6 years
Hence, percentage increase is (3.6 - 1.4)/1.4 x 100 = 2.2/1.4 x 100 which approximates to 157%.

Q21	C

C is the answer here because the passage can only tell us that exercising regularly can improve life expectancy, but we don't have specific evidence of '*exercising more*' helping.

Q22	D

A – this is not necessarily so; we are not told this.
B – this is not a necessary assumption.
C – this is not so, being overweight may increase the risk of illness but this doesn't mean it always will and therefore it will not always reduce life span.
D – this is correct; in order for the conclusion to be sound, we need to be sure that exercise was causing the increase in life span as opposed to fresh air or another factor.
E – this is a stated assumption: it helps '*put off developing heart disease'*.

Q23	D

You need to be able to spot the pattern with regards to the flashes: with a binary system the variables are the number of flashes and the order. For instance, with 1 flash there are 2 choices as shown in the question: either red or blue. With 2 flashes there are 4 choices, red red, red blue, blue red, or blue blue. Hence with 3 flashes there will be 8 choices. Note that the pattern is 2^n where n = the number of flashes.
There are 26 letters in the alphabet, and they will take the following transmissions:
1 flash – A and B ($2^1 = 2$)
2 flashes – C D E F ($2^2 = 4$)
3 flashes – G H I J K L M N ($2^3 = 8$)
4 flashes – O P Q R S T U V W X Y Z (note here there are 12 instead of $2^4 = 16$, but this is because the alphabet has finished)
So, the flashes will take: 2(1) + 4(2) + 8(3) + 12(4) = 82 seconds
But the question also says that there is a 1 second gap between letters, and there are 26 letters with 25 gaps, so 82 + 25 = 107 seconds

Q24	D

A – even if the chances of winning have been affected, this does not tell us that the standard of play has declined
B – the interest of the players is not discussed in the passage; we are told they are '*too friendly*' but this does not mean they are more interested in money than players from other countries
C – just because this generation of competitors are '*too friendly*' this does not mean British players in the past weren't friendly, it doesn't give us any indication about how friendly they were
D – this is a conclusion that can be safely drawn. We are told that '*you can be a millionaire now in six months without even winning*'.
E – this is not inferred at all in the passage

Q25	245

	Red Party	Blue Party
Before GE	2.5x	x
After GE	2.5x - 28	x + 28

In the table you can see that we have represented the blue Party before GE as x and used the information in the question to come up with expressions for the other cells. N.B. the question says that the Red Party's lead was reduced by 56, and as there are only 2 parties this means that the Red Party clearly lost half this number (28) and the Blue Party gained this number.

We are also told that after GE the Red Party has 1.5 times the representatives of the Blue Party; in other words: 2.5x - 28 = 1.5(x + 28)
Solving for x: 2.5x - 28 = 1.5x + 42
X = 70
We know that the total number of representatives is 3.5x (it is the sum of the representative of both the Blue and the Red party, which can be done using the figures before the GE: 2.5x + x = 3.5x). Hence, if x = 70, 3.5x = 245

Q26	D

1 - '*at present the police take DNA samples from everyone who has been arrested*' meaning in order to identify an offender they have to have already offended. As 1 rightly points out, some cases of sexual and violent crime are first offences meaning the offenders will not be in the database hence meaning they can't be convicted using DNA samples. This is a weakness.
2 - '*the police need access to the DNA only of those convicted of a serious offence*' meaning that even if one has not been found guilty of a crime, they may have committed it.
3 – this is not a weakness of the argument, since the argument revolves around the use of DNA sampling it is irrelevant whether cases can be solved without this.

Q27	C

Do not be caught out here, the times in the question have been given in minutes not hours so we need to convert them.
Let the speed of the courier be x, and the speed of the convoy be y.
The distance travelled to get back = overall speed x time
So 1km = (x + y) x 30 seconds and converting to hours gives the following:
1km = (x + y) x 1/120 hours so x + y = 120
Doing the same for the courier's distance to return to the front:
1km = (x - y) x 3 minutes
1km = (x - y) x 1/20 hours so x - y = 20
Solving the two equations simultaneously:
Equation 1: y + x = 120
Equation 2: x - y = 20
2x = 140 x = 70
You may find it tricky to understand why the speeds have been put as x + y and x – y respectively, but try and picture the courier's journey; when he travels to the back he will get there really quickly, not only is he going at his constant speed but the convoy are coming forwards at their speed essentially bringing the back closer to him (hence why the speed is x + y). And when he returns to the front it takes a lot longer; the courier is travelling at his own speed but he is now having to essentially try and combat the speed of the travelling convoy in the same direction (hence why it is x-y).

Q28	E

1 – '*with the pace of climate change set to increase, more areas will be at risk of flooding*'. This can only follow as a conclusion if climate change is the cause of flooding.
2 - '*people who own homes in flooded areas already find it very difficult to sell their houses*' telling us that as people clearly want to sell their homes but can't; that nothing effective is being done to prevent those existing homes from being flooded.
3 – we are '*facing a future of limited geographic mobility*' telling us that people won't be moving around as much hence won't want to move to areas at risk of flooding.

Q29	C

In order to get 6 different numbers, there will be 2 single digit numbers and 4 double digit numbers.
We know that the list has to start with 34, because if you do the alternative which is 3, 43, 74, the 74 is clearly too large as the numbers only go from 1 – 49. And you cannot have 3, 4, 37, 42, 73, 37 which again contains a number that is too large, as well as 2 37s.
We can see that 3 and 7 follow each other twice in this list, and both cannot be 37 as 6 different numbers have been chosen. Therefore, one must be 37, and the other must either be a single 3 or a single 7.
You cannot have 34, 3, 7, 42, 73, 37 as there is 73 which is too large.
Hence, it must be 34, 37, … 7 (we end with a 7 due to the reasoning of the above paragraph)
The ... portion is one of the following 3 choices (it has to contain only 1 single digit as we have already used 1 with the 7 above):
42, 73, 3 – not the one because 73 is too large
4, 27, 33 – the correct answer
42, 7, 33 – not the one because there is another 7 which can't be

You should therefore end up with the following order: 34, 37, 4, 27, 33, 7

Q30	E

1 – this is a flaw, whether speeding accounts for 6% or 60% of accidents doesn't matter. Speed traps will still help to prevent accidents due to speeding.
2 – this is not a flaw. The author doesn't ignore this, it doesn't matter whether the accidents caused by under 25-year olds were due to speeding the author is making the point that more should be done to help young people drive safely through experience and learning.
3 – this is a flaw, '*helping young people to drive safely*' will naturally include obeying the speed limit, but the author goes on to then say that these are '*arbitrary limits*' as opposed to limits needed for safety.

Q31	B

This is a tough visualisation question; it requires you to try and pick up the pieces and move them in your head; hence it is difficult to give a worked solution as different people will "see" different things.
A 3 x 2 x 2 cube will be made of 12 smaller cubes, and F and G contain 8 cubes between them, so we need a piece that has 4 smaller cubes. Hence, we can eliminate A. F already contains a row of 3, so we cannot have another complete row of 3 as this will not fit so we can eliminate E.
If we imagine that G is oriented as it is so 3 of its bases are touching the ground, this leaves space for 1 cube on the bottom. Now imagine that F fits in here with the middle cube protrusion pointing inwards. The only shape that remains to make the 3 x 2 x 3 cube is B.

Q32	E

We are told that the average person makes 14 cycle trips a year. We are also told that cycling accounts for 1% of all trips; hence there are 1400 trips a year. This means there are 1400/52 trips a week (as there are 52 weeks in a year). 1400/52 = 27 to the nearest whole number.

Q33	D

A – we cannot infer this, there is no information about the number of people travelling for under 1 mile, we know about trips under 2 miles, but not under 1 mile.
B – cannot be inferred from the information given. The best estimate we can give for this is knowing that 14 cycle trips take place a year by the average person, averaging out to just over 1 trip a month, which still does not agree with statement B.
C – this cannot be inferred; we are not given any information about this.
D – this can be inferred. If 15% of the population ride a bike at least once a week, 8% ride at least once a month, and 69% cycle less than once a year, this leaves 8% (100 – 69 – 15 – 8 = 8) who ride more than once a year, but less than once every month (therefore less than 12 times a year). This means the range is between 1 and 11 times a year.

Q34	C

A - this simply states the trend indicated by Chart 3, that as you own more cars the number of cycle trips decreases. This is not an explanation.
B – even if B was true, it would not explain the information given by the relationship, it does not explain how a higher income seems to be correlated with a higher number of cycle trips.
C – this adequately explains the matter. If there are lots of people who do not own cars but have a higher than average income, these people would be the ones who make more cycle trips. Because they don't have more cars, this means the trend of more cars and fewer cycle trips doesn't stand.
D – the reason for cycling is entirely irrelevant; we are interested in the number of cars, the number of trips and income.

Q35	B

1 – this is not supported. For males aged 21-29 they made 27 trips per year and do 78 miles per year meaning per trip they did on average 78/27 trips which is less than 3 miles per trip. It is actually 2.98 miles to 2 dp. Whereas, males aged 11-19 make 46 trips a year, and do 74 miles a a year meaning they did 74/46 = 1.61 miles per trip to 2 dp. Clearly, the 21-29 males have not done more than twice this distance per trip as 2.98 miles is less than 3.22.
2 – this is supported. The 11-16-year-old males cycle 46 times per year each compared to 29 trips each by 17-20-year-old males so the younger ones clearly cycle more often. However, they do average fewer miles per trip, the 11-16 year olds do 74/46 miles = 1.61 miles (we did this earlier) and the 17-20-year olds do 59/29 = 2.03 miles to 2 dp. 1.61<2.03 so the second half of the statement is also supported.

2008 Section 2

Q1	D

Active transport takes place against a concentration gradient, i.e. from a region of low concentration to a region of high concentration. D is the only one that follows this.

Q2	C

If Y^{3-} has electron configuration 2,8,8 this means Y has electron configuration 2, 8, 5 as it has 3 fewer electrons as an atom. Hence, if it has 5 outer electrons it is in Group 5 so we can eliminate A, B, E and F. It is in period 3 as it has 3 shells, so the answer is C.

Q3	B

Note that the question asks us for a graph of Y! This means that Y is only going to increase as X decays into Y so we can eliminate A, C and E straight away. We also know that X has a half-life of 20s so if X started at 100% after 20s there would be 50% X and 50% Y. At 40s there would be 25% X and 75% Y. At 60s there would be 12.5% X and 87.5%Y. This makes sense, every 20s the quantity of X is halving. The graph that matches this pattern is B.

Q4	D

$P = 2r^2t$
$P = 2(3 \times 10^{-3})^2 \times (2.5 \times 10^4)$
$P = 2(9 \times 10^{-6}) \times (2.5 \times 10^4)$
$P = 18 \times 10^{-6} \times 2.5 \times 10^4$
$P = 45 \times 10^{-2}$ (N.B the question asks for the answer in standard form so do not stop here and pick B as this is not in standard form).
$P = 4.5 \times 10^{-1}$

Q5	C

The question tells us that homozygous recessive foetus mice will die (genotype rr). We know that crossing 2 heterozygous mice would give the following Punnet square:

	R	r
R	RR	Rr
r	Rr	rr

We are asked for the percentage of LIVE offspring that are homozygous dominant (RR), so rr will have died, so out of the remaining live genotypes: RR, Rr and Rr we want to calculate the percentage that are RR. Each of the genotypes are equally as likely, so 1/3 as a percentage is 33%.

Q6	E

The quickest way to solve these sorts of questions is to set up simultaneous equations:
Taking chlorine: $b = a + 2a + 2y = 3a + 2y$
Taking hydrogen: $b = 2x$ so b:x is 1:2. This means we can eliminate D.
Taking oxygen: $4a = x$ so a:x is 4:1 so we can eliminate C and D.
Substituting $b = 2x$ into the first equation we get: $2x = 3a + 2y$
Substituting $x = 4a$ into that we get: $8a = 3a + 2y$ or $5a = 2y$. The only answer that matches the ratio of a:y as 5:2 is E.
N.B. for speed you could always use the most complex expression $b = 3a + 2y$ and substitute each of the values given in the answers and find the answer that fits.

Q7	B

$$If\ the\ nth\ term\ is\ given\ as: \frac{n}{n+1}\ then\ the\ (n+1)th\ term\ will\ be\ given\ as: \frac{n+1}{(n+1)+1}$$

$$= \frac{n+1}{n+2}$$

When you do nth terms, you essentially substitute n for n+1 (in this case) into the nth term expression.

So to answer the question we need to do the following:

$$(n+1)th\ term\ -\ nth\ term$$

$$\frac{n+1}{n+2} - \frac{n}{n+1} = \frac{(n+1)^2 - n(n+2)}{(n+2)(n+1)} = \frac{n^2 + 2n + 1 - n^2 - 2n}{(n+2)(n+1)} = \frac{1}{(n+2)(n+1)}$$

Q8	A

1 – GPE = mgh = 100kg x 10N/kg x 2m = 2000J so this statement is correct
(Height can be worked out as distance travelled = speed x time = 0.4m/s x 5s = 2m)
2 – The tension in the cable is equal to the weight of the mass. Weight = mg = 100kg x 10N/kg = 1000N so 2 is wrong.
3 – we are told that the mass moves at a constant speed, therefore is not accelerating.

Q9	D

Between 0-11 minutes we can see that oxygen demand exceeds supply, therefore muscles will be respiring aerobically and anaerobically. They respire aerobically using all the oxygen supply they have, but this isn't enough to meet demand so they have to respire anaerobically to make up for this.

Q10	C

We know that cracking an alkane can produce alkanes and/or alkenes and/or hydrogen. So, we can eliminate F. A and D are alkanes (as they fit the general formula of an alkane: C_nH_{2n+2}) so can plausibly be formed. B and E are alkenes (as they have the general formula C_nH_{2n}) so can plausibly be formed. C is not an alkane or an alkene so cannot plausibly be formed.

Q11	D

1 – the electron is released from the conversion of a neutron to a proton, it is not emitted from the outermost electron shell of the atom.
2 – this is false, as we have just explained the neutron changes into a proton releasing an electron in the process, a proton is not changed into an electron.
3 - this is false, based on the above explanation.
4 – this is true, when the neutron is converted to a proton, each have a relative mass of 1, so the conversion does not change the mass number.

Q12	E

To answer this question, you need to think about what happens when we breakdown carbohydrates, proteins and lipids. Carbohydrates break down into monosaccharides (like glucose which won't affect pH). Proteins break down to amino acids (note as an ACID they will affect pH). Lipids break down to fatty acids (again this will affect pH) and glycerol. Hence, E is the answer.

2008 Section 2

Q13	D

To get LMN onto PQR involves a 90 degree rotation, but we need 2 steps that will lead to such a rotation; so recognize that a 90 degree rotation is the same as a 270 rotation in the other direction; and as 2 and 5 sum to a 270 degree rotation this is the answer.

Q14	D

The question asks what change would result in more carbon monoxide being removed i.e. the reaction moving in the forwards direction.
A - adding a catalyst does not affect the position of the equilibrium; only the speed to get to equilibrium so this is wrong.
B, C – increasing or decreasing pressure would mean the reaction would favour both sides equally as there are equal numbers of gaseous moles on each side.
D – decreasing temperature means the equilibrium would move to increase temperature by going in the exothermic direction which is the forwards reaction.
E – adding nitrogen is irrelevant given that it isn't in the equilibrium equation.

Q15	F

X cannot be potential energy as GPE = mgh and the height, mass and g remain constant. It could be acceleration or resultant force. We can therefore eliminate C and D.
Y cannot be mass as the mass of the car will remain constant, so we can eliminate B and E. Y could be drag force (as drag increases in terminal velocity to match thrust). Y could also be velocity as we are told that a terminal speed is reached so eventually the speed becomes constant.
Z cannot be kinetic energy as kinetic energy increases with velocity (recall the equation) so we can eliminate A leaving F as our answer.

Q16	A

Area of a triangle = ½ x base x height
$\frac{4-\sqrt{6}}{2} \times (6+\sqrt{6}) = \frac{24-2\sqrt{6}-6}{2} = \frac{18-2\sqrt{6}}{2} = 9-\sqrt{6}$

Q17	B

Recall the stages of the reflex arc from your knowledge: stimulus, receptor, sensory neurone, CNS with relay neurone going across it, motor neurone, effector (muscle or a gland) and response. Hence 1 is stimulus, 2 is receptor, 3 is CNS, 4 is muscles, and 5 is response and B matches this.

Q18	F

Taking each element in turn we can see what the net effect is on the general formula:
Carbon: going from n to n+1
Hydrogen: going from 2n+2 then it loses 1 Hydrogen and gains 2 so we have left with 2n+3
Oxygen: started with none so O
Nitrogen: started with none so N
Putting this altogether gives $C_{n+1}H_{2n+3}ON$ which is F.

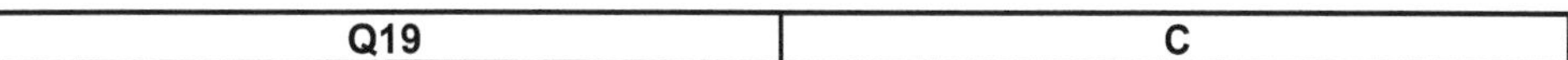

Q19	C

The diagram below shows the bearings; the other 2 we don't initially know can be worked out using the fact that there are 180 degrees on a straight line and 180 degrees in a triangle. We are then asked for the distance between the bottom left corner of the triangle and W. I have called this distance x km. To work this out, we can use trigonometry. The triangle is isosceles meaning we can split it into 2. This is shown below:

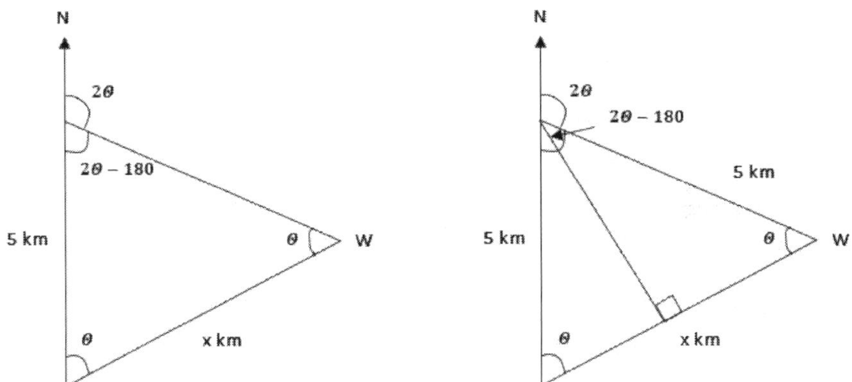

Gives $cos(\theta)$= 0.5x/5. Rearranging for x gives $5cos(\theta)$= = 0.5x Thus, x = $10cos(\theta)$

Q20	F

When the switch is open, we are told that the current in resistor Y is 20mA. There are 12V that can only take 1 route as the switch is open so using V = IR we can calculate that total R = V/I = 12V/20 x 10^{-3} A = 600Ω so this means the resistance in each of the 3 identical resistors is 200Ω.

When the switch is closed, the current will follow the path of least resistance and hence only travel across the upper branch (meaning none goes to Y) and thus the current is split equally between X and Z.

So, when the switch is closed, using V = IR, I = V/R except this time R = 400Ω (as only 2 resistors are encountered on the path of least resistance) and V = 12V. This means I = 12V/400Ω = 0.03A = 30mA so we can eliminate A, B, C and D.

We know that the current across Z is also 0.03A and resistance is also 200Ω so V = 200 x 0.03= 6V.

Q21	B

This question tests knowledge not currently on the BMAT specification.
1 – this is correct, we have double circulation meaning blood flows from the heart twice, once from the right ventricle to the lungs to get oxygenated, then once again from the lungs when oxygenated back to the left atrium then ventricle and out to the body.
2 – although all of the blood goes from the heart to the lungs and back in one complete circuit, from the heart that oxygenated blood does not all go to the kidneys, the aorta branches into several arteries, of which the renal artery is just one.
3 – this is correct; all of the blood from the liver returns to the heart via the hepatic vein that feeds into the vena cava back to the heart.
4 – incorrect. The liver is supplied by the hepatic artery and the hepatic portal vein.

Q22	D

A – this is incorrect; strong covalent bonds hold the structures together.
B – this is incorrect, in graphite each carbon is bonded to 3 others, meaning there are delocalised electrons free to carry a charge.
C – this is incorrect; diamond is incredibly hard and cannot conduct electricity well, but graphite is soft and does conduct electricity.
D – this is correct, combusting any form of carbon with oxygen gives carbon dioxide or carbon monoxide or other oxides.
E – as we already know graphite can conduct electricity, so this is false.

Q23	C

Recall the equation of motion: $v^2 - u^2 = 2as$
We know that the initial speed is given by v, the final speed is 0 (as the lorry comes to rest) and we know using F = ma that a = F/m. The distance travelled is what we want to work out: s.
So substituting this in gives: $v^2 - 0^2 = 2(F/m)s$
Rearranging for s gives: $v^2 m/2F$

Q24	A

Quadratics can be expressed in the following way: (x-a)(x-b) = 0 where expansion gives: $X^2 - ax - bx + ab = 0$. We can take x out of the coefficient portion of - ax – bx giving – x(a+b) so putting this all back together gives: $x^2 - x(a+b) + ab = 0$. we know that ab = 3 and a+b = -5 so substituting tis values into the quadratic expression gives: $x^2 -x(-5) + 3 = 0$ which is $x^2 + 5x + 3 = 0$. This is given by a.

Q25	D

This question tests knowledge not currently on the BMAT specification.
The question tells us that red-green colour blindness is carried by a sex-linked recessive allele on an X chromosome. The colour-blind man has sex chromosomes XY (X coming from his mother and Y from his father) meaning that the recessive allele was carried on the X chromosome in his mother's egg. We can eliminate A, C, E and F for not including his mother. If the man himself has the recessive allele on his X chromosome this means that he will pass it on to his daughter (who will be XX, one X from her mother, one X from her father which contains the recessive allele).

Q26	C

Work out the moles of sulphuric acid that reacted: moles = concentration x volume = 2.0moldm^{-3} x 12.5 x 10^{-3} dm^3 = 25 x 10^{-3} moles.
XOH: sulphuric acid is 2:1 so the moles of XOH must be 50 x 10^{-3}
Using mass = Mr x moles we know Mr = mass/moles = 2.8g/50 x 10^{-3} = 56
However, this is XOH and we are asked for the Ar of X alone, so we need to subtract the Mr of OH (which is 17) from 56: 56 – 17 = 39

Q27	C

We can set up 2 expressions for the distance travelled by the wave and equate them (as the distance the train was when the whistle sounded remains the same in either case).
In steel, distance = speed x time = 4800m/s x t (t being the length of time taken for the wave to travel the distance).
In air, distance = speed x time = 300m/s x (t+1.5)
Equating the two gives: 4800t = 300(t + 1.5)
4800t = 300t + 450
4500t = 450
t= 0.1 seconds
Substituting this value of t back into either equation (for ease here I'm using the steel equation, but you will get the same answer using the air equation) gives:
4800 x 0.1 = 480m which is C.

2008 Section 3

To see the marking grid and mark bands that the BMAT examiners will use to mark your essays, please refer to the BMAT website. *To view the full questions, please see:* https://www.admissionstesting.org/for-test-takers/bmat/preparing-for-bmat/practice-papers/

When you can measure what you are speaking about, and express it in numbers, you know something about it; but when you cannot...your knowledge is of a meagre and unsatisfactory kind. [*Lord Kelvin, 1824-1907*]

This statement claims that you can only have acceptable knowledge of a concept if it is quantifiable. When expressed in numbers, this makes statistics comparable and mathematical calculations can be performed to illustrate further patterns.

Within biology and medicine, the concept of evidence-based medicine comes to mind. To express the efficacy of a drug in terms of dosage and a measured effect on something in the body, such as concentration of a protein in the blood, these two variables can be easily plotted on a graph to observe trends and make changes to dosages depending on what the data indicates is the optimum dosage.

Having quantifiable data also gives the ability to calculate statistical tests, such as in biology where most tests are conducted to leave the probability two variables were correlated by chance as just 5%. Tests such as the student's t-test allow us to compare mean values for data and the Chi-squared test shows us the difference between observed and expected values; something that is particularly important in medicine and biology due to the nature of hypothesis. Advancement comes from drawing up null and alternative hypotheses, and investigation can be shown to be successful enough to be implemented if these statistical tests can be carried out.

You can think about using these ideas and applying them to specific and unique scenarios to really illustrate your point here.

However, on the other side, plenty of topics in biology and medicine do not require quantitative treatment. For example, in the day to day life of a doctor, there will be so many instances of assessing patient wellbeing and their emotional and mental health that could be hindered by a quantifiable scale. Often, it is better to qualitatively assess these individuals as it is more patient-centred. Certainly, in psychology, there has been a history of taking into consideration cultural, religious and ethical standpoints (all of which are qualitative) in order to further research in this area.

Quantitative research is also not required (yet) in fields in which measurement of a variable is impossible quantitatively (as their effect can't currently be measured), but only qualitatively.
Qualitative topics can also include therapeutic medicine or end-of-life care. Within this, doctors are doing what they can within reason to better the quality of life of a patient and this doesn't necessarily include quantitative assessment or treatment.

Life has a natural end, and doctors and others caring for a patient need to recognise that the point may come in the progression of a patient's condition where death is drawing near. [*UK General Medical Council, Good Practice*]

The statement means that healthcare professionals need to understand when natural death is approaching so as to ensure that the patient maintains as good a quality of life before death, and that death is not unnecessarily prolonged through unnatural means. This is relevant to good medical practice because it tries to uphold the pillars of beneficence and non-maleficence. It also retains autonomy for the patient so that they die on terms that are acceptable to them and the professionals around them where possible.

If healthcare professionals don't have a regard for this, they risk essentially pumping someone close to death with drugs and treatments to prolong a life with reduced quality of life. This could lead to patient distress, loss in dignity, feeling like a burden and some could argue that the financial implication in terms of resource allocation may not be fair. For instance, treating to keep someone alive when there is a natural time could be diverting necessary resources from other areas of the NHS. Other risks include lack of closure for the family of the patient and constant distress for them.

Having said this, it is also controversial as to when a "natural death" seems inevitable and becomes the right course of action. For instance, where is the line drawn for treatment to be stopped? In the case of morphine, which has a double effect of alleviating pain and causing organ failure what is the correct course of action? Can a patient's views on their quality of life always be assessed and taken to be genuine? In which case, how can we be sure we are doing right by the patient? Certainly, in some belief systems it could be considered unethical to stop treatment especially if more treatment could be given despite a natural end approaching.

Ultimately, the proximity of a natural death and the awareness of when a natural death appears to be close is very relevant to doctors and other healthcare professionals; whatever the wishes of each party. The legal and ethical rules that we are governed by as well as trying to take into account the patient's wishes must all be married together but there is no denying the relevance to good medical practice.

Authors' Tip:

Euthanasia, end-of-life care and palliative care are all hot topics that are common in medical/dentistry interviews (and in BMAT essay questions!). A good student will have a few solid arguments both for and against euthanasia and will know the differences between active and passive euthanasia, and between euthanasia and assisted suicide. A good starting point to learn about euthanasia, and arguments for and against, is the BBC Ethics website, which can be accessed at the following link: http://www.bbc.co.uk/ethics/euthanasia/

2008 Section 3

Science is the great antidote to the poison of enthusiasm and superstition. ***[Adam Smith, The Wealth of Nations, 1776]***

This statement gets to the heart of what is unique about the scientific method, that it is a fair, comprehensive and reliable source of empirical investigation. This is in opposition to someone having an irrational desire to investigate or assert something, which will not have an evidence basis nor reason or logic behind it.

When Smith is referring to superstition and enthusiasm he could be talking about the apothecaries or doctors of his era, when in the 1700s people still held many irrational beliefs such as how to treat the bubonic plague. The masks and the waving of sage comes to mind here; this was pure superstition and arguably a poison to those who needed real treatment and the aseptic technique.

However, Smith could also be referring to anyone willing to accept an explanation without an evidence basis, for example those who may claim that religion is the only explanation to a phenomenon, yes, to them this may be an explanation but it is also not the only explanation. We have the capacity to use science to work through claims and test these superstitious hypotheses.

You could argue that science is a fantastic antidote to this, mainly because the scientific method is universal, the nature of peer-review, repeatability and reliability gives results that we can generally trust and repeat to confirm.

However, you could argue a different viewpoint entirely, sometimes enthusiasm and superstition are not a poison in the scientific world. There are so many ground-breaking discoveries that were based off of a hunch or some sort of superstition, and arguably science involves a great deal of creativity to push the boundaries of the knowledge we have today when hypothesising about future investigations and areas of investigation. This creativity surely goes hand in hand with enthusiasm and superstition.

You will want to conclude by drawing your own feelings together; since this is a “to what extent” question you need to evaluate your own beliefs and you may want to end on something balanced, that generally speaking enthusiasm and superstition are not helpful in science and that the scientific method and its evidence basis are the necessary antidote; but that in some instances, science needs those very human elements of enthusiasm and superstition to generate ideas, and to provoke intellectual curiosity that is also a big player in some major scientific development today.

BMAT 2009

Section 1

Q1	15

For this question we need to do the following sum: (number of monarchs who have reigned for less than 40 years) – (number of monarchs who have reigned for less than 20 years). 35 monarchs have reigned for less than 40 years. 20 monarchs have reigned for less than 20 years. Therefore 35 – 20 = 15 gives us the number of monarchs who have reigned for 20 years or more but less than 40 years.

Q2	B

The article implies that there are two settings in which one can give birth; the hospital ward which is high tech and provides high levels of pain relief, and at home, with just a midwife, with the facilities provided at each being mutually exclusive (i.e. high levels of pain relief can only happen at the hospital and not at home). Therefore, B is correct.
A is incorrect as the article is objective - it presents the Home Secretary's statement as just a statement without providing the author's opinion.
C is incorrect as no reasons are given for why the Home Secretary has made that statement, nor does the article state that home births are cheaper.
D is incorrect as 'strongly opposed' is too strong for what the article has said.
E is incorrect as such information about progression isn't mentioned in the passage.

Q3	D

This question is relatively simple, although it may take some time. We have to imagine each of the 5 graphs to be the correct one and see if the other 4 graphs have 2 bars wrong relative to it. Starting with A, we can see that it is incorrect as graph C has 3 bars that are different from it. Therefore, both A & C must be wrong. Now, let's take B. E has 4 bars that are different from B, so B & E must be wrong. Therefore, D must be the correct answer.

Q4	B

The passage's main conclusion is: '*Given that the likelihood of a prolonged period of heavy snow in the UK is very low...high cost of investing in preventative measures would be unreasonable*'. Therefore, the answer is B. A is mentioned in the text, but it is evidence for the conclusion, rather than the conclusion itself. ('Given that....' is a clue to identify the conclusion). C is incorrect as that contradicts he passage, D is incorrect for the same reason as C and E is not correct as the text does not imply nor conclude that it is the government who should be the ones giving out compensation for the billions of pound lost.

Q5	E

We know they have five pairs of twins, so that is 10 grandchildren. 3 of the pairs are born in April, so in order to ascertain the minimum number of children, let us assume that the other two pairs of twins are born in different months. That leaves us with 9 months of the year left (with each month having at least one grandchild born in).
So, 10 + 9 = 19 children. However, having 19 grandchildren would mean that it is impossible for them to have exactly twice as many granddaughters as grandsons. Because of this rule, it will also be impossible for them to have 20 grandchildren. Therefore, 21 grandchildren is thus the minimum (14 granddaughters, and 7 grandsons).

Q6	G

1 is correct because the passage suggests that campaigns are not needed because so few people die from it each year but fails to acknowledge that campaigns may be the reason why the death rate is so low, and that without them, the number of users and death rate may be higher.
2 is correct because the passage makes out that horse riding isn't dangerous, by using it as the event to compare ecstasy use with, to make the point that ecstasy use isn't as dangerous as the majority believe.
3 is correct because the passage doesn't state the number of deaths as a proportion of the number of people who do the activity, and instead gives absolute figures.

Q7	C

Let us create an equation to find out the number of times he will need to hire equipment. Let us call x the number of times he needs to hire equipment. As Gold and Silver memberships cost the same: 80 + 1x = 100 + 0.5x
0.5x = 20, so x = 40.
Therefore, the cost of hiring equipment 40 times with a:
Bronze membership is £70 + (£3 x 40) = £190
Silver/Gold membership is £80 + (£1 x 40) = £120, or £100 + (£0.5 x 40) = £120
Therefore, he will save £190 - £120 = £70.

Q8	B

421 residents experienced or witnessed a crime but did not report it. 133 of these did not report it because they thought the crime wasn't important. Therefore, the probability is 133/421, which is greater than 0.25 but less than 0.33

Q9	G

1 is incorrect as the data doesn't tell us about anything about the coming year, nor does it provide information about reporting a crime in the previous year affecting a person's willingness to report another crime in the coming year.
2 is incorrect as we are only provided data about the attitudes of people who did report the crime, and not those of the people who didn't report the crime.
3 is incorrect as the passage provides no evidence/data about people who gave multiple reasons for being dissatisfied with the police response, nor do we know whether any overlap in reasons exists from the data presented.

Q10	A

A is the correct answer because the text tells us that many people did not report crimes last year, and that many of those did not report crimes because they lacked confidence in the police. We also learn that many of those who reported crimes were not satisfied with the speed of or the police response itself, so we can assume that this may be one of the reasons that people did not report crime. The explanations in B, C, D and E are not supported or implied by the text.

Q11	D

This is a visualisation question – if you find these difficult try cutting out the shapes and folding them to see whether you can make a right-angled triangle. D is the correct answer as it will fold twice to make the correct shape (see diagram below). The other answer options will not create a triangle as shown in the question upon two folds.

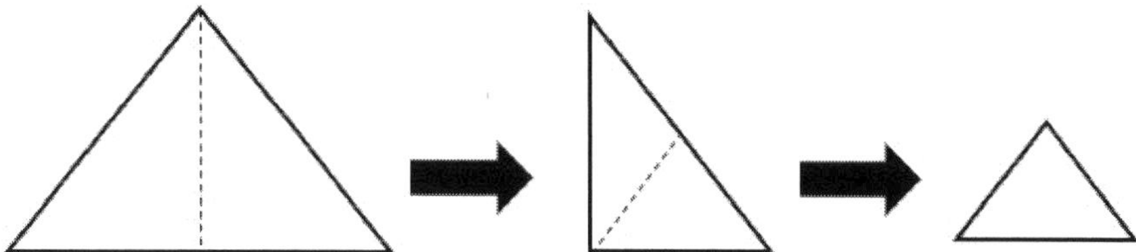

Fold along the dotted lines

Q12	B

'*The government should act now to protect people….make slimming pills subject to the same strict controls as medicines*' is the conclusion of the passage, and therefore we are looking for something that weakens this. B is the correct answer, as it provides evidence that the government is already acting, and therefore it does not need to act now. A, C, D & E do not affect/are not relevant to the conclusion, so neither weaken nor strengthen it.

Q13	E

Go through and see if the combinations in each of the answer options are possible or not.
A is possible; for example, you can have 5 red marbles in the left bag, and 2 red and 2 green in the right-hand bag. If you move a red from the left to the right, and then a red from the right to the left, the right bag will have half red and half green at the end.
B is possible – use the same example as A
C is possible – if the left hand bag starts with 3 red marbles, and the right hand bag starts with 2 green marbles, and one red marble moves from left to right, and one green marble moves from right to left, then the right hand bag will end up with half green and half red.
D is possible – use the same example as A.
E is not possible, the only way that the right hand bag can start with more than two marbles in is if it started off with marbles of more than one colour; if it had more than 2 marbles in to start with which were all the same colour, then swapping only one marble would make it impossible for it to end up with half red and half green.
F is possible – use the same example as C

Q14	A

The passage states that they have incorporated '*colour psychology*' to '*improve the success of interrogation*' [this is the conclusion]. The reason for this is because specific colours have a '*positive, calming, mood enhancing effect*', i.e. they put the person at ease [this is the evidence]. Here, the assumption they make is the link between the evidence and the conclusion, i.e. that the success of interrogation is improved if people are at ease, which is what A says. B, C, D and E are not valid assumptions needed for the conclusion to be true, as they don't link the evidence directly to the conclusion.

Q15	D

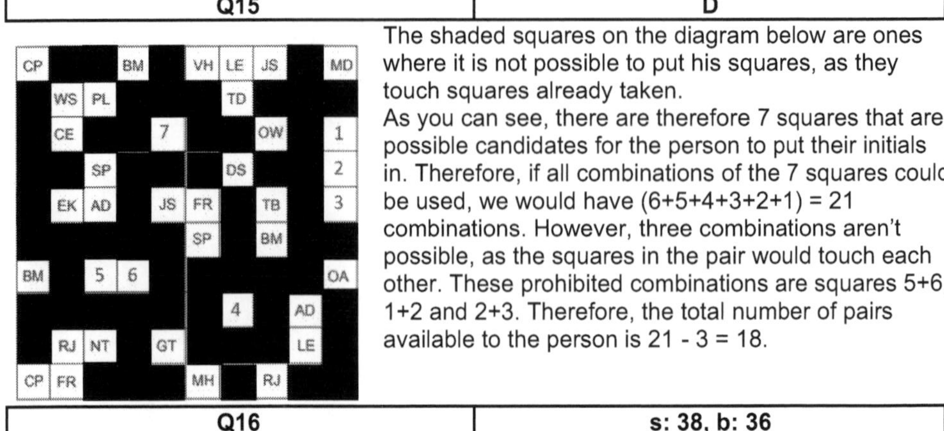

The shaded squares on the diagram below are ones where it is not possible to put his squares, as they touch squares already taken.
As you can see, there are therefore 7 squares that are possible candidates for the person to put their initials in. Therefore, if all combinations of the 7 squares could be used, we would have (6+5+4+3+2+1) = 21 combinations. However, three combinations aren't possible, as the squares in the pair would touch each other. These prohibited combinations are squares 5+6, 1+2 and 2+3. Therefore, the total number of pairs available to the person is 21 - 3 = 18.

Q16	s: 38, b: 36

Figure 2 shows us that the US won 110 medals in total, as each medal (gold, bronze or silver) is equally weighted. Figure 1 shows us that the US won 36 gold medals, so therefore 110 – 36 = 74 medals were silver or bronze. When the medals are weighted, the gold medals will count for 36 x 3 = 108 points for Figure 3. Therefore, using the same weighting we get 112 = 2s + b, where s is the number of silver medals and b is the number of bronze medals. We have two simultaneous equations: (a) 74 = s + b and (b) 112 = 2s + b.
We solve, and we find that s = 38, and b = 36.

Q17	13

Australia does not appear on Fig 1, and therefore it must have won 15 or fewer gold medals. To determine the minimum number of silver medals, let us thus assume that Australia won the maximum 15 gold medals. This would equal a weighting of 45 for Fig 3, and so 89 – 45 = 44 = 2s + b. Australia won 46 medals in total (Fig 2). Therefore, if we say they won 15 golds, 46 – 15 = 31 = s + b. We therefore have two simultaneous equations: 2s + b = 44 and s + b = 31. Solving us this set of equations gives us s = 13.

Q18	B

Let us work out the proportion of gold medal to all medals for all the countries. China: 51/100 = 51%, USA: 36/110 ~ 32%, Russia: 23/72 ~ 31%, GBR: 19/47 ~ 40%. Therefore, Great Britain would have ranked second, behind China.

Q19	F

1 is correct, as Norway has 4.5 points per million population, and a population of 4.6 million, so its total point score is 4.6 x 4.5 = 20.7 = 21. 3 gold and 5 silver = 3 x 3 + 5 x 2 = 19, which is less than 21, so it is therefore possible (as long as Norway also won two bronze medals).
2 is incorrect as Iceland's total point score would be 6.8 x 0.3 = 2.04. Even if the only medals they won were bronze, they would only have been able to won a maximum of 2, and therefore it would have been impossible for them to have won 3.
3 is correct because Slovenia's total points score is 4.5 x 2 = 9. Therefore, it is possible for them to have won 1 gold, 1 silver and 4 bronzes. This would have given them 6 overall medals, a total points score of 9 (3 + 2 + 4 x 1), and one gold medal.

Q20	C

1 is correct as Great Britain's point score would be 98/62 ~ 1.6, and the US' is 220/306 ~ 0.7. Therefore, the UK would rank below Slovenia but above the USA
2 is correct because its point score is 139/145, which is less than 1, which is therefore the equivalent of less than 1 bronze medal (1 point) for every million of its population.

Q21	50g

300 ml of the second drink contains ¾ x 2J = 1.5J
200ml of the first drink contains 1.5J, so in this new 500ml, there are 3J.
We know she needs to have 4J in total, so we need to add an extra J from the powder. As 100g of powder = 2J, 50g of powder = 1J, and therefore only 50g of powder is needed.

Q22	A

1 is correct as we learn that the '*most valuable kind of praise is that which the recipient knows to be appropriate*'.
2 is correct as we learn that '*praise should only be given to the extent that it is deserved*'.
3 is not correct as the argument in the passage does not assume the fact that we should all promote others' self-esteem.
4 is not correct as this is not assumed – we do not learn about the benefits of self esteem to others, nor does the argument need to assume this to hold true.

Q23	E

The best way to solve this question is to identify the month in which each sample was taken. Since the 124th month of this clinic was a September, A was taken in July (254th month), B was taken in May (264th month), C was taken in March (274th month), D was taken in January (284th), and E was taken in November (294th month). All the samples were taken on the 31st day of the month; November does not have 31 days; therefore, E is not a number of a sample taken at this clinic, and therefore is the correct answer.

Q24	E

1 is not correct as we only know data about pregnancy, as opposed to the sexual activity of those who do drink, and who don't drink. Additionally, the data only provides information about girls, whereas 1 mentions young people, which includes girls AND boys.
2 is not correct as this cannot be inferred from the data provided in the passage, as there is no evidence to support the assumption that alcohol is the main reason why these girls had sexual intercourse and became pregnant.
3 is incorrect as the data does not say 40% of all girls under the age of 16 have consumed alcohol, merely 40% of girls who became pregnant were found to have consumed alcohol/been under its influence during sexual intercourse.

Q25	A

Look at the data point second from the right. It has the second highest score on the x-axis, and the lowest on the y-axis. Look through the table at the top and find in which data sets this could occur. You will see it is possible with the x axis being absenteeism rate, and the y axis being percentage achieving 5 or more A* to C grades, with that aforementioned data point being Shelley.

Q26	E

The passage tells us about the Rebel's large blue butterfly which imitates ant sounds to enable it to get food from the worker ants and be better protected when the ant colony is disturbed. This is paraphrased in E which is the correct answer. A is incorrect because although the ant sounds may harm the survival of individuals, the passage doesn't suggest that it harms the survival of the entire species. B is incorrect as the Rebel butterfly is only used as an example, and there is no mention that it is the most notable or only example. C is incorrect as the passage doesn't suggest whether this is unusual or common in the insect world, and also makes it clear that the slaughtering of their own young is not intentional. D is not correct as we do not know the reason why ant sounds developed.

Q27	B

Tim is unable to get a free meal on the Tuesday 9th (6 meals after Monday 1st), which means that each meal must cost 9 tokens. This is because he would lose 2 tokens every day. On Monday at 2pm he would have 11 tokens, on Tuesday at 2pm he would have [(11 + 7) – 9] = 9 tokens, on Wednesday at 2pm he would have [(9 + 7) – 9] = 7 tokens etc until Monday 8th at 2pm where he would have [(3 + 7) – 9] = 1 token, so on the Tuesday 9th in the morning he would have 8 tokens (1 + 7 from Monday 5pm) left, which is insufficient to have a free meal. So:

Day	Number of tokens left at 2pm
Wednesday 10th	(8 + 7) – 9 = 6
Thursday 11th	(6 + 7) – 9 = 4
Friday 12th	(4 + 7) – 9 = 2
Monday 15th	(2 + 7) – 9 = 0

Therefore, on Tuesday morning he would only have 7 tokens (0 + 7), which would be insufficient for a meal.

Q28	B

The passage's conclusion is '*So if the Kepler telescope finds that such planet exists we can at last be confident that there is life on planets other than Earth'*, based on the fact that the telescope can identify planets within the *habitable zone*. The assumption is the statement that links the evidence with the conclusion; here the assumption is that an Earth sized planet in the habitable zone means that life will definitely exist there, which is what B says. A is wrong because the passage only mentions 'life' generally and makes no mention to what kind of life form would be present. C and D are to do with the telescope itself and do not link the evidence to the conclusion, while E is wrong, as it can be seen to contradict the passage.

Q29	D

For this question, you need to look at the placement of the black squares relative to an edge and see if this placement is the same in any of the other tiles, which would have just been rotated. As you can see below, we have 7 different tiles.

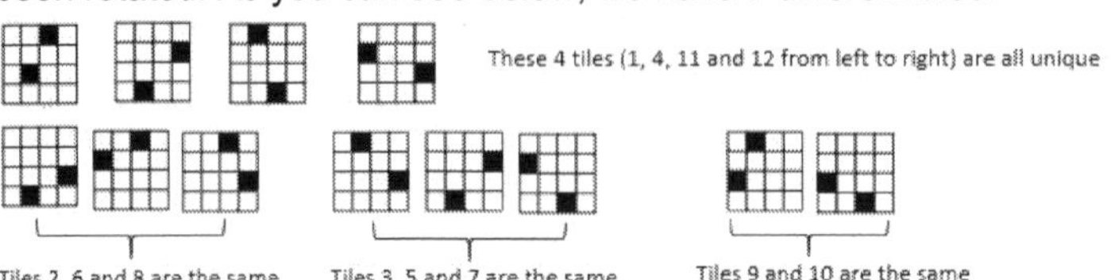

Q30	D

The passage's conclusion is '*While....the more systematic and organised the studies we conduct, the more likely they will produce valid explanations that can be used to support decisions'* – D says this (it says common sense explanations will be less likely to be valid than scientific ones, which is suggested by the conclusion)

Q31	D

The lift will first go to floor 10, then back down to floor 7, then down to floor 4, then down to floor 0, then to floor 14, and then finally to floor 16. Therefore, it will make 5 stops before it reaches floor 16 [the stops are at floor 10, floor 7, floor 4, floor 0 and floor 14]

Q32	C

You should see just by inspection that the biggest percentage change is for the potatoes.

Item	Change
Cattle	490.4 to 439.7
Pigs	89.9 to 70.2
Potato	**81.2 to 117.1**
Wool	7.7 to 7.4
Vegetables	34.5 to 38.3

Q33	C

Look for the sector which saw growth from 1994 to 1995 and decline from 1996 onwards. The figures for 1995 and 1996 will be similar. Looking at the table, we can see that Livestock matches this trend, with the figures for 1995 and 1996 being incredibly similar (1036.1 and 1033.5 respectively).

Q34	D

A cannot be inferred as we are unable to infer what the farmers changed their production to.

B is incorrect as the £ output of pigs increased from 1995 to 1996, while the £ output of cattle decreased during the same time period. C is not correct as although income was higher in 1998 than in 1980, this does not mean that this was due to a very strong pound in the 1980s, and we are provided with no evidence to prove this is the reason.

D is correct because from 1997 to 1998 farm crop output decreased, whereas horticulture output increased, while '*volumes of production had not changed*'. We learn from the commentary that because of the strength of the pound in 1998, lower prices were experienced for farmers who exported crops out of the UK. Since there is a decrease in farm crop output, we can assume this was caused because of a greater proportion of far, crops being sold abroad (a/o to horticulture which saw an increase).

E is incorrect as we do not know about other factors that could have affected the £ output, such as more/less potatoes could have been produced in certain years, which would have affected £ output.

Q35	E

% change in sheep from 1997 to 1998 = (237.4 – 245.1)/245.1 = ~8/245 = ~3.2%

All the exported sheep lost 5% in value, whereas the ones that were not exported did not lose any value. There was a 3.2% drop in total value due to the 5% drop in value of those exported meaning that 3.2/5 = 64% is the percentage of sheep that were exported. Note, since 3.2% is greater than 2.5% (half of 5%), more than 50% of the sheep must have been exported, so A-D must be wrong, and E is the correct answer.

2009 Section 2

Q1	C

Call the recessive allele r, and the dominant allele R. Therefore, A has genotype RR and B is rr. Therefore, both C and D will have genotype Rr. If E is homozygous recessive, then it will have the genotype rr. If E is heterozygous it will have the genotype Rr. Let us draw Punnet squares for both crosses, which will help us solve the question.

i) Rr (D) vs rr (E)

	r	r
R	Rr	Rr
r	rr	rr

50% chance of offspring being homozygous recessive

ii) Rr (D) vs Rr (E)

	R	r
R	RR	Rr
r	Rr	rr

25% chance of offspring being homozygous recessive

Q2	E

Only unsaturated compounds (those with double bonds) can take part in addition polymerisation (AP) reactions, such as alkenes (general formula: C_nH_{2n}) or haloalkenes (alkenes where hydrogen atoms are substituted with halogen atoms). 1 is a halogenoalk<u>a</u>ne, 2 is an alkene, 3 is a halogenoalk<u>a</u>ne, 4 is a haloalkene and 5 is also a haloalkene. Therefore, only 2, 4 and 5 can take part in AP reactions.

Q3	C

The resultant force is 300N upwards (as 900-600 = 300). Therefore, we can rule out A, B and E. We can then use Newton's second law to work out the acceleration.
F = ma
300N = 60kg x a
a = 5.0ms^{-2} so C is the correct answer.

Q4	C

The probability of getting a red ball is $\frac{x}{x+y+z}$, and the probability of getting a blue ball is $\frac{y}{x+y+z}$. Since there is replacement, the probability of first getting a red ball, and then getting a blue ball will be $\frac{x}{x+y+z} \times \frac{y}{x+y+z} = \frac{xy}{(x+y+z)^2} = C$. Remember we multiply probabilities her because of the 'AND' rule.

Q5	E

A is not correct due to environmental factors affecting phenotypic expression, for example think of two twins; all of their features will not be identical, for example, one may be slightly taller than the other.
B is not correct as fraternal twins exist – they come about when two eggs are fertilised, and both get implanted in the uterus; these twins are not identical.
C is not correct as identical twins are members of a clone but arise naturally.
D is not correct as the result of mutations is genetic variation, and not clones.
E is correct, the definition of clones is that they are genetically identical.

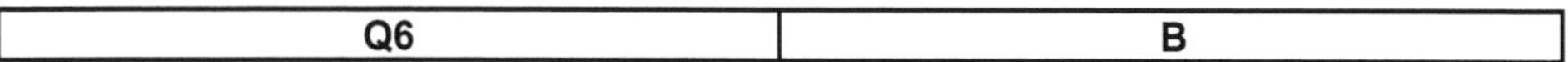

Q6	B

SiO_2 is the only substance listed that forms a giant covalent structure; the others all have simple molecular structures.

Q7	E

Think of all the equations that involve voltage such V = IR, P = IV, E = VQ = IVt. Only E is correct (it comes from P = IV, so V = P/I); the others are all incorrect.

Q8	B

For this question, we need to form two triangles. We need to work out the length of the diagonal (call this c) of the base, which can be done through Pythagoras. So, $c^2 = 1^2 + 1^2$, so $c = \sqrt{2}$. Therefore, half of the diagonal would be $\frac{\sqrt{2}}{2}$.
We can then work on our second right angled triangle:

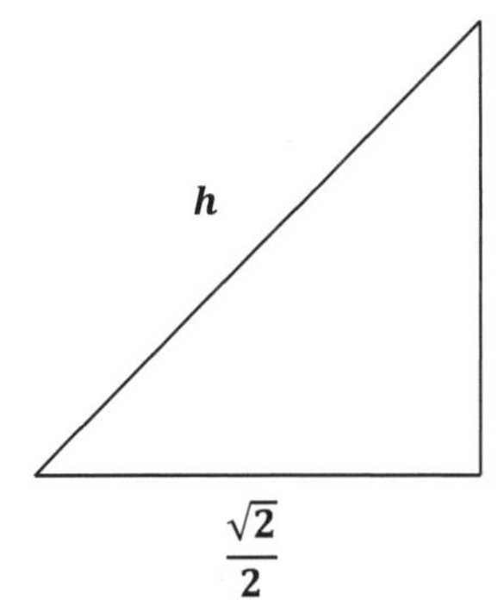

We want to work out h, which we do by using Pythagoras again.

$$h = \sqrt{(\frac{\sqrt{2}}{2})^2 + 1^2} = \sqrt{\frac{2}{4} + 1} = \sqrt{\frac{3}{2}}$$

Q9	D

This questions tests knowledge not on the BMAT specification
A is correct as for both light and heavy drinkers, the greater the number of mutant alleles, the greater the risk.
B is correct as heavy drinkers have a greater risk value for all numbers of mutant alleles.
C is correct as drinking increases the risk value more than the number of mutant alleles.
D is incorrect (**and so is the correct answer to this question**) because drinking alcohol increases the risk more than the number of alleles (a heavy drinker with 0 alleles has a 4 times higher risk than a light drinker with 0, whereas the increases in risk due to number of alleles are a lot smaller – a 0.3 increase per allele in a light drinker).
E is correct as having 2 alleles in a heavy drinker results in a 1.5 increase in the risk, compared to a heavy drinker with 1 allele, whereas having 2 alleles in a light drinker results in only a 0.3 increase in the risk, compared to a light drinker with 1 allele.

Q10	E

The carbon : carbon dioxide molar ratio is 1:1, as there is only one carbon-based reactant, and only one carbon-based product as complete combustion takes place. 4.77g of CO_2 (Mr 48) is produced, which is 4.77/48 = ~ 0.01 moles. Therefore 0.1 moles of carbon must be in the original compound. 0.1 moles of carbon is 1.2g of carbon (mass = moles x Mr), and therefore the percentage of carbon in the original compound is $\frac{1.2}{2.0}$x 100 = 60%, which is nearest to E.

2009 Section 2

Q11	C

As only detector 1 detects the radiation, we know that the type of radiation is beta, so we can rule out A, B, E and F. We need to be careful when working out the half-life. After 16 hours, the count rate stabilises, so we can assume that that background radiation accounts for 20 counts/min. Therefore, the initial count rate at time 0 is 200 counts/min (220 – 20). We want to see how long it takes for the count rate to fall to 120 (as 200/2 = 100, and we need to add 20 for the background radiation, as the graph/best fit line includes background radiation). The sample reaches a count rate of 120 counts/min after 2.4 hours, so that is the half-life.

Q12	C

Write out the equation in terms of mathematical operators, instead of diamonds.

We get: $\left(\frac{2^3}{3}\right)$ ◈ $2 =$: $\left(\frac{8}{3}\right)$ ◈ $2 = \frac{\left(\frac{8}{3}\right)^2}{2} = \frac{\frac{64}{9}}{2} = \frac{64}{9} \times \frac{1}{2} = \frac{64}{18} = \frac{32}{9}$

Q13	B

We need to work out which process needs oxygen to work (i.e. which processes are passive, and which are active. Active processes need energy to occur, and so need oxygen for aerobic respiration to produce that energy/ATP). Only B is an active process (active transport), and so would be the only one disrupted by a low oxygen blood concentration, as respiration to produce energy/ATP would not occur (or occur fast enough/in sufficient amounts). A and C are diffusion processes (and a low oxygen concentration would actually facilitate oxygen movement due to increased oxygen conc. gradients), D occurs by ultrafiltration, and E and F work by osmosis. All these processes are passive, and so don't need energy from respiration to occur, and therefore do not need oxygen in order to occur.

Q14	B

A more reactive element will displace a less reactive element from one of its compounds. 1, 5 and 6 cannot occur because a less reactive element cannot displace a more reactive one. 2, 3 and 4 can occur as the more reactive element is displacing a less reactive one.

Q15	D

This is a speed-time graph, so the distance is equal to the area under the graph. Each rectangle in the grid is equal to 600m (as we need to work in seconds as that is the SI unit, and 1 minute equals 60 seconds)
Counting up the rectangles, we see that there are 8 full rectangles, so 8 x 600m = 4.8km. The top left rectangle (labelled a on the diagram) and the bottom right rectangle (labelled b on the diagram) can be merged to form a full rectangle, so that is approximately another 600m. We have two half rectangles left (labelled c and d on the diagram), so we roughly have another 600m.

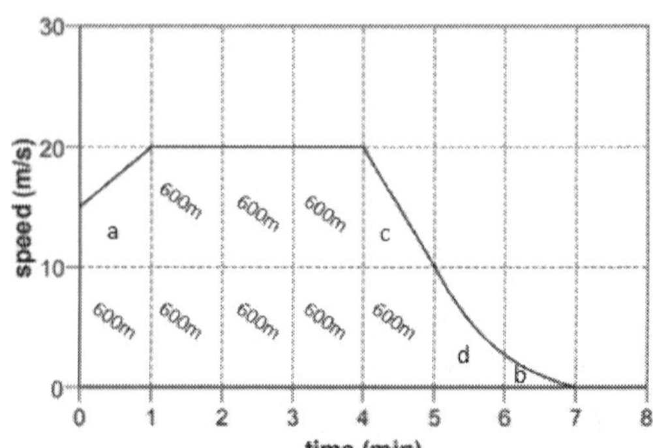

So, we have 4.8km (in full rectangles) + 600m + 600m = roughly 6.00km, which is D

Q16	F

$$\sqrt{\left(\frac{2\times10^3+8\times10^2}{\frac{1}{2500}+3\times10^{-4}}\right)} = \sqrt{\left(\frac{2000+800}{\frac{4}{10,000}+\frac{3}{10,000}}\right)}$$

$$= \sqrt{\left(\frac{2800}{\frac{7}{10,000}}\right)} = \sqrt{\frac{2800}{7}\times\frac{1000}{1}} = \sqrt{400\times1000} = \sqrt{400,000} = \mathbf{2000}$$

Q17	F

All 4 are correct: 1 and 2 are correct because competition can both be interspecific (between other same species), and intraspecific (between the same species). 3 and 4 are also correct because some species are selected for (evolution), and some are selected against (extinction) i.e. those with more advantageous characteristics evolve, whereas those with less advantageous ones are selected against and eventually go extinct.

Q18	D

We need to use simultaneous equations to solve this question.
b = 2c (for hydrogen). b = 2a + 2 (for nitrogen). 3b = 6a + c + 2
Therefore, we can put c in terms of a so we only have two variables: 2c = 2a + 2, so c = a + 1
We can also but b in terms of a, since b = 2c, and so b = 2(a + 1) = 2a + 2
Therefore [substituting our values into nitrogen's original equation]:
3(2a + 2) = 6a + a + 1 + 2, so 6a + 6 = 7a + 3, so a = 3.
Therefore, b = 2(3) + 2 = 8.

Q19	B

KE = GPE
KE = ½ mv^2 = ½ x 5 x 20^2 = 1000J
GPE = mgh, so 1000 = 5 x 10 x h, so h = 1000/50 = 20m.

Q20	D

The area of a cylinder is $\pi r^2 l$, so the area of this cylinder is $\pi r^2(2r) = 2\pi r^3$, as the length is the same as the diameter of the sphere, which is 2r.
The area of the sphere is $\frac{4}{3}\pi r^3$.
Therefore, the fraction of the space inside the cylinder taken up by the sphere is:

$$\frac{\frac{4}{3}\pi r^3}{2\pi r^3} = \frac{\frac{4}{3}}{2} = \frac{2}{3}$$

Q21	D

Oxygen diffuses from the alveolus into the capillary because there is a high concentration of oxygen in the alveolus, and a low concentration of oxygen in the capillary. Carbon dioxide diffuses from the capillary into the alveolus as there is a high carbon dioxide concentration in the capillary and a low carbon dioxide concentration in the alveolus.

Q22	D

In reactions 1 and 4 bonds have to be broken; in reaction 1 the H-H and the I-I bonds are broken, and in 4 the H_3C-Br bond is broken. In reactions 2 and 3 no bonds are broken, instead bonds are only formed, and so reactions 2 and 3 are the quickest.

Q23	A

The total mass of the train is 5,000 + 5,000 + 20,000 = 30,000kg. The acceleration of the train is 15,000N/30,000kg = $0.5ms^{-2}$ (using F = ma). The tension force for each carriage is 5000kg x $0.5ms^{-2}$ = 2500N (again using F = ma).

Q24	A

$$y = 5\left(\frac{x}{2} - 3\right)^2 - 10$$

$$\frac{y+10}{5} = \left(\frac{x}{2} - 3\right)^2$$

$$\pm\sqrt{\frac{y+10}{5}} = \frac{x}{2} - 3$$

$$\pm 2\sqrt{\frac{y+10}{5}} = x - 6$$

$$x = \pm 2\sqrt{\frac{y+10}{5}} + 6$$

Q25	F

1 is incorrect as insulin helps to control the blood sugar content of the body.
2 is incorrect as homeostasis needs both the endocrine (hormonal) and nervous systems.
3, 4 and 5 are correct (5 – sweat glands and hair on the skin help control body temperature).

Q26	C

The CH_2 part always has the same mass, and has Mr of 14. Therefore, the BrCl must have a Mr of 114 (128 – 14), which means that the Cl is Cl^{35} and the Br is Br^{79}. The chance of the chlorine being Cl^{35} is 75% (as it is three times more common than Cl^{37}), and the chance of the bromine being Br^{79} is 50% (as Br^{79} and Br^{81} exist in equal amounts). Therefore, the chance that CH_2BrCl has an Mr of 128 is ¾ x ½ = 3/8

Q27	E

From the first graph we can work out that the wavelength is 30m, as two waves are shown, and the distance is 60m. From the second graph we can work out the frequency; 3 waves take 0.6 seconds, so each wave takes 0.2 seconds, so in one second there will be 5 waves passing a particular point, meaning the frequency is 5Hz.
Speed = frequency x wavelength = 5 x 30 = 150m/s

2009 Section 3

To see the marking grid and mark bands that the BMAT examiners will use to mark your essays, please refer to the BMAT website.

You must be honest and open and act with integrity. *GMC Good Medical Practice 2006*
To see the full question, please see:
https://www.admissionstesting.org/Images/20768-past-paper-2009-section-3-.pdf

The GMC argues in the above statement that doctors and other medical professionals should tell the truth, and always the full truth, be approachable and acknowledge their mistakes, and be principled (they should hold themselves to high standards and adhere to ethical principles and medical guidelines).

Honesty, openness and having integrity are key traits in a medical professional:

- A doctor must always be honest in order to respect a patient's right to **autonomy** or self-determination. They must always provide all the necessary information about a surgical procedure, e.g. a heart transplant, and be honest and open about any risks involved, so the patients are able to give **informed consent.**
- A doctor should always act with integrity, so standards are upheld, and so patient care and wellbeing isn't compromised. For example, a doctor (as part of their duty of **non-maleficence**) shouldn't break confidentiality unnecessarily, as this could affect patient care and lead to a potential breakdown in the doctor-patient relationship.
- All three traits are essential in doctors, so trust in the medical profession is maintained, ensuring patients feel confident and safe when asking for medical help.

There may be certain circumstances where a doctor may be justified in not being perfectly honest or open, and in these cases, it is done purely to put the patient's best interest first.

- Sometimes, further disclosure of a patient's illness may cause them further harm. For example, a patient with mental health problems, such as suicidal ideation, was to be told about the details of another of their medical conditions, their mental health could be further damaged in a serious manner.
- When administering a **placebo** drug, it wouldn't be in the patient's best interest for the doctor to make them aware that the drug is merely a placebo, as this may defeat the point of administering the placebo in the first place and this could reduce trust in the doctor and break the doctor-patient relationship.
- When breaking bad news – for example, when a doctor is explaining to a patient that they are terminally ill, being less honest and open about the specifics of the disease could be justified as the doctor's priority should be in reassuring the patient, and seeing how they can improve the patient's quality of life.
- A doctor may not be entirely honest or open with family members, in order not to break confidentiality, especially if the patient has requested that their family not be told to the specifics.

A good doctor should possess the traits of honesty and openness and should act with integrity at all times, However, there may be certain instances where full disclosure is not beneficial to the patient, and a good doctor should therefore be able use their professional judgement to know when they should be completely open and when they should be less open.

2009 Section 3

Science is a way of trying not to fool yourself. ***Richard Feynman, 1964***
To see the full question, please see:
https://www.admissionstesting.org/Images/20768-past-paper-2009-section-3-.pdf

Science is an objective field of study, with subjectivity not playing much of a role, if any, in generating scientific knowledge. In this way, the statement may argue that scientific truth is generally irrefutable. Fooling oneself is convincing oneself that a belief/statement/observation/opinion/fact is true when it is actually false (whether proven to be or not). It is essential for a scientist not to fool themselves in order to maintain its objectivity and to avoid/minimise bias thus maintaining the integrity of scientific endeavours.

Scientists are humans, and are therefore guided by many emotions, such as passion, anger, fear and hatred to name a few. Therefore, it is very easy for scientists to overlook the truth and believe falsehoods based on their emotions.

Additionally, when people find an explanation reasonable or logical, they normally accept it to be true, and this can sometimes lead to scientists fooling themselves – not everything that is logical turns out to be true. Humans also jump to conclusions rather quickly and are able to create false patterns and relationships from unrelated data sets and are quick to ignore alternative explanations. Scientists should therefore be wary of this ad sufficient evidence/proof should be the prerequisite to determining whether a theory/statement is actually true.

Scientists should guard against mistakes in their experiments by ensuring they follow the scientific method to generate new knowledge, and should only be satisfied that their findings are the 'truth' when they have been supported by sufficient evidence, and not just logical reasoning.

Peer review is also a key method to ensure the validity of scientific findings. It allows for the methodologies of scientists to be critiqued and compared and allows bias to be picked upon and allows any flaws in the scientific process to be identified.

Authors' Tip:

Objectivity in science is essential to maintain its integrity as a way of knowledge. To learn more about objectivity in science, please see: https://en.wikipedia.org/wiki/Objectivity_(science). Avoiding bias is also key to producing accurate and reliable scientific knowledge. The following article explores the three types of bias in science, and how they can be avoided https://pubmed.ncbi.nlm.nih.gov/25714762/.

It is an obscenity that rich people can buy better medical treatment than poor people.
To see the full question, please see:
https://www.admissionstesting.org/Images/20768-past-paper-2009-section-3-.pdf

The statement argues that It is unfair that those who are wealthier can receiver better medical treatment than those who cannot afford it. This is because:

- Medicine is a basic, universal human right and everyone should be able to get sufficient, quality treatment that they need, regardless of their economic status. This was one of the core principles that the NHS was founded on.
- Some people would view it as unfair that people are able to skip waiting lines and receive better treatment simply because they have more money.
- If poor people are unable to receive the treatment that they need, it can exclude certain segments of society from progressing, as health is a key factor in education, employment etc.

The statement makes many assumptions, some of which include:

- It assumes better is always more expensive. There are good doctors in both public and private systems, and undoubtedly there will be some doctors in public healthcare systems that are better than some doctors in private systems, as a better doctor can be seen to treat the patient with more care, and put more effort in (as opposed to by how much they are paid).
- For many conditions, whether or not a person is in private or public healthcare, they will receive the same drugs/medication, for example, a cancer patient would receive the same chemotherapy drugs; private may not always be better.
- It also assumes that only the rich can afford better healthcare; as private healthcare becomes cheaper, and private healthcare is included as a benefit in many jobs, far more people have access to private healthcare.

People may say that those with the money should be able to access better healthcare should they wish because:

- Medical care in many countries is a business; it is a person's right to choose whether they want to pay for better treatment. For example, wealthier people are able to buy more expensive food, and send their children to private schools, even though both education and food are basic rights, which are also provided in the public sector.
- The key issue is improving the basic provisions, so everyone receives quality basics.
- A private healthcare system co-existing with a public healthcare system may actually be beneficial for the public system. Private healthcare takes pressure off public healthcare systems, meaning it is better equipped to provide quality services to those who can't afford private treatment.

Freedom of choice means that people should be allowed to pay for better healthcare if they so deicide. However, I agree with the statement in the fact that poorer people shouldn't be deprived of essential healthcare just because of their economic status; the UK system prevents this from occurring; perhaps the real issue is we should ensure that everyone has access to quality healthcare

BMAT 2010

Section 1

Q1	A

Jay has a BMI of 22 and a height of 150cm. Reading along the table we know his weight is 49kg. Charlie's BMI is 24 and his/her height is 156cm tall; hence reading along the table we know his/her weight is 58kg. We know that the sum of their weights is 172kg. So, this mean's Alex's weight is 172kg – 58kg – 49kg = 65kg.
Finally, reading off the table, at 162cm tall and 65kg in weight, Alex's BMI is 25.

Q2	C

A – this may be true but doesn't affect the argument because it is not to do with the reasoning of it.
B – this again may be true but the type of influence on a citizen's psychological health could be positive, in which case it is not a flaw.
C – the argument says that if the Government subsidises the arts to a point where they can flourish, that will lead to an economically robust society. C rightly points out that if the precursor to a flourishing arts sector is a strong economy then this reasoning doesn't hold; C because a strong economy may come before, not after a flourishing arts sector.
D – this doesn't matter. The argument has already said the societies with flourishing arts sector '*tend*' to be more egalitarian but the use of '*tend*' implies that some may be viewed otherwise.

Q3	C

By looking at the axes, we can see that for Test 1, whoever scored the white diamond came 5th. For Test 2, they came 5th as well. (N.B the way you can see this is going along the axis from the top-right most point, for instance taking the x-axis first, you can count the number of black diamonds that were further from the origin than the white diamond; and repeat for the y-axis).
Ranking the test scores from 1 to 12 shows us that Erin came 5th in both tests.; clearly with the largest scores ranking higher.

Q4	C

A – this is not true; the passage states that it is better to fight spam at the source, but this doesn't mean all problems should be fought in this method
B – this is not drawn; the passage simply expresses the emissions of spam emails in terms of car emissions.
C – this is a conclusion. '*More effective spam filtering could reduce the amount by 75%*' which does support C.
D – this is not the case; the passage says '*a better strategy would be to fight spam athlete source*' so the filtering system doesn't necessarily need to be improved as much as possible if the better strategy would be to deal with the source of the spam.
E – the use of the term '*never*' is very strong and does not match anything we are told in the passage.

Q5	D

72 cakes need to be made in batches of 12, so 6 batches will be made.
There is a pattern with how long it takes the middle batches to be made. The first batch will take 40 (prep) + 25 (cooking) + 5 (cooling) = 70 minutes. However, the second batch can be started as soon as the 1st batch has been prepped, so 25 minutes of second batch prep takes place until the first batch need taking out of the oven. The oven then needs cooling for 5 minutes but the remaining 15 minutes of prep has to take place. 25 + 5 + 15 = 45 minutes of prep for the remaining 5 batches.
70 + 5(45) = 70 + 225 = 295 minutes = 4 hours and 55 minutes.

Q6	B

1 – doesn't matter because the argument is a model of a hypothetical scenario.
2 – this is a weakness because the model has begun after the 50 years with double the '*pre-industrial levels*' which may be too high a starting point if carbon dioxide levels have been reduced by then.
3 – other predictions that are not specific to this model are irrelevant.

Q7	B

To have a score of –05 the first number could be 0, 1, 2, 3, or 4 to fit in the score limit of 501. But if 3 lights are permanently on, then the digital look of 0, 1, 2, 3 or 4 can only be up to 3 lights difference from 8.
0 is 1 lights difference.
1 is 8 lights difference.
2 is 3 lights difference.
3 is 4 lights difference.
4 is 8 lights difference.
Hence only 0 or 2 could be the different numbers, giving scores of 005 or 205.

Q8	A

A – this is most challenged: '*traditional sociological explanation is that boys and girls...play with different types of toys*' but '*growing scientific evidence suggests...preferences may have a biological origin*'.
B – the first line confirms this, so the statement does not present a challenge.
C – the second line confirms this, so the statement does not present a challenge.
D – animal behaviour is not mentioned in the first paragraph so cannot be challenged.

Q9	A

A – this is a challenge to the statement that the monkeys showed preferences that varied in accordance with their sex. Just because the more aggressive sex monopolised the toys doesn't mean that the monkeys differed in their preferences. The female and male monkeys found the toys that were most attractive to them and there is no indication of them having a preference.
B – this doesn't actually have anything to do with preference of the toys; rather it talks about how long they are interested in the toys for.
C – food has nothing to do with toys.
D – we aren't talking about other species besides monkeys; hence this would not present a challenge to the inferences about vervet monkeys.
E – this is about their behaviour but not with regards to preferences on toys hence is unrelated to the question.

Q10	A

The claim made in paragraph 2 is that the two sexes did not differ in their preference for the neutral toys, and this was made by an experiment that measured *'how much time they spent with each'* toy.
A – this refers directly to the method of study so is correct; in order for the claim to be accepted, time as a reliable indicator of interest must be assumed.
B – this does not need to be accepted. The study was done on moneys and showed that they *'showed the same-sex typical toy presences as humans'* but this doesn't require them to have alike genetic make-up because it is a correlation.
C – this is not true; the paragraph explicitly states that these are *'stereotypically feminine toys'* and hence this statement doesn't need to be assumed.
D – this is not a necessary assumption. The study doesn't attempt to explain why the interest or preference is there for different types of toys so this does not need to be assumed.
E – this definitely does not need to be assumed to show data in this study that *'stunned the scientific world'*. Stunning implies this type of experiment has not been done before to the community's knowledge, but that would be a study that had previously been conducted with using stereotypically feminine or masculine or neutral toys. However, the statement only refers to an experiment about preference for different toys which is not as specific as the investigation in question.

Q11	D

1 – showing these photos alone does not reliably infer that humans and vervet monkeys respond in the same ways as humans because these are only two monkeys (a small sample size) and we don't know whether they were just given the toys to play with individually; not that they actually chose them.
2 – this also can't be reliably inferred. The photos showed are taken at one instance in time and are not an indication of preference over time. They are also unreliable due to the reasoning above.

Q12	C

A 3 x 3 grid has 9 squares in it, and four types of tile will be used, so altogether there will be 36 squares. We are told that the proportion of squares of each colour needs to be equal so 36 squares divided by 3 different types of square (black, white and grey) gives 12 of each colour.
To answer this question, one way is to use trial and error. We are given 5 squares and told we can only use 4 of them. So, excluding A to E one at a time and counting the number of each colour of squares (making sure they add up to 12 each) will tell us which one will need to be excluded.
Excluding A – total black: 13, total grey: 10, total white: 13
Excluding B – total black: 14, total grey: 12, total white: 10
Excluding C – total black: 12, total grey:12, total white, 12 hence is the ANSWER
Excluding D - total black: 11, total grey: 12, total white: 13
Excluding E – total black: 10, total grey: 10, total white: 16

Q13	E

The conclusion is given in the last line: '*since there will be negative stories in the press either way, we should ignore these stories and not worry about them*'.
A – this is not directly related to the conclusion so is wrong.
B – this is a subjective statement also not directly related to the conclusion.
C – this is not directly related to the conclusion.
D – the degree of difficulty of the exam is irrelevant to the argument presented.
E – this sums up the problem with the components of the conclusion: just because there will be negative stories doesn't mean they need to be ignored.

Q14	D

It would take a very long time to try and use systematic trial and error so I would advise you to try and pick number changes from the display with the fewest number of elements to one of the larger number of elements as this is likely to have a large number of element changes. 1 is clearly the display with the fewest elements (2) and going across you can see that:
From 1 to 0: 4 elements change
From 1 to 2: 5 elements change (you can now eliminate A, B and C)
From 1 to 3: 3 elements change
From 1 to 4: 2 elements change
From 1 to 5: 5 elements change
From 1 to 6: 6 elements change (this is the answer as nothing else is larger)
From 1 to 7: 1 element changes
From 1 to 8: 5 elements change
From 1 to 9: 4 elements change
Doing as much of this in your head will help you to cut down time, but this is a tricky question so come back if you have time.

Q15	D

A – we cannot infer this; the information is about deaths not ownership and riding.
B – we cannot infer this either; no reasoning is given for the discrepancy in figures.
C – this is subjective and casts aspersions on the nature of each of these incidents; which isn't detailed in the passage.
D – this is correct. In total, 2500 children were killed or seriously injured as pedestrians or child cyclists (1300 boy pedestrians + 700 girl pedestrians + 500 child cyclists = 2500). Of this figure, 1300 boy pedestrians + more than 400 male child cyclists = 1700 boys. This means 2500 – 1700 = 800 girls were killed or seriously injured. The ratio of 1700 boys : 800 girls indicates that the boys are more than twice as likely to be killed or seriously injured.
E – this cannot be inferred; we do not know that the reason more boys die is because they have less knowledge on road safety.

Q16	D

A – this cannot be. We know that the 3 on the die should be opposite to 4, but A doesn't show 4 opposite 3, as we know 3 is next to the 6 in its horizontal orientation.
B – this is also wrong; although the die is possible with 2 rotations in the same direction, the position is not possible with 2 rotations in different directions like the question asks.
C – this is not possible. Clearly, the 6 and the 3 are not arranged in this manner on the die in the question so this is obviously wrong.
D – this is correct; rotating the die in the question 90 degrees upwards and 90 degrees to the right gives the die in D.
E – this is also incorrect. It is a possible die but needs more rotations than 2.

Q17	C

The conclusion is that the safety of the artefacts is maintained because had the British Museum given 1 of these artefacts away, it would've been looted at the nation museum of Iraq.
A, B – this does not affect the safety of the artefact.
C – this is the flaw. The reasoning is that just because 1 museum was looted it doesn't mean that all will be.
D – this is not related to the conclusion of the passage.
E – this is not a flaw, because the argument does not try and convince us all artefacts are safe, it just tries to tell us that the ones in the British museum are safe.

Q18	D

The H is actually a tessellating pattern: imagine that the cards can fit together as shown with 2 H ends fitting into the middle part of the other H (as the 4cm width accommodates 2 x 2cm ends). We can see that the total number of Hs is 15.

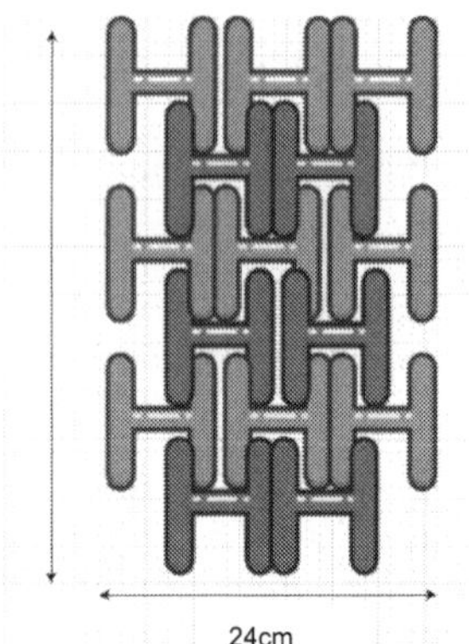

Q19	217

In 2005 the number of passengers at UK airports was 228 million and we need to correct this figure by counting domestic passengers only once per flight. The number of domestic passengers was 10% of 228 million ("nine in ten air passengers at UK airports in 2005 were travelling internationally" so 1 in 10 or 10% were domestic). Counting these passengers only once per flight instead of twice means halving this figure, leaving us with 11.4 million domestic flights.
Hence the corrected figure will be 228 million – 11.4 million = 216.6 million which rounds to 217 million (the question asks for the figure to the nearest million).

Q20	C

There were 34 million movements between Spain and the UK in 2005: out of a total of 228 million passenger movements in 2005. This is a proportion of 34/228 = 0.15 to 2 dp.
The number of total passenger movements in 1980 was about 60 million (reading off the graph) so 0.15 x 60 million = 9 million, to the nearest whole number.

Q21	F

1 - in 1980 there were about 60 million passengers, in 2005 there were 228 million; so in the 25 years between there was an increase of 228-60 = 168 million years.
In 1955 there were 5 million passengers, and as we know in 1980 there were 60 million passengers; so in those 25 years there was an increase of 60-5 = 55 million years.
N.B. the statement refers to the increase per annum, but you can see that there are 25 years between 1955 and 1980, and 1980 and 2005. This means we don't need to divide each one by 25 because the proportion will remain the same.
We can see that an increase of 55 million to 168 million is over a three-fold increase, so the statement is correct.
2 – Heathrow and Gatwick have 68 million + 33 million passengers between them = 101 million. We know that there are 228 million passengers in the UK so 101/228 x 100 = 44% to the nearest percent. This means the statement is correct.
3 – the current number of passengers in 2005 is 228 million. The growth over the next 25 to 500 million is an increase of 272 million. Hence, that is a per annuum increase of 272 million/25 which is clearly over 10 million per year. Hence, this statement is also correct.

Q22	D

The conclusion is that the sharp fall in passenger numbers '*will not necessarily prevent the Department of Transport's prediction*' due to the reasoning that the 1990 drop recovered. Hence the conclusion is justified.

Q23	E

The total number of possibilities is given by: 14+13+12+11+10+9+8+7+6+5+4+3+2+1 = 105. This is done by seeing that 1 can go with 14 other numbers, 2 can go with 13 etc.
The total number that have 3 different digits are listed below:
1 cannot go with anything else, it would have to go with a two-digit number but 10 –15 all had a 1 in them.
2 can go with 10, 13, 14, 15 (4 options)
3 can go with 10, 12, 14, 15 (4 options)
4 can go with 10, 12, 13, 15 (4 options)
5 can go with 10, 12, 13, 14 (4 options)
6, 7, 8 and 9 could go with 10, 12, 13, 14, 15 each (so 4 x 5 = 20 options)
This is a total of 36 options.
36/105 = 12/35

Q24	C

A – this is not a necessary assumption; the critical point of differentiation between space impact and super-volcanic activity is the presence of the cooling of the atmosphere and acid rain so even if volcanic activity caused the large-scale fires and earthquakes it would have other telling signs indicating this was the cause and not space impact.
B – these are symptoms of volcanic activity (the primary cause) so does not need to be assumed.
C – this is correct. The argument jumps from only giving the two options of origin as space impact and super-volcanic activity to then saying as no evidence was present to support super-volcanic activity, space impact by default became the explanation.
D – this is not underlying, the argument states this itself.
E – this is not an assumption nor does the argument ever use it as such. The reference to change in marine and land ecosystem is as a result of hypothetical super-volcanic activity.

Q25	A

If we need to exchange on of the cards to come highest, that means we need to calculate the scores of the other hands as they are:
4 of diamonds, 7 of diamonds: 22 (same suit so doubled)
5 of clubs and 8 of spades: 13
2 of hearts and 9 of clubs: 11
And our hand is 2 of spades and 7 of hearts: 9
In order to finish in the highest position, a card needs to be exchanged from the highest scorer; so, a 4 of diamonds or 7 of diamonds needs to be exchanged. The 7 of diamonds can be exchanged for the 2 of hearts to obtain a final hand of 7 of diamonds and 7 of hearts: 14.

Q26	A

A – this is the conclusion. '*people think they should be entitled to full medical care 24 hours a day*'.
B – this is not even mentioned as an alternative so cannot be the conclusion.
C – this is not the case; the implication of the phrase '*no matter how trivial the problem is*' implies that they can potentially detect the severity of a medical problem, but simply choose to seek care anyway.
D – we do not know that this is the case and is certainly not the conclusion as we are given no information as to the number of people seeking care for non-urgent and urgent medical problems.
E – this is not the conclusion, there is no indication that this is the presented solution and the argument doesn't actually present one; it simply ends by saying '*minor problems should be dealt with at day surgeries*' but this is not explained further.

Q27	C

Phil has already scored 20 so simply needs to score a further 10.
To be confident of winning he must score 10 in the next 2 goes. Remember that the accuracy is 1 section either side of the intended section.
By exploring each of the answers in turn you can solve this:
A - if Phil aims for 4, he could score 4, 1 or 9 and taking the worst possible scenario of 1 means he would have to aim for a section where each adjacent section and the section in question was 9 or greater, to ensure he gets to 30. However, no such section is placed here.
B – if Phil aims for 7, he could score 7, 3 or 5 and taking the worst possible scenario of 3 means he needs to aim for a section where each adjacent section and the section in question was 7 or greater to ensure he gets to 30. No such section is placed in this way.
C – if Phil aims for 9, he could score 9, 4 or 6 and taking the worst possible scenario of 4 means he needs to aim for a section where each adjacent section and the section in question was 6 or greater to ensure he gets to 30. This is plausible, aiming for 6 is a guarantee as the score could end up being 6, 9 or 11 so Phil would definitely score at least 30.
D - if Phil aims for 10, he could score 10, 5 or 8 but we already know the sections have to be different and Phil has already got an 8 so he can't risk scoring there again because that will not guarantee getting over 30 as he would've violated the game's rules.
E - if Phil aims for 11, he could score 11, 2 or 6 and taking the worst possible scenario of 2 means he needs to aim for a section where each adjacent section and the section in question was 8 or greater to ensure he gets to 30. No such section is placed in this way.

Q28	A

1 – this would strengthen the argument because if the readers saw that the article contained truthful, sympathy inciting accurate information about the boy's *'difficult and violent upbringing'* but still decided to call for tough measures based off of the name of the article alone.
2 – this would not strengthen the argument that the *'name alone had influenced public opinion'* because it suggests that the contents of the articles influenced them, not the name.
3 – this again doesn't strengthen the argument because it suggests as above that the contents reflected sentiments in favour of harsher measures on the boy as opposed to the name alone.

Q29	C

The range of the possible weights is 597 – 603kg. Looking at the weights given, it is clear that they are all close to 200kg, which would make sense as we need 3 of them to get in the range. So, writing the weights in relation to 200kg gives us –27, -18, -12, -3, +7, +19, +24 and we need to find a combination of 3 of these that will leave us with an answer in the range –3 to +3. This is achieved by doing –27 +19 +7 = -1 and –18 –3 +24 = +3. Hence –12 which corresponds to 188 is the answer as it is the one left over.

Q30	B

A – this is an assumption; the argument is that reducing class sizes hasn't worked in the USA, so it won't work here and what matters is the quality of the teacher. Hence, if more teachers were needed their qualifications would be lower hence, they would be less likely to be a good teacher.
B – this is not an assumption here. The only mention of money is the $50 billion in California, but it is not the money that is being criticised, it is how the money was used. For instance, the author clearly wants more good teachers, and this potentially means setting up an expensive scheme here to improve matters.
C – this is assumed because the author has said '*evidence from the USA*' has confirmed that reducing class sizes is not a good idea; but then goes on only to reference California as a state where they only moved up in the rankings by 1 position.
D - this is assumed; in saying that '*countries whose children do well at school are those that recruit their teachers form the brightest graduates*' this assumes that it is the bright graduates who have improved pupil performance.

Q31	D

A – this clearly cannot be, although the white and black squares as well as the cross and the blank face are in the right place, the circles are symmetrical to the net shown in the question so no rotation could make them the same. They are non-superimposable.
B - this is wrong, we can clearly see that in the die in the question the black square is opposite to the blank square, but in B they are adjacent.
C - in the net in the question the cross and the blank square would be opposite each other, but in C they would actually be next to one another, so this is wrong.
D – this is the correct net; it matches the one in the question.
E – this is wrong, in the net in the question the black square and the white circle are adjacent to one another, but in E they are opposite one another.

Q32	C

The information is set out as a distribution so the average earnings of the poorest 20% will be in the middle of $16203 and $17338 which is about £16500 and the average earnings of the richest 20% is in the middle of $50,656 and $162,029 which is about $105,000. So, the ratio relative to 1 is 105,000/16500 = 6.36 to 2 dp. Hence this is approximately 6:1

Q33	C

If overall the average income is $40,000, we can multiply it by 10 to get a total for the amount earned by the whole country: $400,000. Out of this, $162,029 is earned by the richest 10%. 162029/400,000 x 100 = 40%

Q34	C

The tax of 20% on 20% of the top earners is equal to:
0.2 x $162,029 = $32,405.80
0.2 x $50,656 = $10,131.20
So, the total is $42,537 which is then split evenly among the remaining 80% so the bottom 10% would receive 1/8 of this which is $5317.13
So, their new average earnings would be their existing earnings plus the money from the taxation of the rich: $16,203 + $5317.13 = $21520 which is closest to C.

Q35	B

1 – the right-hand graph shows that there are 2 plottings for those with a higher average income (richer) who are clearly healthier on the index of health.
2 – this can be concluded from the left-hand graph. Less variability of income corresponds to lower levels of income inequality and we can see that with lower levels of income inequality people are healthier on the index of health.

2010 Section 2

Q1	E

Temperature change is detected by the hypothalamus. Eliminate A, B and C. Arterioles dilate (vasodilation) in order to increase the surface area of the blood vessel in an attempt to conduct more heat away to cool the body down. Eliminate D and F. For fullness, hair erector muscles relax because the hair does not need to stand up to collect air beneath as an insulator, the body needs to cool down not warm up. The capillaries do not move in any case.

Q2	E

When calculating empirical formula you may find it easier to use a format similar to the table below. Hence the formula is: I_2O_5

	Iodine	Oxygen
Mass (g)	63.5	20.0
Ar	127	16
Mass/Ar	0.5	1.25
Ratio	2	5

Q3	A

Note that what is being measured is the mass of u-234, and we can see that over the duration of the experiment this reaches a constant mass of 16.0mg. Hence, all the protactinium in the sample must have decayed into u-234. Hence, the half-life would have been when half of the protactinium had decayed, i.e. there were 8mg of u-234 and 8mg protactinium. This happened at 1.2 minutes.

Q4	C

We know that the containers will both contain the same amount of water meaning the larger container will have half of its capacity left. Hence $p = 0.5$ so eliminate A, D and E. For the smaller container, imagine filling two containers (one large and one small) with the same volume of water. The amount the smaller one's capacity is filled will clearly be greater than that of the larger one, hence $q > 0.5$.

Q5	C

1 – this is incorrect; insulin allows the conversion of glucose to glycogen so the glucose concentration will fall; not rise.
2 – this is correct; recall that oestrogen thickens the uterus lining from your notes.
3 – this is also correct; recall the action of adrenaline and that it increases heart rate and breathing rate among other changes.

Q6	D

Step 1: work out the moles of carbon reacting in stage 2. moles = mass/Mr = 12.0g/12 = 1 mole.
Step 2: work out the moles of CO_2 produced in stage 3. We can see in stage 2 that the ratio of C:CO is 1:2. We already worked out that 1 mole of C reacts, so this must produce 2 moles of CO. The question tells us all of the CO produced in stage 2 reacts in stage 3. So, the ratio of CO: CO_2 in stage 3 is 3: 3 which is actually 1:1. This means that the moles of CO_2 produced is 2.
Stage 3: work out the mass of CO_2: mass = moles x Mr = 2 x (12 + 32) = 88g

Q7	A

The amplitude is half of the distance between the peak and trough of a wavelength. Here, that difference is 6 so half of 6 is 3, so we can eliminate C, D, E, F, G and H.
Frequency = 1/time period
The time period is the time taken for 1 cycle; reading off the graph this is 12 hours. 12 hours needs to be converted to seconds as for frequency to be given in Hz the time period must be in seconds. So, 12 hours x 3600 is the time period.
This makes the frequency = 1/(12 x 3600) which is clearly A.

Q8	C

The total number of combinations over 2 goes is $(\frac{1}{4})^4$ because each spinner has a probability of landing on any segment of ¼, and there are 2 spinners spun twice each: 4 spins total.
The total number of combinations resulting in ending up where you started are 16, listed below:

L1 R1	R1 L1	U1 D1	D1 U1
L2 R2	R2 L2	U2 D2	D2 U2
L3 R3	R3 L3	U3 D3	D3 U3
L4 R4	R4 L4	U4 D4	D4 U4

16 x 1/256 = 16/256 = 1/16

Q9	B

This question assumes knowledge not currently tested on the BMAT specification.
During the process of evolution, natural selection will favour individuals with an advantageous allele. Whenever you have learnt about natural selection it has always been with regards to a specific advantageous allele, individuals do not benefit from an advantageous gene pool (a whole population may). Geographic distribution is irrelevant here.

Q10	D

1 – this is not produced; it is a reactant!
2 – This is produced by incomplete combustion.
3 – This is produced by complete combustion.
4 – This is produced by complete combustion.
5 – This is not produced by fuel combustion.
6 – This is not produced by fuel combustion.

Q11	C

Radon begins with a mass number of 219 and an atomic number of 86. It loses 3 alpha particles, each with a mass number of 4 and an atomic number of 2, producing a net loss of 12 from the mass number and 6 from the atomic number. Then. it loses 2 beta particles, which each cause the atomic number to increase by 1, so together will have the net effect of increasing the atomic number by 2.
Mass number: 219 – 12 = 207
Atomic number: 86 – 6 + 2 = 82

2010 Section 2

Q12	C

The mean of the first group is given to us: $54 = \frac{total\ time\ of\ group\ 1}{20}$ so

$total\ time = 20(54) = 1080$

The mean of the second group: $T = \frac{total\ time\ of\ group\ 2}{P}$ so $total\ time\ of\ group\ 2 = PT$

The new mean when the first and second group have been added together: $mean = \frac{total\ time\ for\ group\ 1\ and\ 2}{total\ number\ of\ people\ in\ group\ 1\ and\ 2} = \frac{1080 + TP}{20 + P} = 56$

Rearranging this for P gives:

$$1080 + TP = 56(20 + P)$$
$$1080 + TP = 1120 + 56P$$
$$TP - 56P = 40$$
$$P(T - 56) = 40$$
$$P = \frac{40}{T - 56}$$

Q13	F

1 – transmitter molecules are produced in the pre-synaptic membrane, not the receptor
2 – the signal is transmitted by diffusion, not osmosis! Osmosis refers to water
3 – this is incorrect. The transmitter molecules move across the synapse to attach to receptors to then trigger an action potential, not the other way round.
4 – this is correct.
5 – this is correct.

Q14	A

1 – this is correct, the charges balance.
2 – this is correct, there is a neutral overall charge on the LHS, and neutral charge on the RHS. If a 1- negatively charged ion loses 1 electron, the atom itself is left.
3 – this is incorrect, there is a 4- charge overall on the LHS, and neutral charge on the RHS.
4 – This is incorrect, there is a 3- charge overall on the LHS, and neutral charge on the RHS.
5 – this is incorrect. The iodine atoms are not balanced, there are 2 on the LHS, and 1 on the RHS.
6 – this is correct, the overall charge is 0 on the LHS and 0 on the RHS.

Q15	B

Assume for this question that the wire is carrying no resistance.
When P is open and Q is closed, the current will follow the path of least resistance (bottom part of the parallel circuit through switch Q) hence Y receives all current and all voltage.

When P is closed and Q is open, the current is now forced to be split between the two rows on the parallel circuit (as it can no longer go through Q). As X has more current now (current at all) it gets brighter.
We can visualise this now as one series circuit (the 4 bulbs in parallel on the LHS need to be viewed as 1 component in series with Y) Y receives less voltage than it did previously as in series the voltage is split between the 2 components, and as we now have 2 parts Y must receive less voltage than it did before. So, with less voltage and the same current, as P = IV this bulb will get dimmer.

Q16	C

AB:BC is 4:x. AD = 4 +x – 4 = x
The ratio of AD:DE is x:x+3
The ratio of AB:BC is the same as AD:DE as these are similar triangles.
This means

$$\frac{4}{x} = \frac{x}{x+3}$$
$$4(x+3) = x^2$$
$$4x + 12 = x^2$$
$$x^2 - 4x - 12 = 0$$
$$(x-6)(x+2) = 0$$
$$x = 6 \text{ or } x = -2$$

Ignore $x = -2$ *as length BC cannot be negative*
So, if x = 6, then DE is x + 3 = 6 + 3 = 9

Q17	E

R and X are clearly homozygous recessive (rr) as they are the only ones to have the recessive disease.
P and Q are heterozygous (Rr) because they carry recessive alleles without having the disease.
Crossing P and Q gives a 1/2 chance of being a carrier:
N.B. it is not ¾ because we can eliminate rr as we are told that P and Q do not have the condition, the only people that do are R and X and, for fullness, RR is not a carrier.

	R	r
R	RR	Rr
r	Rr	rr

This means the chance of S and T being a carrier is 50%.
However, for U, we already know that U's offspring X is homozygous recessive. The only way homozygous recessive offspring is formed is if both parents are carriers or have the condition and are recessive themselves. We know U does not have the condition so U must be a carrier, hence the percentage for U is 100%.

Q18	B

A – Mg^{2+} has a 2+ charge, $2H^+$ have a 2+ charge, $2PO_4^{3-}$ has a 6- charge, overall, this is a 2- charge which is not the possible as the formula will have a net charge of 0
B – Mg^{2+} has a 2+ charge, $4H^+$ have a 4+ charge, $2PO_4^{3-}$ has a 6- charge, overall, this is a net charge of 0 hence is the answer.
C - Mg^{2+} has a 2+ charge, $3H^+$ have a 3+ charge, PO_4^{3-} has a 3- charge, overall, this is a 2+ charge.
D - Mg^{2+} has a 2+ charge, $6H^+$ have a 6+ charge, $2PO_4^{3-}$ has a 6- charge, overall, this is a 2+ charge.
E - $2Mg^{2+}$ has a 4+ charge, H^+ have a 1+ charge, PO_4^{3-} has a 3- charge, overall, this is a 2+ charge.
F - $2Mg^{2+}$ has a 4+ charge, $2H^+$ have a 2+ charge, PO_4^{3-} has a 3- charge, overall, this is a 3+ charge.

2010 Section 2

Q19	B

We know acceleration on a distance – time graph is shown as a curve, but R and S are straight lines, showing no acceleration so we can eliminate R and S.
Hence, out of the two velocity-time graphs, acceleration is given as the gradient of the graph. The gradient of P (using the figures already outlined by the hashed lines) gives gradient = 10-0/24 = 10/24 = 0.417 ms^{-2}
The gradient of Q = 59 – 10/20 = 2.45ms^{-2} which is closest to the answer.

Q20	A

The surface area is (2 x the area at either end of the cylinder) + the area of the rectangle wrapped round it = the volume of the cylinder:

$$2\pi r^2 + 2\pi rh = \pi r^2 h$$

We can divide all terms by $\pi$and r as they are common to all:

$$2r = rh - 2h$$

$$h(r-2) = 2r$$

$$h = \frac{2r}{r-2}$$

Q21	B

1 – this is correct, the only meiosis that takes place in animals is in the production of our gametes which takes place in our reproductive organs
2 – this is correct. Mitosis forms genetically identical daughter cells called clones.
3 – this is incorrect, meiosis results in 4 nuclei
4 – this is incorrect, mitosis results in 2 nuclei
5 – this is correct; asexual reproduction produces clones with identical genetic information whereas meiosis leads to genetic variation

Q22	C

Percentage yield = actual yield/theoretical yield x 100
To work out the theoretical yield we need to start be working out the moles of benzene:
Moles = mass/Mr = 3.9g/(6x12) + (6 x1) = 3.9g/78 = 0.05 moles
Benzene: nitrobenzene is 1:1 so 0.05 moles of nitrobenzene are formed theoretically.
Hence, the theoretical mass of nitrobenzene = Mr x moles = [(6 x 12) + (5 x 1) + 14 + (2 x 16)] x 0.05 = 123 x 0.05 = 6.15g
So, the percentage yield = 3.69g/6.15g x 100 = 60%

Q23	G

Power = energy transferred/time
The energy transferred here is GPE into KE and GPE = mgh = 5kg x 10N/kg x 5m = 250Joules
The question tells us that "each second" this energy is transferred; so, power = 250J/1second = 250W. Thus, we can eliminate A, B, C, D, E and F.
As we know the GPE is transferred to KE and that KE = ½ x mv^2 we know that the 250J of GPE = 1/2 x 5kg x v^2
Rearranging for v^2 = 2 x 250J/5kg = 500J/5kg = 100 so v = 10m/s

Q24	C

This a rather long question so skip it and come back at the end if you have time.
Let the side length of the largest square be 1. So, the area of the largest square is also 1.
To work out the side length of the fourth square we can use Pythagoras on each square:
On the second square: The side lengths a and b are 1/3 and 2/3 respectively.

$$a^2 + b^2 = c^2$$

$$so\ c = \sqrt{a^2 + b^2} = \sqrt{(1/3)^2 + (2/3)^2} = \sqrt{1/9 + 4/9} = \sqrt{5/9} = \sqrt{5}/3$$

On the third square: the side lengths a and b are (⅓ x $\sqrt{5}/3 = \frac{\sqrt{5}}{9}$) and (⅔ x $\sqrt{5}/3 = \frac{2\sqrt{5}}{9}$) respectively. So $a^2 = 5/81$and $b^2 = 20/81$

$so\ c = \sqrt{a^2 + b^2} = \sqrt{\frac{25}{81}} = \frac{5}{9}$

On the fourth square, the side lengths a and b are (⅓ x 5/9 = 5/27) and (⅔ x 5/9 = 10/27) respectively.

$$so\ a^2 = \frac{25}{27^2}\ and\ b^2 = \frac{100}{27^2}$$

$so\ c = \sqrt{a^2 + b^2} = \sqrt{\frac{125}{27^2}}$

The area of the fourth square is therefore $c \times c = \sqrt{\frac{125}{27^2}} \times \sqrt{\frac{125}{27^2}} = \frac{125}{27^2} = \frac{125}{729}$

Q25	E

Note that the question asks for statement that are true about both the hormonal and nervous system!
1 – while this may be the case for the nervous system, it is not the case for the hormonal system, which as you know relies on hormones.
2 – This is correct; both hormones and nervous impulses act on target structures.
3 - the nervous system is a lot faster than the hormonal system so this is correct.
4 – this is incorrect; transmitter molecules used in the nervous system can be chemicals.
5 – this is correct; in releases of hormones such as adrenaline the CNS is involved in stimulating the pituitary gland to lead to the release of adrenaline.

Q26	B

Here, just count the total number of corners (as these are the carbons on skeletal structure) and you will count 17. Then add on the 3Cs from the groups that are branched off, there are two CH_3 s and 1 CO_2H. 17 + 3 = 20

Q27	D

The work done in this question is two-fold, first is the work done against gravity, the second is work done against friction.
Taking the first case, work done against gravity is equal to GPE.
GPE = mgh
Height can be worked out using the fact that this is a 1 in 20 slope and we are told the car has moved 50m. We have been told that for every 20m the car gains 1m in height so 50/20 = 2.5m gained in height.
So mgh = 800kg x 10N/kg x 2.5m = 20,000J = 20kJ

Taking the second case, work done against friction = Force of friction x distance travelled
This is equal to 500N x 50m = 25000J = 25kJ
Summing all the work done gives 20kJ + 25kJ = 45k

2010 Section 3

To see the marking grid and mark bands that the BMAT examiners will use to mark your essays, please refer to the BMAT website.

Anyone who has a serious ambition to be a president or prime minister is the wrong kind of person for the job. To see the full question, please see:
https://www.admissionstesting.org/Images/20766-past-paper-2010-section-3-.pdf

The reasoning behind this statement requires us to examine the attributes of someone who has a serious ambition to be a world leader. These types of people may stop at nothing to become leader, thus may be involved in corruption, power and money grabbing and doing whatever they can to further their own career. Serious ambition could lead to sabotaging other candidates, rigging the voting system and misleading the general public with false propaganda. I'm sure you know of a few pertinent examples of this kind of behaviour if you felt the need to exemplify your thoughts. Contrasting this with the leadership, compassion and fairness that we believe should be upheld by world leaders tells us that these types of people will lose those traits that we value so greatly on their conquest to become president or prime minister. This is why the statement argues that these types of people will not be the right kind of person for the job; they will instead have morals that do not align with the tolerant views of a democratic society.

However, there are some strong arguments against this reasoning. The first that comes to mind is that if a candidate going for president or prime minster does not have serious ambition then how will they be able to convey the passion and enthusiasm required to win over the electorate? How will they have a good understanding of what the job involves, with physical, moral and emotional sacrifices for the good of the country? Serious ambition is also needed to build together a team to support your campaign; in most countries a leadership contest or a general election campaign requires a lot of funding; and serious ambition is needed to secure the support of the benefactors of your party.

Further to this, once one has assumed their role in office, the decisions to negotiate, decide the future of and implement change are almost always met with challenge. Again, serious ambition within each element of the job is needed to bring about this change.

But many would agree that ambition is needed to a degree, we all thrive off ambition as it allows us to visualise an end-goal and gives us the vision from which we can manifest in reality. You may think that a healthy balance of ambition is needed to provide the motivation necessary to hold this sort of public office but restrained so as to comply by rules and regulations to promote fairness at all times.

People injured whilst participating in extreme sports should not be treated by a publicly funded health service. To see the full question, please see: ***https://www.admissionstesting.org/Images/20766-past-paper-2010-section-3-.pdf***

The reasoning behind this statement is that those who participate in extreme sports put themselves at a very high level of risk of injury, and essentially shouldn't be treated using taxpayer money because they knowingly did so. The money that the NHS receives should be spent on those who need treatment and who haven't exposed themselves knowingly to this sort of risk. Arguably, spending money on treating these patients diverts funds from those who need treatment for illness that is entirely out of their control; such as some genetic disorders.

The statement suggests however, that the alternative is for these individuals to seek private healthcare, which is not affordable for all people doing extreme sports. In addition, those who do extreme sports pay taxes like everyone else, hence they contribute to the funding of the NHS so they too should be entitled for treatment.

In addition, it is not just those with unavoidable illness that are treated on the NHS. Arguably self-inflicted diseases caused by excess smoking or drinking are treated on the NHS and it is also part of not casting judgement upon others; and treating everyone equally (which forms part of the NHS constitutional values). Ethically speaking, this is what a doctor ought to do; treat all patients as the Hippocratic Oath also states. In addition, if we take the line of reasoning from this argument, we will end up restricting what treatment can be funded on the NHS through trying to judge what has been knowingly done/self-inflicted; which many in society would find unpopular and unfair. Often, there are multiple issues with a patient's physical and mental health that leads to problems such as excessive drinking meaning it is unfair to brand their illness as self-inflicted.

In terms of the public perception of personal risk taking, nearly everything we do is taking a risk; from crossing a road to extreme sport. This scale is difficult to quantify and therefore it is unfair to brand others as too much of a risk taker. We are all individuals, weighing up our own safety and well-being when we decide to undertake something. This autonomy is a pillar of ethics that must be respected; so although clear sign-posting of risks must be made clear, it is unfair to go further in trying to influence people that are complying with extreme sports under the law. For those who believe that those who do extreme sports should not have treatment on the NHS, you may argue that more should be done to try and change their perception of risk taking and equality of treatment.

Authors' Tip:

These kinds of questions are relatively common in interviews and in the BMAT Section 3. It may be helpful to consider arguments for and against treating smokers, those with obesity and other self-inflicted conditions on the NHS, trying to link each point with one (or more) of the 4 pillars of medical ethics (beneficence, non-maleficence, autonomy and justice). An important ethical principle to consider here is the **slippery slope argument**, and where do we draw the line on what is self-inflicted?

2010 Section 3

Question 3 was written to widen access to the exam paper, as in the past, students hoping to study Veterinary Medicine would also have to take the BMAT. VetMed students no longer take the BMAT, and so in its current iteration (2017 onwards), there are none of these questions, so the authors have not included worked essays for these and recommend that you only attempt these after having attempted all the previous ones.

Science only tells us what is possible, not what is right.

To see the full question, please see: ***https://www.admissionstesting.org/Images/20766-past-paper-2010-section-3-.pdf***

Science is the pursuit of knowledge through empirical means; but this knowledge is objective in the sense that it isn't inherently good or bad. Hence, science cannot tell us what is right or wrong because that is a moral matter and its outside the remit of science. It is humans who make these decisions about morality. Science is the basis for which we can make these later subjective statements.

However, some people argue that science does help us to judge what is right and wrong because we can measure effects of different variables. The scientific method allows us to collect and interpret data, for instance we can measure the efficacy or toxicity of a drug and inferring whether it is right or wrong to give a drug with a certain dosage to a patient based off of this information. In medicine, this is particularly important because in evidence-based medicine is used to make so many decisions about policy, rationing, and levels of treatment; all of which are subjective elements.

We know decisions about what is right and wrong can be informed by science because of the use of examples such as the one above. What you may wish to think about is not the extent of involvement but actually the responsibility of those researchers conducting the experiments and the companies interpreting these results. Because science is objective, it is easy to pick and choose which elements you want to display, by which humans will make decision about the moral use of the results at their own discretion. This is the subjective responsibility where what is right and wrong is decided.

BMAT 2011

Section 1

Q1	D

This is a question to be done using the process of elimination. Match each bar graph to the datasets in the table, and you will be left with one graph that does not fit any. In this case A is cloud cover, B is chance of rain (note the 50 on Tuesday and 50 on Wednesday), C is average wind speed and E is maximum temperature.

Q2	E

None of the statements given can be reasonably drawn from the paragraph. A is wrong as the paragraph provides no causative link between whale numbers becoming depleted and modern life. B is wrong as the effects of sea-based wind farms are not discussed. C is wrong as the modalities do not match; '*are trying to adapt*' is not the same as '*will adapt*'. D is wrong for similar reasons to A.

Q3	C

A deluxe room is $80/night, but we don't want meals, so the room cost per night is ($80-$15)/night = $65/night. So, for 6 nights it will be (6 x $65) = $390. We also want to hire a car for the whole stay which is $5 + (6 x $5) = $35. So, the total is $390 + $35 = $425.

Q4	E

This passage assumes that children who interact with each other and children who play computer games are mutually exclusive (i.e. no child who plays computer games interacts with other children). This is the flaw of the passage, as no evidence is provided to establish this link.

Q5	F

This is a visualisation question. If you have difficulties with these types of questions, try cutting out the cube's net and building it to help build confidence and visualisation skills. In this question, 1 is the same as the right-hand mirror, and therefore cannot be a reflection, and 2 is a rotation of the left-hand mirror, therefore ruling both of those options out.

Q6	C

Here, the passage assumes that it was learning for the test that is the cause for this development in the part of the brain associated with memory, and not any other factors present within the population who choose to become taxi drivers, which is paraphrased by C. A, B and D are not assumed by the passage.

Q7	A

First, have a look at the range. C, E, F have smaller ranges than 5600 miles, so are not suitable. Next, have a look at the passenger requirements. All the remaining planes are able to carry between 163 and 177 passengers. To find out the most fuel-efficient plane, we need to use this formula: (fuel consumption of empty plane + fuel consumption of 163 passengers). Just by looking at the table, A is the obvious answer as it has the lowest fuel consumption for an empty plane (3.0) and the lowest additional fuel consumption per passenger (0.01)

2011 Section 1

Q8	D

For these types of questions, go systematically through the options, deciding whether they are true or false. A is false as the chart mentions the gender pay gap, as opposed to absolute pay. B is false as there is no information mentioned about the willingness of employers. C is false as there is no data for each age, we only have data for the range of ages. D is correct therefore by elimination, but also because a woman earns more than 20% less than a man in those age categories, which is what D states.

Q9	C

From the formula given we know that:
22.8 = 100 x (m- £16,000/ m), where m is male pay.
0.228m = m - £16,000
0.772m = £16,000
m = 16,000/0.75 (use 0.75 as it is easier to calculate, but BEWARE, that the answer will be larger than needed, as we have reduced the denominator)
We get £21,300 but from above, we know this is too large, so the answer must be £20,700.

Q10	C

The assumption made in the paragraph is related to the '*motherhood penalty*' - that it is being a mother, and looking after their children that is the only reason deterring them from taking high positions. This is what C says.

Q11	D

Again, work through the options. D, here is the only correct option using the data given, as we know that women in their 40s working part time earn 41.2% less than their male counterparts. £15 is roughly 41% greater than £8.82 (use £15 and £9 for this calculation, as they are nicer to work with).

Q12	D

For these types of questions, we recommend drawing out all the different types of tile. Working our way across the first row we can see that these are the only kind of tiles:

Once you think you have drawn all the different kinds of tiles, quickly go through the rest of the diagram to double check you have not missed any.

Q13	B

B is a clear correct answer for this question, as a problem with the gene (mutation) leading to a problem with speech shows us that it is this gene that is responsible with language.

Q14	C

Central has two points, meaning they have drawn two matches, and lost two matches. Western has one point, meaning they have drawn one match and lost three matches. Northern has 8 points, meaning they have won 2 and drawn two. Southern have 5 points meaning they have won one and drawn 2 and lost one. If we count up the draws, we can see that we have an odd number of draws. However, we see that we have got 3 wins and 6 losses. Therefore, Eastern must have won 3 and drawn 1 (to ensure the number of draws is equal and that number of losses = number of wins), and therefore Eastern must have 10 points.

Q15	B

1 is incorrect as it does not address the argument.
2 is correct as it assumes that a constitutional right is mutually exclusive from a human right.
3 is incorrect as there is no mention in the text of willingness of prisoners to vote.

Q16	D

Depth is volume/area. Go down the table, quickly using estimations to work out the depth for the lakes. Using this calculation, you should see that Baikal has the greatest depth at roughly 0.75km (I used 24,000 and 32,000 as my estimations).

Q17	C

1 is incorrect as the argument is not built upon the number of people who have eaten the beef, it is based on the fact that those who have eaten it will be susceptible to two further outbreaks.
2 is incorrect as a group in PNG with M-V combination later inherited the disease.
3 is correct, as the argument focuses on the combinations of the variants (line 3) as opposed to the individual variants themselves.

Q18	B

Jasper is 43, and Ruby is 35.
Therefore, Jasper will earn £240 + £110 [this is 22 x £5] + £120 [this is 6 x £20] = £570
Ruby earns £40 more, so earns £610.
£510 = £240 + £70 [this is 14 x £5] + (£20 x y), where y is the number of years Ruby has worked in Grindstone.
Therefore, we get: y = £200/£20 = 10 years
10 years is 4 years greater than 6, therefore B is correct.

Q19	A

This question asks about the financial viability of drilling compared to not drilling. Work out the profit x chance column and add up the values for drilling and not drilling. For drilling you will get -$72,000 + $320,000 + $380,000 = $628,000
For not drilling you will get $200,000 + $300,000 = $500,000. Therefore, drilling is more favourable than not drilling = A

Q20	D

Again, work through the options systematically.
A is incorrect, as we have worked out above a medium strike will provide $320,000, which is a profit. B is incorrect, as the lowest sale of drilling rights is $500,000. A medium strike is $320,000 which is less than $500,000, and so would not be a better outcome than selling. C is incorrect as the probability of making a loss is 10% compared to 90% of making a profit. D is correct as the probability of a medium strike is 80%, and the probability of a sale is 60% + 20% = 80%.

Q21	F

1 is correct, a medium strike would only bring a loss of $100,000 dollars as costs are ($800,000 + $500,000) but profit is only $1,200,000. 2 is correct as the chance of making a profit is 10% ('big strike'). 3 is correct as reducing costs by 25% to $600,000, would mean that overall, $100,000 profit is made.

Q22	E

Using our figures from q19, we know that drilling on average will give us $628,000 and not drilling will give us $500,000. Paying the insurance would mean we would only get $428,000 [this is $628,000 - $200,000], not paying the insurance would be $328,000 [this is $628,000 - (0.03 x $10,000,000)]. So, the order is 3,1,2.

Q23	D

The numbers 2,4,6,7 and 8 haven't been used. On the right hand side, remaining numbers have to sum to 10 (so 8 + 2), at the top numbers have to sum to 12 (so 6 + 4 + 2) and on the left numbers have to sum to 13 (6 + 7). Looking at the combinations therefore the top left must be 6 and the top right must be 2. We can then fill in the remaining gaps, giving us D as our answer.

Q24	A

Petermass will play '*only if Fredericks isn't fit*'. However, this does not mean that if Fredericks isn't fit, Fredericks will definitely be playing, simply that the only chance of him playing is when Fredericks isn't fit. Therefore, only Jed's statement is correct.

Q25	C

The new larger mix contains (120ml + 45ml) = 165ml oil + (60ml + 45ml) = 105ml vinegar. (270ml in total)
The original one will contain then 45ml oil and 45mil vinegar.

After the second mixing, the original container will contain (45ml + ⅓ x 165ml) oil + (45ml + ⅓ x 105ml) vinegar = 100ml oil + 80ml vinegar
The other container will contain 110ml oil + 70ml vinegar. Therefore, C is correct.

Q26	C

The conclusion of the argument is '*planets like this must be really common*' which is C. The other information in the passage, such as the subsequent lines are additional evidence to strengthen this conclusion, with preceding information providing context to the conclusion.

Q27	A

The question asks whether you can make a 4x3 rectangle or a 6x2 rectangle with three of these pieces, which is not possible with any of these shapes. If you have difficulty with these questions, try cutting the shapes out and seeing whether you can fit them together (this is a very helpful way to practice these questions!)

Q28	C

We need to know 1 because fuel efficiency will allow us to see whether hydrogen buses are better. 3 is needed as it is relevant to the argument, which uses carbon dioxide output as a measure of environmental efficiency. For the same reason, 4 is needed. 2 is not relevant to the argument presented.

Q29	D

Charles will therefore travel the 3km distance in 20 minutes as well as the distance Claire travels in 20 minutes, which is 3km. Therefore, Charles will have to travel 6km in 20 minutes, giving a speed of 18km/hr.

Q30	B

Here we have an effect (pulsars) and a potential cause for that effect (sterile neutrinos), so B is correct as sterile neutrinos could be a potential cause. There is no definitive proof, so we cannot say that it must be the cause (A), or have no alternative explanation, so we cannot say that it is the best explanation (C). Additionally, there may be another cause of pulsars that we do not know of, so D is not correct.

Q31	C

This is another visualisation question. We know that there are 20 cans remaining. From our view from X, we know that there must be 6 cans left in the white areas (and that 6 have been removed). Therefore, there must be 14 cans in the middle columns (shaded), and so a maximum of 4 cans can be removed from the shaded area. A, B, E, F are all possible combinations because there are sufficient cans in both areas. D is possible if the very middle two columns have one can each (thereby having only removed 4 cans from the central area). Therefore, by elimination, only C is not possible, as 6 cans would have been removed, and at a maximum, only 12 cans could be in the middle section (shaded), when we actually need 14.

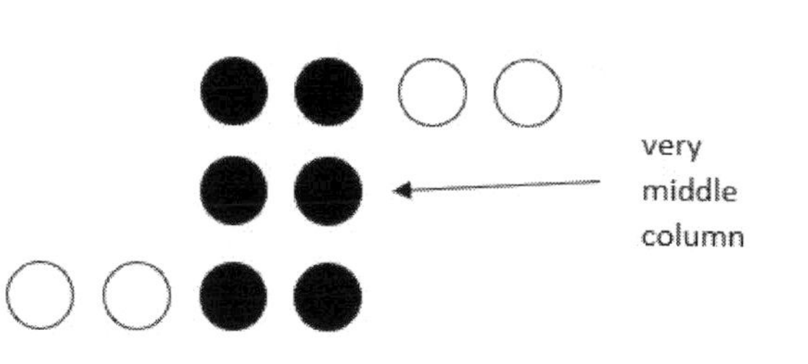

Q32	C

In 2006, each person saw their doctor on average 5 times, so in effect the doctor would have to make 1500 x 5 appointments = 7500 appointments. 7500/250 days = 30 consultations a day, so C is the correct answer. (Note: I rounded 5.26 to 5 to make calculations easier, which is why 30 is not an answer option available - I chose the answer closest to 30)

Q33	D

In 1995, nurses performed 0.8/3.29 of the consultations, which is around 0.2. In 2006, this was 1.8/5.26 which is around 0.35. [(0.35-0.2)/0.2] x 100 = 75% which is closest to 67% so D is the answer.

Q34	C

The number of male appointments exceeded female appointments in the older age categories, so the female : male ratio would be lower in those age groups. In the younger age groups, the reverse is true. Line C shows this and so is correct.

Q35	C

A,B and D are all reasonable answers. D is the only one that is not, as ageing is not an explanation, as the graph contains all age groups. For example, a person who was 20 in 1996, will be 31 in 2006, both age ranges are present in both graphs, so ageing is not an explanation.

2011 Section 2

Q1	F

This question tests knowledge not currently on the BMAT specification
We can see that the three columns are glands, hormones and functions. Looking through the answer options we can see that F (carbohydrase) is neither of these - it is an enzyme. If all the answer options had been glands, hormones or functions, the best way to answer this question would be to work your way through the table, filling the gaps, and seeing which answer option has been left out.

Q2	B

If a metal is in group 3, its valency is +3 charge. If a non-metal is in group 6, its valency is -2. We can then use the swapping method for determining formulae which will mean that the formula is $X_2 Y_3$

Q3	C

We need the formulae: GPE = mgh and KE = ½ mv^2. Both cars have identical masses, and so will have identical masses (let us call the mass m)
P; GPE = 250m, KE = 200m
Q; GPE = 500m, KE = 50m
Therefore, we can see that C is correct.

Q4	C

For these questions, it is helpful to have a good command of algebra and a good understanding of the laws of indices. You should know that $y^{-1} = \frac{1}{y}$and $(ab)^3 = a^3b^3$
$3x(3x^{-1/3})^3 = 3x(27x^{-1}) = 3x(\frac{27}{x})$ = 81

Q5	F

Mitosis is the division of a diploid cell to produce two genetically identical diploid daughter cells (no variation). Meiosis is the division of a diploid cell to produce 4 genetically different haploid daughter cells (causes variation). Therefore, only 3,4 and 5 are correct.

Q6	D

Increasing the temperature, increases the frequency of collisions per second, and means more collisions occur with energy greater than or equal to the activation energy (i.e. with more energy). Therefore 1 and 2 are correct. Temperature does not affect orientation, so 3 is not correct.

Q7	E

Work through the statements until you find one that is true. A is incorrect because that is not the definition of nuclear fission, which is the splitting of a radioactive nucleus. B is incorrect as the half-life is the time taken for half of the sample to decay. C is incorrect as the number of neutrons is the mass number - atomic number. D is not correct, because nuclear power is generated using fission, not fusion (RTQ carefully). E is correct, as beta emission results in the changing of a proton into a neutron and an electron which is ejected, so the number of particles in the nucleus (nucleons) remains constant.

2011 Section 2

Q8	D

At 9:45, the minute hand touches the 9, whereas the hour hand is ¾ of the way between the 9 and the 10. Therefore, the angle is ¾ of the angle between 9 and 10. A clock is circular so has 360°. The number of degrees between each hour is 30° (360/12). So ¾ of 30 is 22.5°.

Q9	C

This question requires a good understanding of the specification content. 4 is the only incorrect statement, as individuals with less advantageous adaptations still will breed, just they are less likely to breed than those with advantageous adaptations.

Q10	D

Each Carbon can make 4 bonds. On the right is the full diagram. There are 12 carbons, and 18 hydrogens, so the Mr is (12 x 12) + (18 x 1) = 138.

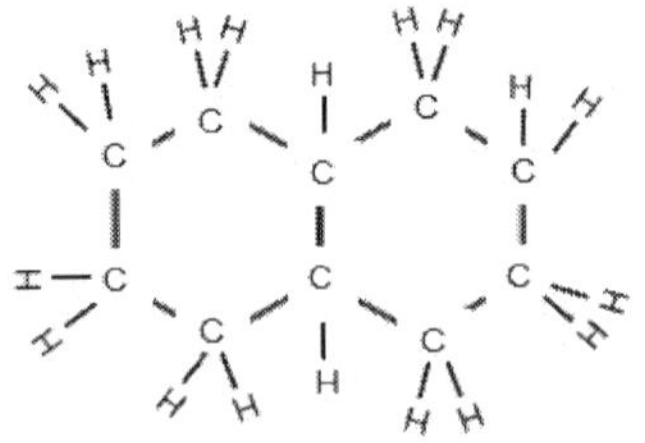

Q11	B

When the switch is open, the circuit is incomplete as no current can flow (this is because the diode only allows current to flow in one direction through it from right to left, whereas the current in this circuit flows clockwise (look at the battery!). When the switch is closed the current can go around the diode, and so the current = voltage/resistance, which is 6V/3Ω = 2A.

Q12	D

For complex inequalities such as these, assign values to each letter. Using trial and improvement, we can then work out which of the following statements is true. Choosing numbers such as w = 6, x = 4, y = 1, z = 2, we can see that A and C can't be true. w = 1, x = 6, y = 2, z = -3, we can see that B and E can't be true. Therefore, only D can be true.

Q13	E

In an active muscle, aerobic respiration will be taking place at a high rate, so there will be a high CO_2 concentration in the plasma. Therefore, lots of oxygen will be required to feed the muscles, so there will be a high O_2 concentration in red blood cells. Gas exchange occurs through diffusion, not osmosis. Because of respiration, there will be a low oxygen concentration in the muscle, so E is our answer.

Q14	C

Covalent bonds form between two non-metals and involve the sharing of electrons. Metals can't form covalent bonds with non-metals, and instead form ionic bonds, so NaCl and Na_2O are the only ones that do not have covalent bonds.

Q15	B

For these question types we need to know the following formula:

$$v^2 = u^2 + 2as, so\ 0 = 300^2 + (0.6 \times 2)a, so\ a = \frac{300^2}{1.2} = 75000$$

We then use Newton's second law to work out the force.

$$F = 0.05kg \times 75{,}000 = 3750N = 3.75 \times 10^3 N$$

Q16	E

For the BMAT it is expected that you can sketch simple graphs, such as those in the question. To save time, sketching in these sorts of questions will allow you to quickly and visually see the intersections between the lines. (the diagram shows a sketch that you should be able to do in the BMAT) From sketching the graphs, you should see that 3 and 4 do not intersect. (Alternatively you could have worked this out algebraically, 3 has a maximum point at (0,1), and at x = 0, the graph of 4 has a y coordinate of 6, and the gradient is shallower than that of 3, so the graphs won't intersect).

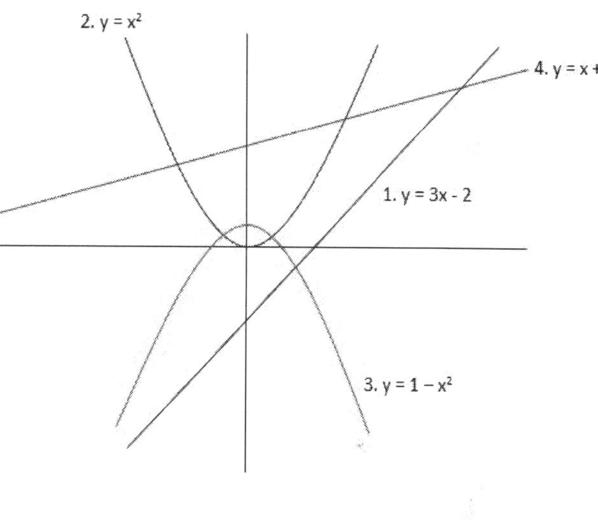

Q17	D

Let us call the recessive allele g and the dominant allele G. 1 is possible if P, Q, R and S are all gg and T and U are Gg or GG. 2 is possible as if T is Gg or GG, the G allele could have been carried in the sperm to U, making it also have the genetic condition. 3 is possible, because mutations could have led to U having the genetic condition.

Q18	E

A good way to solve these questions is to set up algebraic equations for each element. We know that a = x, and that b = 2y. We also know that 3b = 6x + y + 2. (from balancing to oxygens). From b = 2y, we know that 6y = 6x + y + 2, so 5y = 6x + 2. See if any of the options satisfy the equation, which E does.

Q19	A

As voltage increases across a resistor at a constant temperature, current increases at the same rate. Since both quantities are directly proportional, the resistance stays constant as V = IR.

2011 Section 2

Q20	B

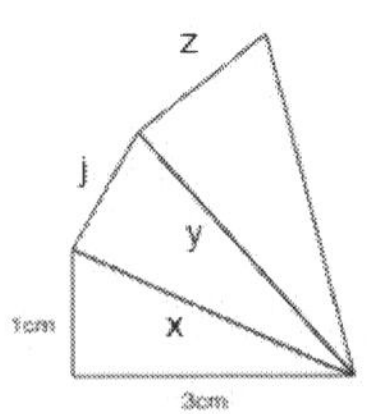

$x = \sqrt{(1^2 + 3^2)} = \sqrt{10}\ by\ Pythagoras'\ Theorem$

$j = \frac{\sqrt{10}}{3}\ by\ similar\ triangles$

$y = \sqrt{((\sqrt{10})^2 + (\frac{\sqrt{10}}{3})^2} = \sqrt{10 + \frac{10}{9}} = \sqrt{\frac{100}{9}} = \frac{10}{3}$

$z = \frac{10}{9}\ by\ similar\ triangles$

Area = ½ x base x height = $1/2 \times \frac{10}{3} \times \frac{10}{9} = \frac{50}{27}$

Q21	D

This question tests knowledge not currently on the BMAT specification

P is a haploid cell, so must be a type of gamete (either a sperm or egg cell). Q is a normal body cell and R must be a cell without a nucleus or a RBC. Only D fits all three options, so is correct.

Q22	D

In 478kg of ore, there is (0.7 x 478) = 335kg of PbS

The % of lead in PbS is $\frac{207}{207+32} = \frac{207}{239}$which is around 0.875

So, 0.875 x 335 = 293, which is closest to D.

Q23	C

When light travels through glass, its speed slows down, but its frequency stays the same. Because of the equation v = fλ, the wavelength therefore decreases. Answer option C is therefore the only correct one.

Q24	B

The probability of getting two sixes = probability of getting a six on the fair die x probability of getting a six on the unfair die

$\frac{1}{18} = \frac{1}{6} \times P(getting\ a\ six\ on\ the\ unfair\ die)$, therefore P(getting a six on the unfair die) = ⅓

Therefore, the P of getting a 1 on the unfair die is (1-⅓)/5 = 2/15

P(getting a two) = P(getting a 1 on the fair die) x P(getting a 1 on the unfair die) = 2/15 x ⅙ = 1/45

Q25	D

If the homeostatic system was less responsive, it would mean a higher raised level would be needed before the body's homeostatic system would recognise that there was an imbalance, so 2 would be higher.

Q26	E

We know that it burns in an excess of air, so complete combustion will occur. When C undergoes complete combustion, carbon dioxide is formed, not carbon monoxide, so D is incorrect. When S undergoes complete combustion, SO_2 is formed not sulphur or hydrogen sulphide or carbon sulphide, so A, B and C are wrong. Therefore, E is correct.

Q27	B

There is a beat every 1.2 seconds, as 60/50 = 1.2. However, when the beat is heard the left foot is put down, so the time difference is only 0.6 seconds as the soldiers at the rear put their left foot down when those at the front put their right foot down. Distance = speed x time, so 330 x 0.6 = 198m = B

2011 Section 3

To see the marking grid and mark bands that the BMAT examiners will use to mark your essays, please refer to the BMAT website.

'Democratic freedom means there should be no restriction on what may be said in public.'

To see the question in full, please see: https://www.admissionstesting.org/Images/20765-past-paper-2011-section-3.pdf

Democratic freedoms are liberties granted upon all people in a democracy (a type of society where common people hold political power) and are symbolic of equality for all, examples of which include freedom of speech and freedom to practice religion. The statement means that there should be no limits on what a person may say, or what opinions they choose to express in public.

- Freedom of speech should not mean that you should say extreme, hateful or racist things that cause harm to others, therefore restrictions on this type of speech should be put in place to encourage mutual respect, tolerance and a more just society. If there were no restrictions in society, extreme/radical ideas would be more easily propagated.
- If false or misleading information is said in public about individuals and businesses, this can potentially be very damaging to their reputation. To protect the rights of these individuals and businesses, restrictions should be in place to stop this, and as seen in certain democracies through libel and slander legislation.
- Fake news can be damaging and can incite hatred, fear and panic, and result in physical harm to the individual. Specifically, fake news and extreme ideas are most likely to affect vulnerable groups of society such as children, who are more likely to believe these ideas and act upon them. Therefore, restrictions should be imposed for the protection of society.

- Free speech is needed to allow people to stand up against oppression. It can create a more tolerant society, as differing viewpoints can be openly acknowledged, expressed and discussed. Free speech is also needed for the development of a society (socially, artistically etc.), with countries who limit freedom of speech historically having stunted development trajectories.
- In order to have a just and equal society, a balance needs to be struck between complete free speech and a fair, safe society. In this situation, it may be useful to use a utilitarian point of view - some form of limitations should be placed on speech that causes harm to others (John Stuart Mill's harm principle - which states that state intervention isn't allowed unless one is behaving in a way that causes 'harm to others'). However, the definition of 'harm' is questionable and not always clearly explained or defined. The question becomes who gets to judge/define harm, and due to the subjective nature of such judgements, arbitration won't always be consistent.
- However, we must ensure that these restrictions aren't the start of a slippery slope, where further restrictions on other actions are eventually put in place.

2011 Section 3

'The art of medicine consists of amusing the patient while nature cures the disease.' (*Voltaire*)
To see the question in full, please see: https://www.admissionstesting.org/Images/20765-past-paper-2011-section-3.pdf

This statement means that medicine is more involved with simply reassuring or distracting the patient, using key social and interpersonal skills. These include empathy, kindness and good communication skills to alleviate the patient's worries while nature and time solves the patient's ailment.

- In some circumstances, e.g. cancer, patients would die if nature was allowed to take its course. Medicine can save cancer patients' lives or extend their life such as through the use of chemotherapy.
- Medicines, such as specific drugs (e.g. isoniazid for TB), can cure diseases, while vaccines (preventative medicine) can ensure that patients live longer, healthier lives and ensure society is protected through herd immunity. Medicines can also be used to prevent certain diseases from getting worse such as in the case of HIV which requires PrEP to prevent it from developing into AIDS.

- Sometimes, a doctor's job is to allay a patient's worries, while nature (the body's immune system) sorts the problem out, such as in the case of the common cold. Additionally, using a placebo drug is sometimes effective - in this case, the doctor would simply be 'amusing the patient', while the patient recovers naturally, as no 'medical' intervention is given.
- While this statement may have been true at the time of Voltaire's writing in the 18th century when medical technology was somewhat rudimentary, nowadays medicine can cure far more illnesses, and provide a far better quality of life to many more patients. However, doctors in practising this 'art' of medicine, still need to use far more skills than scientific ones alone - interpersonal skills such as empathy, leadership, teamwork and communication are still of paramount importance when interacting with patients.
- The best doctors will be those who combine the 'arts' of empathy and reassurance with the 'science' of performing physical interventions quickly when needed.

'A scientific man ought to have no wishes, no affections - a mere heart of stone.' (*Charles Darwin*)

To see the question in full, please see: https://www.admissionstesting.org/Images/20765-past-paper-2011-section-3.pdf

This statement means that those who work in scientific fields should be emotionally detached from their work to ensure that their work is impartial and not subject to external bias from personal emotion. It could be argued that objectivity should be maintained in science because:

- Science is based on empirical observation and the scientific method, which does not require emotion (emotion/affection could in fact affect the accuracy of an experiment!)
- If scientists are driven by money, or other motivations, it may lead them to produce superficial research, or not present the whole truth in order to meet their desired outcome.

- Oftentimes, scientific enquiry stems from personal wishes; scientists may yearn to find cures to particular diseases because their loved ones have been affected by this condition. If a scientist is personally interested in a subject, and desires to study/research this area, they will be more motivated to do so and more likely to solve the problem.
- Without personal wishes and affections, science could become unethical. If scientists were not guided by a system of ethics and moral obligations, scientific enquiry runs the risk of being unethical (this system of ethics is why genetic experiments to create designer babies are not currently happening in the UK) and could be used in a detrimental way, as opposed to for the betterment of humanity.

- A scientist needs wishes and affections to start the process of scientific inquiry, and have passion, drive and desire to study and research to advance science.
- However, these wishes and affections need to be controlled so that they do not negatively affect the outcome of the scientific endeavour or reduce the accuracy or precision of the science.

Question 4 was written to widen access to the exam paper, as in the past, students hoping to study Veterinary Medicine would also have to take the BMAT. VetMed students no longer take the BMAT, and so in its current iteration (2017 onwards), there are none of these questions, so the authors have not included worked essays for these and recommend that you only attempt these after having attempted all the previous ones.

BMAT 2012

Section 1

Q1	D

Firstly, in order to calculate roughly 20% of Bondia's area divide the total, 26513 by 5 giving 5263. Eliminate all islands less than this figure leaving Connery, Dalton and Moore. 10% of Bondia's population is approximately 862871 people. The only island with a population of less than this figure out of Connery, Dalton and Moore is Dalton. Hence D is the answer.

Q2	C

A isn't necessarily correct because the passage points out pale-skinned people may get burnt if they get more sun. B is incorrect because the passage doesn't state anywhere that vitamin D is best obtained from sunlight, it simply cites it as an example of how one could obtain more sunlight. C is correct because it essentially paraphrases the wording of the first sentence of the second paragraph: '*pale-skinned people...vitamin D supplements by the government*'. D is incorrect because skin cancer isn't mentioned at all in the passage. E is incorrect because although darker skinned people may be vitamin D deficient there is no mention of them being more deficient than pale skinned people in the passage.

Q3	F

The easiest way to answer this question is to test the number of each patterned tile when removing each cross-shaped pattern; which should be 5 as 25/5 is 5 and we need to have equal numbers of each tile. Starting with black first to eliminate easily:
Removing A gives 6 black tiles, which is immediately incorrect because we need to have 5 of each tile.
Removing B gives 5 black tiles.
Removing C gives 3 black tiles.
Removing D gives 6 black tiles.
Removing E gives 5 black tiles.
Removing F gives 5 black tiles.
So looking at B, E and F, checking this time for white:
Removing B gives 6 white tiles.
Removing E gives 5 white tiles.
Removing F gives 5 white tiles.
Looking at E and F this time for dotted tiles:
Removing E gives 3 dotted tiles.
Removing F gives 5 dotted tiles. Hence F is the correct answer.

Q4	B

A is incorrect because the passage states the fossil fuel source for the National Grid could power electric cars. B is correct because it paraphrases the third sentence: '*If you make extra demand...only fossil fuels, which produce emissions of CO_2, can provide the extra capacity.*' The use of the word '*only*' in the passage is linked to the use of the word '*yet*' in the statement for B. C is incorrect because the passage does not state that wind will '*never*' provide more electricity than it does at present. D is incorrect because it directly contradicts the first line in that the electric engines are '*more economical*' and thus would produce less emissions than a petrol engine.

Q5	E

To do this, subtract the area of all of the garden features from the total.
Firstly, the total is 12 x 18 = 216m^2.
The pond is 3 x 3 = 9m^2.
The length of the total veg is 18 - 3 - 1 - 1 - 1 - 0.5 - 0.5 = 11. The width is 3m so the veg area is 33m^2.
The lawn length is 12-3(pond length)-1-1-1 = 6. Its width is given so 6 x 3 = 18m^2.
The length of the shrubs is 18-1-3-1-0.5-1 = 11.5 The width is given as 4m.
Thus, the area is 11.5 x 4 = 46m^2.
So 216m^2 - 46-18-33-9 = 110m^2
We know that 4 slabs will be needed per m^2 so 110 x 4 = 440 which is E.

Q6	E

This is a good example of correlation not being causation. The argument ends with the conclusion that '*discussing these issues will help their children read well*' whereas the evidence shown above in the argument describes patterns of correlation between more discussion and better reading skills. The conclusion goes a stage further - that is unfounded.

Q7	A

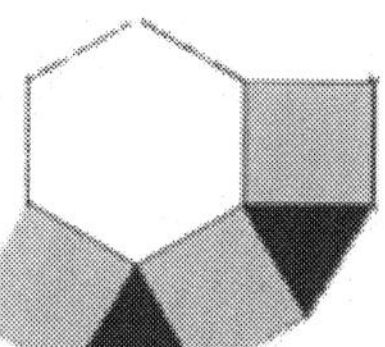

This is a very time-consuming question. Only attempt at the end of the section. If you break down the pattern given taking the bottom left hexagon and its surrounding shapes you will notice that in order to eliminate the other hexagons and their surrounding shapes you are left with this shape: From the repeating unit we can see that the ratio of shapes is 1 hexagon: 2 triangles: 3 squares

Q8	C

Sum the number of cases for organisation 4 over the two years: this gives 3. The total number of patients over each of the years is (11549 + 30432) = 41981. Thus, we do [(3/~42000) x 100000] = 300/42 = 7.14 hence C is the correct answer by rounding.

Q9	D

The largest proportion of cases can be found by scanning down the 2009 cases column and finding the highest number of cases. This is 26 from organisation 3. Summing the total number of cases in 2009 gives 69 so 26/69 = 0.38 hence D is correct.

Q10	B

16163 is the number of patient days for 11 months so the number of patient days per month is ~1470. Multiplying this as the rate is constant for 12 months gives 17640. 1 case divided by 17640 then multiplied by 100,000 gives the rate of infection. This is 5.669 so B is the correct answer.

Q11	E

A and C are false inference as we don't know how the total hospital figure per organisation is split into large and small hospitals. B has data contrary to the statement so is definitely false. D is not true because it could be the case that for organisation 5, all of the cases of CdI were at the TC hospital, not the DC one; meaning a DC hospital wouldn't have had a case.

Q12	B

Nicola will take the 9:15 from the airport as it is the first bus on Thursday. The journey takes 50 mins so she will arrive at 10:05. Looking at the departure times from the centre, Nicola must be back before 17:00 meaning the latest bus she can take is the 15:20 as the 16:30 would cause her to return 20 mins too late. So, if she takes the 15:20 then she has from 10:05 to 15:20 in the centre, which is 5 hours and 15 mins.

Q13	D

A is false, the argument makes no reference to the Arctic ice melting being the *'only'* source of unusual weather. B is not correct because the unusual weather could've been caused by other phenomena than the melting Arctic ice. C uses the word *'must'* which is not the same as the use of the conditional *'can' used* in the last line of the argument. Hence by elimination D is correct.

Q14	D

Considering A, the triangle points to the thin end of the black rectangle but doesn't do so on the net so A is false.
B makes the same failing.
On the net the black rectangle is directly adjacent to the cross. However, on C the cross has the thin end of the black rectangle at its midpoint as opposed to the fat end as on the net so C is wrong.
For E the black rectangle is horizontal when it should be vertical if the net was folded up so this can also be eliminated. This leaves D.

Q15	C

A would support the argument so is false. B would also strengthen the conclusion that if oxytocin has never been used on children then it could potentially be damaging for children's health as the effects haven't been measured properly. C would weaken the argument because it suggests that in such low quantities the oxytocin hasn't got damaging effects, contrary to the conclusion. D may be true but isn't specific at all to weakening or strengthening the argument so is incorrect. E also strengthens the conclusion by adding to the list of negative things oxytocin does.

Q16	C

Find the repeating unit which we can say is 1/6th of the area i.e. the 5 x 5 portion of the floor that repeats. This has 25 tiles which when multiplied by 4 conveniently gives 100. We can see that when we multiply the individual tile patterns by 4, the first contains no black quarters, the second contains 1 black quarter, the third 2, and the fourth all 4. There are 5 of the first type giving 0 black quarters. There are 4 of the second type giving 4 black quarters. There are 12 of the third type giving 24 black quarters. There are 4 of the fourth type giving 16 black quarters. Adding all the black quarters gives 0 + 4 + 24 + 16 = 44. So, 44/100 quarters are black which is 44%.

Q17	G

Statement 1 is false as the passage states lower staffing levels '*may contribute*' to the increase of deaths but statement 1 says improving staffing '*would*' reduce death rates. It assumes correlation is causation.

Statement 2 is false because the enhancement of community and primary care services on the weekend just means less hospital deaths and more deaths within these services i.e. at home at the weekend which isn't a conclusion that can be drawn.

Statement 3 is false because in the case of emergency admissions, it isn't feasible to admit fewer patients because then patients who need emergency care would die thus increasing the death rate.

Q18	A

Make columns for the bounds as so:

Dishwasher: 75% to 85%
Tumble Dryer: 35% to 40%
Neither: 0% to 5%

Add for the upper and lower bounds and subtract 100% from each column:

Lower: 75% + 35% + 0% - 100% = 10%
Upper: 85% + 40% + 5% -100% = 30% hence A is correct.

Q19	B

The number of category A calls is 2.23 million. The number responded to within 8 mins was 74.9% meaning that ~25% of calls were responded to but not within 8 minutes as 100% - 74.9% = ~25%. So 25% of 2.23 million can be done by dividing by 4 and this gives ~0.56 million calls hence B is correct.

Q20	D

The information states that category A calls made up 33.7% of calls, and category B made up 39.8% of calls. By subtracting from 100% this means category C made up about 26%. Thus, in order of the size of the slice of the pie from biggest to smallest:

Category B then category A then category C. Matching this to the answer key gives D. Note C is not correct because the size of category A and category C appear equal in the pie but this is not the case as we know.

2012 Section 1

Q21	B

B is correct because the passage states that '*Of these, 6.61 million calls (81.8%) resulted in an emergency response*' that implies that the other 1.47 million calls didn't result in an emergency response.
For the record, C and D can be eliminated quickly because we don't know whether these calls are genuine emergencies which means they could be; and that a Category C call doesn't necessarily mean no response; it just means the response time standards are determined locally.

Q22	A

We know that in 2011 the number of category A incidents warranting an emergency response within 8 minutes was 74.9% of 2.23 million (1.67 million) whereas it was 74.3% of 2.08 million (1.55) in 2010. This is a difference of 0.12 million. Use approximations of 75% for each percentage calculation to speed this process up.

Q23	B

Numbering the patterns from left to right is helpful. With regards to the patterns with 3 black squares, we can see that pattern 4 and pattern 12 are the same as you can rotate 4 90 degrees to get 12. We can also see that pattern 7 and 11 are the same as you can rotate 7 90 degrees to obtain 11. Focusing now on the ones with 2 black squares, patterns 1, 3, 8 and 10 are the same. Pattern 2 and pattern 9 are the same as well. This leaves pattern 5 which is entirely unique because it is symmetrical instead of a rotation of an alternative pattern which makes it distinct. Counting these up gives us 5 distinct patterns:
4, 12
7, 11
1, 3, 8, 10
2, 9
5

Q24	E

A, C and D can be eliminated because they weaken the argument. B is problematic because the lack of training and resources could be interpreted as a negative effect of water cannons because it would make them more usable by members of the public as opposed to the police. Therefore, E is the only sensible option because it directly strengthens the argument posed.

Q25	C

A rough guess would indicate that the range of scores to investigate is 2-18, i.e. simply having 2 points.
2 can be scored by a 2, 2, miss
3 can be scored by a 2, miss, 2
4 can be from a 4, 4, miss
5 can be from a 4, 6, miss
6 can be from a 6, 6, miss
7 can be from a 6, miss, 4
8 can be from a 4, miss, 6
9 can be from a 6, miss, 6
10 can be from a 2, 2, 6
11 cannot be made
12 can be from a 4, 4, 4
13 cannot be made
14 can be from a 6, 4, 4
15 cannot be made
16 can be from a 6, 4, 6
17 cannot be made
18 can be from a 6, 6, 6

Q26	D

D is the answer because it follows the same format as the conclusion of the argument: i.e. to simplify, the final line of the argument is:
If A is C, then F (which is defined as C earlier) is A .
D matches:
If F is E, and S is E, then F is S.
As you can see, the pattern of the letters is identical in both cases hence the reasoning matches.

Q27	C

It takes 3 months to pay for furniture, as stated in the question; in the order of ½ , ¼, and the remainder, which we can say is ¼ as the total must be 1. As the shop has been closed for May and June, this means the figure for June, $2000 must be the remainder of the payment from April; i.e. a quarter of the price. So what was bought in April must be $8000. Now we have dealt with June's table figure, let's move on to the other months as in the table. So the figures in red show what has been sold between January and June, and it is important to remember this because we don't need to continue the table any further to the left with more remainders of sales pre-January as we have already answered the question. Summing the final column gives us $20000.

Item	January	February	March	April	May	June	**Total**
1)	-	-	-	$4000	$2000	$2000	$8000
2)	-	-	$2000	$1000	$1000		$4000
3)	$4000	$2000	$2000				$8000
4)	$1000	$1000					
Total	$9000	$3000	$4000	$5000	$3000	$2000	

2012 Section 1

Q28	G

All 3 points are weaknesses of the argument because they accurately show flaws in the reasoning of the argument. The first identifies that travel damages the environment but that the argument has not accounted for the possibility of damage arising anywhere but from the ski industry. The second statement makes the strong pot that the consumption of energy is relative to other sectors within the resort industry which is entirely plausible. The third point includes the word *'may'* and goes on to suggest that environmental damage isn't necessarily all from the root cause of energy consumption which is also highly plausible.

Q29	C

Let n = the number of people at the concert
$0.4x \times 15$ = price for the 40% of x who originally paid £20 but had a £5 refund so ended up paying £15 total
Therefore $0.6n \times 20$ is the cost of the remaining non-fancy dressed people, paying full price tickets. It is 0.6 as 0.6 + 0.4 = 1
So $0.4x \times 15 + 0.6n \times 20$ = 12240
$12n + 6n = 12240$ so n = 680
40% of 680 is the number of people with refunds, and this amounts to 272.
The refunds were £5 each so 272 x 5 = £1360

Q30	C

1 is incorrect because it makes a blanket statement that is not necessarily true because one could receive fees and still give a fair judgment of new medical treatments. 2 is also incorrect because it is a possible scenario that the companies that sponsor authors do not wish to influence the article contents at all. 3 however is correct because it is a necessary assumption that the author makes in order to reach the conclusion that *'the public need to know what weight they should put on these articles when they are assessing evidence from various sources.'*

Q31	C

'Jill knew regardless of the outcomes, there would be no ties and she would finish in third place' so she has to have a sufficient number of points above 4th place and below 2nd place. This amounts to 7 points, as if another scored 6 and she scored 0 and the difference between them was 6, they would be tied. Hence it has to be the smallest number greater than 6 which is 7. If the last placed player scored the highest possible, this means they scored 6 in the 10th round. This means that we need to consider the 9th round; all points need to add up to 90 and be 7 points apart each so that regardless of the outcome the result is clear. So, we shall subtract 7 from each of the answers and test from biggest to smallest:
Starting with E, if 4th place gets 23 in the final round then they must have got 17 in the 9th round. This means that 3rd got 24, 2nd got 31 and 1st got lowest 32 to avoid a tie. However, summing these numbers gives 104 which is too high.
For D, if 4th place gets 21 in the final round, they get 15 in the 9th. So, 3rd gets 22, 2nd gets 29 and 1st gets lowest 30 to avoid a tie. Summing these gives 96 which is too high.
For C, if 4th place gets 19 in the final round, they get 13 in the 9th, so 3rd gets 20, 2nd gets 27 and 1st gets lowest 28 to avoid a tie. Summing these gives 88 which is the first answer within 90 so is the answer.

Q32	A

Deaths per vehicle in 1930 would be 7000/2.3 million (which is about 1/328) and today it is 3180/27 million (which is about 1/9000). Let's invert the fraction so that simplification at this stage is a lot easier. The sum we want to do is 1/9000 divided by 1/328 which is the same as saying 1/9000 multiplied by 328. This gives us 328/9000 and doing this gives an answer of 0.036 which rounds to 0.04 in the answers as we used imprecise numbers for ease.

Q33	D

A is incorrect because roads can still be unsafe even if no injuries are sustained. B is incorrect because it is already mentioned in the text and the question asks us to find an additional reason. C is incorrect because accident reporting is not the same as the actual number of accidents taking place so for all we know this number could be very high and thus show that roads aren't safe. D is correct because if hospital reporting is more accurate and as the figures show in the text if hospital admission figures remain about the same this means that there are fewer accidents as time goes by as the initial figure would've been most likely under-reported. E is incorrect because severe trauma in the first place is indicative of unsafe roads.

Q34	C

The data we need is in the third paragraph where it says the 10-year safety target is *'40% of the 1994-8 average - 319,928 casualties'*. Here we need to do a simple calculation: 40% of 319,928. We can round this to 320,000 and multiply it by 0.4 and obtain 128,000.

Q35	A

The DfT figures for death and serious injury is 59.4 per 100,000 and hospital admissions are 91.1 per 100,000 so hospital admissions are higher. This means that our reason must align with this. A must be correct because this is the only way the DfT would have figures lower than hospital admissions. B is wrong because if the roads were not getting safer then the DfT statistics would also be higher for death and injury. C is wrong because this implies hospital admissions decrease when we can see that hospital admissions were higher than DfT statistics anyway. D and E are wrong because they imply that the DfT figures would be higher than the hospital ones which, like for C we know is not the case.

2012 Section 2

Q1	F

We know that homeostasis is the maintenance of a constant internal environment despite internal or external changes so all 4 are correct as these are all changes of an internal or external nature.

Q2	D

Percentage yield is the actual yield/theoretical yield multiplied by 100. So, to work out the theoretical yield we need to work out the reacting moles. The moles of 1-bromobutane is mass/Mr which is $\frac{2.74}{(4 \times 12) + (9 \times 1) + 80}$ which is 2.74/137. We can see that 274 is double 137 so dividing 2 by 100 gives 0.02 moles. The ratio of moles is equal in the equation so 0.02 moles of butan-1-ol is produced. $theoretical\ mass = moles \times Mr$ so $0.02 \times [(4 \times 12) + 10 + 16)$which is 0.02 x 74. This comes to 1.48 so putting this back into the equation gives (1.11/1.48) x 100 which is about 75%.

Q3	B

We know that from X to Y an alpha particle has been released because it is a $_2^4A$ and this has been released from X. If the mass number, then remains the same from Y to Z but the atomic number changes this means that a beta particle has been released $^0_{-1}B$. This means that P has to be N - 4 and Q has to be R - 1 as we know that in releasing an electron the atomic number increases by 1 as a neutron is converted into a proton in the process.

Q4	A

This can be solved easily by working from the largest circle to the smallest. Set up the following equation to obtain just the shaded area:

$(2d)^2\pi - (\frac{3d}{2})^2\pi + d^2\pi - (d/2)^2\pi$

Expanding gives $4d^2\pi - 9\pi d^2/4 + d^2\pi - \pi d^2/4$

Solving gives $5\pi d^2/2$

Q5	B

This question tests knowledge not currently on the BMAT specification.
Carbon monoxide will affect the red blood cells, bronchitis will affect the bronchi, emphysema will affect the alveoli, and nicotine will affect the brain. The only row that matches this is B.

Q6	C

This question tests knowledge not currently on the BMAT specification.
Similar to fats, the head is hydrophilic and will face outwards in a micelle, and the tail is hydrophobic thus will face inwards.

Q7	F

We know there cannot be any alpha radiation because when the paper is placed between the source and detector there is virtually no change in the radiation counts. However, there is beta because when aluminium is used the beta is blocked from passing through. Gamma can pass through the aluminium and is responsible for the counts in the table. Hence F is the answer.

Q8	E

Simple algebra is needed to rearrange this for R in terms of G.
Firstly subtract 5 from each side:

$$G - 5 = \sqrt{7(9-R)^2 + 9}$$

Square both sides:

$$(G - 5)^2 = 7(9-R)^2 + 9$$

Subtract 9 from both sides: $(G-5)^2 - 9 = 7(9-R)^2$
Divide both sides by 7: $[(G-5)^2 - 9]/7 = (9-R)^2$

Square root both sides: $\sqrt{\frac{(G-5)^2-9}{7}} = 9-R$

Rearrange for R: $R = 9-\sqrt{\frac{(G-5)^2-9}{7}}$ which is answer E.

Q9	A

Only 1 and 2 are correct because as the receptors can't detect the stimulus the reflex arc can't be followed so no reflex action is taken. The patient could take appropriate action if they could see the application of the stimulus because they could identify the pain causing stimulus, not by pain but by sight. 3 and 4 however are incorrect because both say that the patient could sense pain, which is wrong. If the neurons that detect stimuli (i.ie the receptors) are unable to do so then pain can't be sensed.

Q10	D

It may be easier if you find these questions hard to quickly substitute in the numbers from the answers and eliminate the incorrect answers. Doing this will show D to have the correct values for the stoichiometry in the equation.

Q11	D

The work is calculated by multiplying the force by the amount of movement of an object so we can eliminate Diagram 1 from any answers, the person isn't moving at all. This tells us the answer must be C or D. In Diagram 2 and 3 there is work as there is movement. However, in Diagram 2 work isn't F x d as labelled because these are perpendicular and the forces must be parallel like in Diagram 3 for them to be the ones from which the work done arises.

Q12	E

$$\sqrt[3]{\frac{2 \times 10^5}{(5 \times 10^{-3})^{-2}}} - \sqrt{(4 \times 10^3) - (4 \times 10^2)}$$

Expand the lower half of the first fraction: $\sqrt[3]{\frac{2 \times 10^5}{(25 \times 10^{-6})}} - \sqrt{(4 \times 10^3) - (4 \times 10^2)}$

We know that the rules of indices are such that $10^5/10^{-6}$ is 10^{11} so we can rewrite the first fraction. We can also rewrite the second half by expanding it out:

$$\sqrt[3]{\frac{2}{25}10^{11}} - \sqrt{4000 - 400}$$

$= \sqrt[3]{0.08 \times 10^{11}} - \sqrt{3600}$
$= \sqrt[3]{8 \times 10^9} - 60 = 2 \times 10^3 - 60$
$= 2000 - 60 = 1940$

2012 Section 2

Q13	E

1 is correct as the zones of inhibition for Q and R are the same. 2 is incorrect because the zones of inhibition suggest there is no resistance as the bacteria is being killed. 3 is also a possibility so E is the answer.

Q14	F

The formula has to contain 3 Coppers so it is either 2 of $CuCO_3$ or $Cu(OH)_2$ and 1 of the other. Trying both ways gives the answer:
2 of $CuCO_3$ and 1 $Cu(OH)_2$ gives $Cu_3C_2H_2O_8$ hence E is the answer.
1 of $CuCO_3$ and 2 $Cu(OH)_2$ gives $Cu_3CH_4O_7$ but this isn't an option in the answers.

Q15	B

N.B. convert 12cm to 0.12m
Frequency = wave speed/wavelength = $3 \times 10^8 / 0.12 = 30 \times 10^7 / 12 \times 10^{-2} = 2.5 \times 10^9$.
The wavelength of the microwaves through this is wave speed/frequency = $2 \times 10^8 / 2.5 \times 10^9 = 0.8 \times 10^{-1} = 0.08$m which is 8cm

Q16	C

Firstly, we need to drop a line from C so it hits AB at a perpendicular. If we label the relationships on the triangle this will be helpful. We can see that tan B = ⅔ by labelling the diagram. Then we can use the fact that tan A = ⅙ but as the opposite here is already 2 this means the adjacent must be 12 as 2/12 = ⅙. So this allows us to calculate AB as 12 + 3 = 15. Halving this to obtain AM as 7.5 as it's the midpoint is useful because it means MB is also 7.5cm so M to the bisector is 4.5. Thus, tan of theta is 2/4.5 which is 4/9.

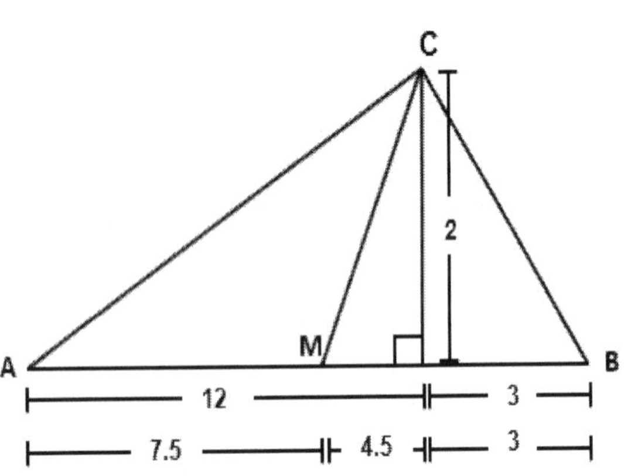

Q17	C

ADH is a hormone thus it travels in the bloodstream so 1 is correct. More ADH leads to more reabsorption of water so a more concentrated urine so 2 and 3 are incorrect. Less ADH means less water reabsorption so could lead to dehydration so 4 is correct.

Q18	D

Sodium, aluminium and magnesium are all above vanadium in the reactivity series so can be used to get vanadium from its ore. Electrolysis will also liberate vanadium from its chloride. However, iron is below Vanadium in the reactivity series as it is below zinc so this tells us iron will not release vanadium from its ore.

Q19	D

When lamp X breaks the current can't flow down that branch so all of it must go down the other, meaning the current measured at Ammeter 2 is higher. However, the total resistance has decreased because the circuit is now series and has lost a component and so Ammeter 1 that measures the same voltage with a lower resistance will therefore have a lower current following Ohm's Law (V = IR)

Q20	B

The question says that the '*balls are arranged to give the smallest possible probability for the player to win*'. This means that the contents of the bags must be as follows: Bag 1 - 2 red, 2 yellow. And Bag 2 - 1 blue, 2 yellow, 2 red.

Bag 1: The ways to win with this bag are to choose two reds, and two yellows. Remember, the balls are not replaced, so the probability of picking a same coloured ball decreases for the second ball.

P (two reds picked) = $\frac{2}{4} \times \frac{1}{3} = \frac{2}{12}$

P (two yellows picked) = $\frac{2}{4} \times \frac{1}{3} = \frac{2}{12}$

P (wins with bag 1) = $\frac{2}{12} + \frac{2}{12} = \frac{4}{12}$

Bag 2: The only way to win is to pick two reds, again remember the balls are not replaced.

P (two reds picked) = $\frac{2}{4} \times \frac{1}{3} = \frac{2}{12}$, so P (winning with bag 2) = $\frac{2}{12}$

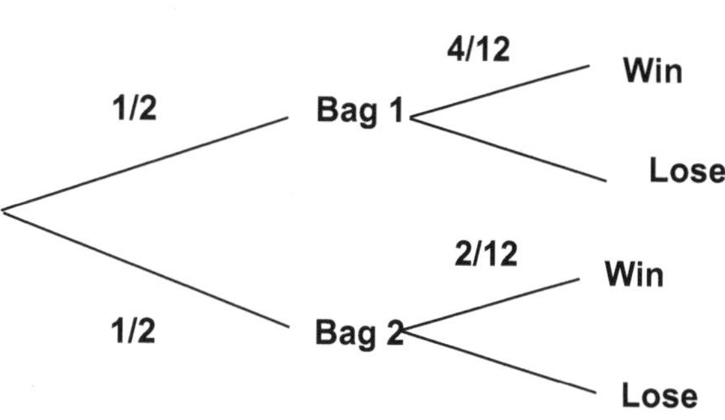

However, as the player is equally likely to choose either bag, we must halve the probabilities of getting two balls of the same colour from each bag. (think of it as a tree diagram).

So the total probability of winning is:

$(\frac{1}{2} \times \frac{4}{12})$*[bag 1]* + $(\frac{1}{2} \times \frac{2}{12})$*[bag 2]* = $\frac{3}{12} = \frac{1}{4}$

Q21	D

1 is not correct because if you have genetic crosses of varying criteria (e.g. 2 heterozygous individuals) none lead to a 3:0 ratio even if the homozygous dominant offspring died. You can try it and check! 2 and 3 are correct because a big sample size would normally help a pattern become as reliable as possible and chance means that probabilities could be such that any outcome however unlikely could take place.

2012 Section 2

Q22	B

This question tests knowledge not currently on the BMAT specification.

1 is not a normal product, it doesn't make sense for HeOH to be a thing, as He would be unlikely to have a 1+ charge to cancel the OH^- and He is also inert because of its full outer electron shell so is unlikely to bond in the first place.

$^{3}_{1}T = {}^{0}_{-1}\beta + {}^{3}_{2}He$

2 is correct because it is plausible for $4HTO = 2H_2O + O_2 + 4He$

3 is not correct because the following equation remains unbalanced:

$HTO = H_2O + H_2 + He$ You cannot balance this because there is a 1:1 ratio for HTO to H_2O and H_2 which can't be fulfilled.

Q23	D

The cyclist's GPE loss = mgh = 100kg x 10N/kg x 100m = 10^5J so we can eliminate A, B and C. The total resistive force will equal the force done from work as the forces are balanced; which we know already from the GPE loss. We can rearrange the equation work = Fd for F so F = work/d.

N.B. Don't get caught out; the slope is a 1 in 10 slope, so if the total height change is 100m, then the total distance travelled on the road is 1000m.

Finally, we can substitute in the numbers; F = 10^5/1000m = 100N hence D is correct.

Q24	A

We have 2 scenarios we need to consider here; the first is before any alterations are made and will be called Round 1:

Here we have the total cost of a certain proportion of wood and metal where w = amount of wood, m = amount of metal and we know these are proportional to d^2 and d respectively.

Putting this in an equation gives the following:

Round 1: $3wd + md^2$

Round 2 describes the condition of the question: '*if the diameter of the sign is doubled, then the total cost of the materials will be tripled.*'

This means the following:

$3(2d)w + m(2d)^2 = 3(\text{Round } 1)$

$6dw + 4md^2 = 9wd + 3md^2$

Rearrange: $md^2 = 3wd$ Divide both sides by d: $md = 3w$ rearrange for d:$d = 3w/m$ and represented as a ratio this is: 3:1 where the metal represents a quarter or 25%.

Q25	E

If U is recessive and no other people in the family can be recessive this means that U's parents S and T must be heterozygous because this is the only situation from which recessive offspring can be formed when no parents can be recessive themselves. For S's parents therefore, one of P and Q must also be heterozygous, because although Rr can be formed from crossing homozygous dominant and recessive, for this condition only U can be recessive. But, one of P or Q could be Rr and one could be RR and still give rise to a Rr offspring. R therefore can be RR so the total is 3 heterozygous for the first condition of the question.

For only R and U being recessive, we know S and T must be heterozygous regardless, so that's 2 already. For R to be rr it means that P and Q have to be heterozygous also, this is the only way to produce rr offspring without being recessive themselves as individuals. This is a further 2 totalling 4.

Q26	E

Begin by writing an equation to see what happens to the moles:
$C_2H_4 + H_2 = C_2H_6$
When the Nickel is added, we are told the temperature increases to 150⁰C which will increase pressure. However during the course of the reaction the pressure will actually decrease because as the reaction goes to completion, we go from 2 moles of reactants to 1 mole of products, and as we know molar quantities take up the same volume regardless of Mr when they are gaseous so 1 mole will exert less pressure than 2 moles.

Q27	G

P and R are both false because although X and Y are 5mm apart, this doesn't mean the wavelength is this value. In fact, it can't be because in air, sound travels at approximately $330ms^{-1}$ not $25ms^{-1}$. Q is wrong, the amplitude of a wave is the maximum distance from equilibrium, which is the distance from the midpoint of XY to either X or Y; in other words 2.5mm not 5mm. S is correct, frequency = 1/T $= \frac{1}{0.2 \times 10^{-3}}$ =5kHz

2012 Section 3

To see the marking grid and mark bands that the BMAT examiners will use to mark your essays, please refer to the BMAT website.

"Doubt is not a pleasant condition, but certainty is absurd" (Voltaire)

To see the question in full, please see: https://www.admissionstesting.org/Images/136626-past-paper-2012-section-3.pdf

The statement hits at a deep philosophical point about our perception of the world, we cannot possibly be certain about anything according to Voltaire and this could potentially be because we are fallible and limited humans and we therefore cannot be arbiters of certainty. Voltaire recognises that humans find doubt unpleasant because he may think that we prefer when there is an answer without doubt; i.e. something indubitable. This could be because it provides greater clarity, assurance and a basis from which we can build knowledge.

- In our day to day lives, it is of paramount importance that we regard some things as certain. Furthermore, to not be certain about something can be unproductive and even dangerous. For example, if a patient had a blood test and one of the readings came up as showing a deficiency, what would be the use in doubting the certainty of a result because certainty is absurd? To doubt may hinder the treatment of the deficiency and seems to have a potentially detrimental effect.
- In scientific fields, doubt may not always be helpful, and certainty is often needed for development. For example, if scientists (or mathematicians) were never certain about the axioms upon which science and maths are built, then science would not have been able to advance/develop in the way that it has.
- The famous rationalist philosopher Descartes came up with the following famous maxim: '*cogito ergo sum*' meaning I think therefore I am. He claimed this was the one indubitable thing we could say about ourselves as humans. Many have agreed with him or found common ground with this thought; and not considered such a thought absurd.

- Voltaire raises a very important point about the importance of retaining doubt because he rightfully assesses that humans don't have the faculties to assess certainty arguably. Even things we hold true such as the structure of an atom, cannot be considered certain in the same way that the plum pudding could not have been considered certain or indubitable. Is it not productive for humanity to doubt? Is that not how we evolve because we haven't accepted the certainty that has preceded us? If we were certain the earth was flat, what would life be like today?
- However, maybe you'd like to comment on the effect of Voltaire's statement on our day-today lives. How helpful is this maxim to us? Does holding doubt constantly not bring its own problems and as Voltaire says himself, this is unpleasant so why should we doubt?

'There is something attractive about people who don't regard their own health and longevity as the most important thing in the world.' (Alexander Chancellor)
To see the question in full, please see: https://www.admissionstesting.org/Images/136626-past-paper-2012-section-3.pdf

Chancellor regards the altruism of an individual to think of others before themselves as a good quality. There is a sense of the community over the individual.

- It seems logical that we would put our own health and longevity first as we are mortal humans and as evolutionary biologist Richard Dawkins argues in his "Selfish Gene" we do seem predisposed to only care for ourselves. If this is evolutionarily beneficial then surely nothing is more important than our own health and longevity. You could link in the "survival of the fittest" argument.
- It is also considered very logical in jobs such as being a doctor to look after oneself before treating others. How are you expected to provide adequate care for others if you yourself haven't prioritised your own health? This will improve your mental health, clarity and ability all of which have secondary effects of being helpful to others.

- Chancellor's comments to you may be stretching for a social and altruistic goal that simply isn't feasible and may not be the most productive way of being. Although the altruism may be "attractive" it could be argued that the opposite approach of looking after oneself may be more beneficial to humanity as a whole
- However, it could equally be argued that we have gone too far to the selfish route of simply caring about ourselves, and thus Chancellor may be making a well observed comment that we ought to be more caring towards others; as evidence of selfishness can be seen in the rise in homelessness and the rich-poor divide.
- It could be a good compromise to consider the middle route of considering the health of yourself AND those around you as the most important thing in the world.

Authors' tip

Knowledge of the scientific method, and other aspects of the nature of science, are helpful in answering questions like these. UC Berkeley's '*Understanding Science*' site is a good starting point to learn about the nature of science.

2012 Section 3

'The scientist is not someone who gives the right answers but the one who asks the right questions.'
To see the question in full, please see: https://www.admissionstesting.org/Images/136626-past-paper-2012-section-3.pdf

This statement identifies the importance of scientific intellectual curiosity as potentially more important than answering the questions this has raised. Many would argue that everything needs to be questioned to make sure that our investigations are based on good foundations that have survived questioning. We take peer review and evidence-based research very seriously and that too requires questions from the community to validate or authenticate or challenge the views of scientists and this leads to the positive evolution of ideas so that we (hopefully) gain more knowledge. It is also known that the very basis of most investigations begins with a hypothesis which is essentially a question.

- Questioning is all very well and is also arguably the easier path to take. To question something is as simple as using the 5 W's but this action in itself doesn't lead directly to progress. It is the answers that do and obtaining these are a lot less straightforward thus they are more important.
- An unanswered question is not necessarily helpful and the answer represents the true scientific progress.
- Without the right answers, one may ask how science will progress. It is all well and good asking questions, such as 'What is the structure of a ribosome?', but if the answer is not gained, how will one be able to develop a greater understanding of other related phenomena, such as protein synthesis?

- The "right questions" imply that we need to focus on areas of science that are potentially missed on purpose or avoided because of their complexity or daunting nature. In these circumstances, we should surely take the approach to question as much as enters our scope as scientists and try and think about the less answered parts of science to ask questions.
- Having said that, some scientific discoveries such as penicillin were an accident; it didn't require a carefully planned hypothesis but its result did provoke questioning that resulted in an answer of how penicillin works. In this way maybe one could argue that it isn't' necessarily the "right question" but just questions in general about science.
- Because it is empirically verifiable that means the knowledge obtained can be measured, by us as arbiters as opposed to a rational fact that is arguably indubitable. So we can see more evolution within empirical fields like science and this makes the right questioning very important.

Question 4 was written to widen access to the exam paper, as in the past, students hoping to study Veterinary Medicine would also have to take the BMAT. VetMed students no longer take the BMAT, and so in its current iteration *(2017 onwards)*, there are none of these questions, so the authors have not included worked essays for these and recommend that you only attempt these after having attempted all the previous ones

BMAT 2013

Section 1

Q1	A

Carla doesn't work on Monday, therefore both Amy and Bob must work on Monday, as '*exactly two [are] on duty on a single day*'. Therefore, Bob works Monday, Tuesday and Friday and is off Wednesday and Thursday. Now work through the answer options to see which one can be correct:
A - If C works T, W, Th, then A will work M, W, F which is possible, so A is correct.
B - If C works T, W, F then only one person will be working on Thursday, which isn't possible.
C - If C works T, Th, F then only one person will work on W, which isn't possible
D - If C works W, Th, F then A will have to work M, T, W and Th which isn't possible
E is incorrect as '*None of the operators work for four consecutive days in a week*'.

Q2	C

The passage concludes that the criteria used cannot give a good judgement of whether a planet is habitable or not, as using the new criteria, Earth would be '*almost too hot for liquid water*' and not habitable. However, the passage says Earth is habitable, creating doubt over the true accuracy of the criteria. Therefore, C is the best answer as it sums up the passage's conclusion the best.

Q3	C

To have the birthday on the same day as the week as someone else's, the difference in the days between the two birthdays must be a multiple of 7. Therefore, only C is correct as 281 - 218 = 63 which is a multiple of 7.

Q4	C

The conclusion of the passage is '*Therefore, the secret to losing weight is painfully simple - do more and/or eat less*' which is summarised by C.

Q5	D

Price on first day - £12   Number sold: x which is <60
Price on second day - 0.75 x £12 = £9   Number sold: 2x
12x = money made on first day
2(9x) = 18x = money made on second day
18x-12x = £342, so 6x = £342, so x = 57
2x + x = total number of Spruggles sold = 57 x 3 = 171 = D

Q6	C

The Clovis-First Theory suggests that the Clovis were the first people who settled in America, in 11,500BC. C is correct because if a settlement was found that was dated in 12,000 BC (i.e. 500 years before the Clovis), then that would severely challenge the Clovis-First Theory. Although the other answers could weaken the theory, only C would '*seriously challenge*' it.

2013 Section 1

Q7	A

Simon and Dylan must have surnames Hyde and Rush (because their first name has 5 letters, so their surnames can't). Therefore, it is Simon Hyde and Dylan Rush.
Liam must have the surname Shore because Doyle and Floyd both have 'l''s in them
Eric cannot be Doyle because they both have 'e''s.
So, it must be Eric Floyd, and thus Ian Doyle.

Q8	D

The first paragraph embodies a sarcastic tone, so the answer is clearly D. B and C are incorrect because the '*No, really?*' refers to the children and not to blondes or chocolate. A is incorrect because of the sarcastic tone of the paragraph.

Q9	A

The evidence suggests that in the process of gaining money, we've become sadder, which is what A says. The benefits of wealth or children are not mentioned so B and C are wrong, and D is wrong because it implies a causal relationship, which isn't mentioned in the text.

Q10	D

1 - The psychologist says that the more time you spend on your job, the less time you will have with your children. This does not mean that people who work shorter hours will spend more time with their kids, as they may be doing other things.
2 - Just because as we seem to get wealthier, we are more miserable/stressed does not mean that 2 is correct, as the transcript talks about one end of the spectrum (the wealthy).

Q11	B

The evidence used in the paragraph is based on the author's own account of a family that he knows - i.e. it is based on an anecdote. It is not conclusive, as one family's experience may not be representative of everyone's, there are no statistics, it is relevant as it provides evidence for the topic at hand, and it is not hearsay, because the author is '*intimately involved'* with the family.

Q12	B

For this question, it is best to work systematically through the set of cards and see if you can find a pair. Starting with the card on the top left, look and see if any cards have the symbol for the Moon on the top, or silver. The top right card has silver at the top, but they are not a match because copper does not match with sun. We can therefore rule out these two cards. Work in a similar fashion through the eight cards, and you will see that there is one pair (on the right).

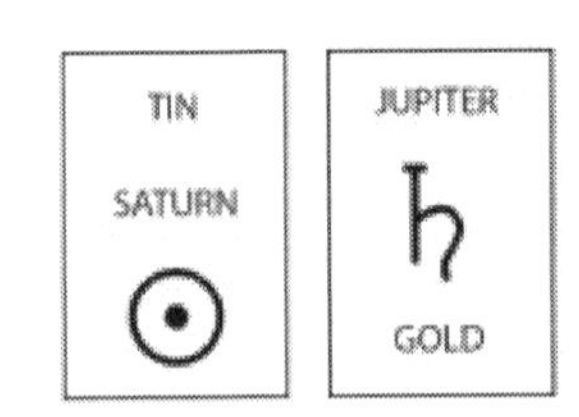

Q13	D

Again, for these types of questions, identify the conclusion of the text, and see which answer options best fits. The conclusion here is '*In the interests of providing the most desirable outcomes, it is clear that placebos should be used as a treatment offered by the NHS'*, which clearly shows that it is D. The other answer options are not entirely relevant to the argument.

Q14	B

What we know about the PIN so far is that it is: 4 - - 0/four - - zero
Because the numbers are in alphabetical order, we know that the middle gaps cannot be eight or five. The total number of letters so far is 8, yet the numerical sum is 4. Therefore, the total number of letters of the middle two must be 4 less than the numerical sum.
The digits we have remaining are: one, two, three, six, seven, nine.
Therefore, we can see that the only two numbers that fit our rule above are nine and two.
Therefore, the answer is 7, as there are 4 digits in nine and 3 in two.

Q15	B

The major evidence that the author's argument is constructed upon is '*Sport is what people do to counter the stress and pressure of work*' - B directly counters this, therefore weakening the argument. A & C merely support the passage, while D doesn't weaken the argument (although it opposes it).

Q16	C

Jenny could be born in January, June, or July.
Alice could be born in April or August.
Michael could be born in March or May.
However, it says that Jenny and Alice's birthdays are 2 months apart, so Jenny must be born in June (since August and April are both 2 months apart from April). Michael's birthday must be in March, since it is the only M starting month that is 5 months away from one starting with A (August). Therefore, Alice must be born in August. Therefore, the answer is C as June is 3 months apart from March.

Q17	D

For these types of questions, it is often useful to first identify the error in reasoning in the paragraph. This paragraph claims that old age causes a lack of sleep, and that old age results in a worse memory, and so therefore it must be the lack of sleep that '*must account for the impairment in memory which often occurs with ageing*'. Therefore, weaknesses that can be identified are weaknesses with the link between lack of sleep and impaired memory (i.e. statements that present different reasons for the link between age, lack of sleep, and impaired memory) which are options 1 and 3.

Q18	B

There are 4 different values at play here: the hour, the minute, the day and the month. The month (09) will be the same for each display, and therefore we need not consider the month. Since there are 31 days in September, there will be 5 days that are square numbers (1, 4, 9, 16 and 25), since there are only 5 square numbers below 31. However, the question asks for times when there are <u>different</u> numbers on the clock, so we remove the 9th, leaving us 4 days.
Not counting 9, there are only 3 hours that are square numbers (1,4 and 16), and only 6 minutes that are square numbers (1, 4, 16, 25, 36 and 49). Now we can write out the possible combinations.
01.09 = 04:16, 04:25, 04:36, 04:49, 16:04, 16:25, 16:36, 16:49
There will also be 8 possible times on 04.09 and 16.09 as 16 is a day, hour and a minute.
However, on day 25, there will be 12 possible combinations as 25 is not an hour, as below:
25.09 = 01:04, 01:16, 01:36, 01:49, 04:01, 04:16, 04:36, 04:49, 16:01, 16:04, 16:36, 16:49
So, 8+8+8+12 = 36 = B.

Q19	B

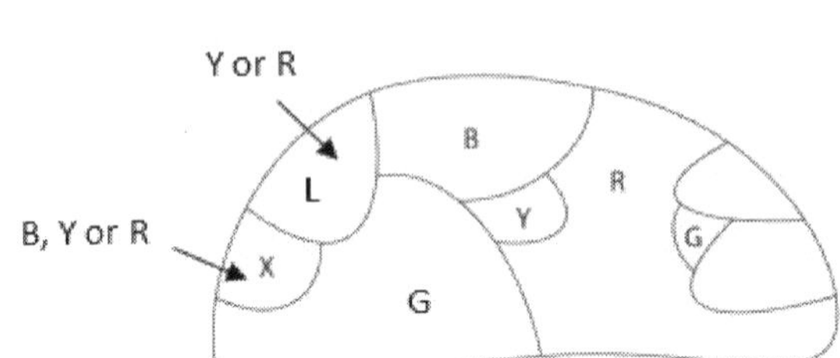

The bottom left area must be green as it borders a blue, a yellow and a red region. The area marked L must be yellow or red since it borders a blue and a green region. Therefore X, could be blue, yellow (if L was red) or red (if L was yellow).

Q20	C

If the circle is placed within one of the squares on the chess board, no extra colours would be needed (i.e. if the square was within a white circle, it would be black and vice versa). If the circle was bigger than one square, then one extra colour would be needed, so that the circle wouldn't be the same colour as either the black or the white square.

Q21	A

Two colours will always be sufficient as no matter where you place the three lines, each region will only share a border with one or two other regions (which will be the opposite colour). In the BMAT exam, draw lines on the diagram provided to help you visualise this, or draw out many different shapes with three lines, until you spot the pattern.

Q22	B

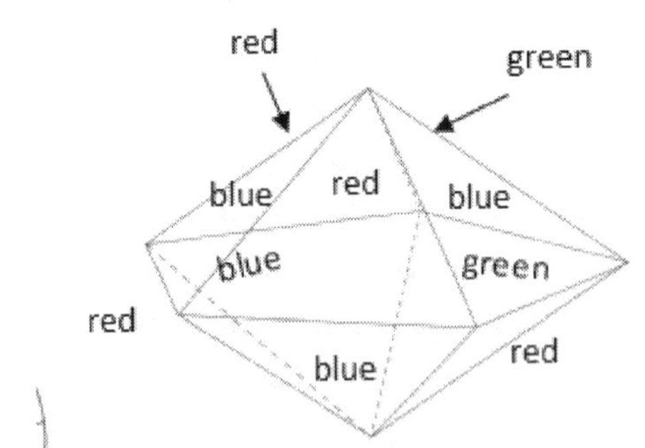

This question is a visualisation question, which I suggest you attempt by assigning a colour to one face and working from there. I assigned the central triangle the colour red, and the triangles to the left and right blue. Working from there, if you assign the triangle to the left of the left blue triangle red, the triangle to the right of the right blue triangle, must be a third colour (it can't be red, as the triangle to the left of it is red). See the diagram for more clarity. The same thing occurs for the bottom triangles.

Q23	D

Work from right to left in a systematic way till you have identified all the different kinds of tile, which can be seen below. In total there are 8 tiles.

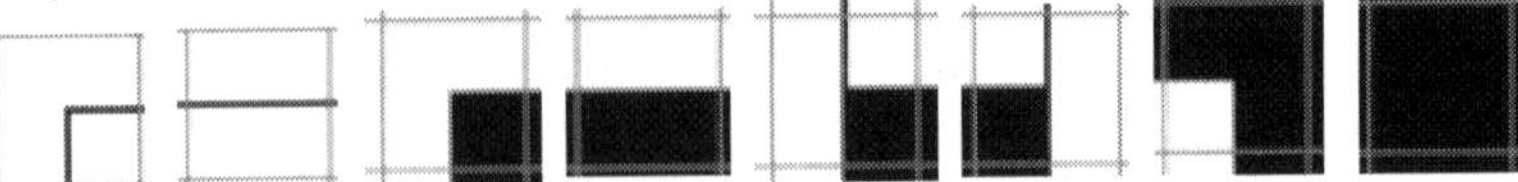

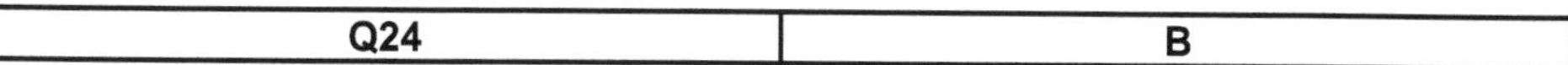

Q24	B

The above argument concludes that we ought to reduce the consumption of alcohol and one method to achieve this is to make alcohol more expensive. Option B is an example of evidence where decreasing the price has increased consumption, and therefore we can assume the inverse to be true, strengthening the argument the most. The other options don't focus entirely on reducing consumption in society.

Q25	B

The two clocks are 41 minutes apart. This strange phenomenon must occur when one clock shows a time between 19:00 and 19:59, and the other clock between 20:00 and 20:59, because between other hours either a 0 or a 1 will be common to both clocks.
Let us call the minutes xy and pq for ease. So, we have 19:xy as the slow clock and 20:pq for the fast clock. X, y, p, q must be drawn out of 3, 4, 5, 6, 7 and 8 (not surprisingly, these are also the answer options). The latest time for xy can be pq can be 39 (as 41 onwards would give times 41 minutes earlier also starting with 20:--, and 40 can't be used because a 0 is already used in 20:--). Thus, p must be a 3. And the earliest time for xy can be 34 (as the earliest the fast clock can be is 20:15, to avoid repeating digits). Thus, x must be a 5 (since p is a 3).
Therefore, y and q must be chosen out of 4, 6, 7 and 8.
If y was a 4 then q would have to be a 5 (due to the 41-minute time difference), this is not possible so y = 6 and q = 7 or y = 7 and q = 8. Therefore, 4 is the only number not to be used.
The time of the slow clock is 19:56 or 19:57 and the fast clock is 20:37 or 20:38

Q26	A

P will hit 5, Q will hit 7, R will hit 4 and S will hit 1. If you find visualisation difficult, it would be best to guess this question, move on and only come back to it at the end if you have time.

Q27	C

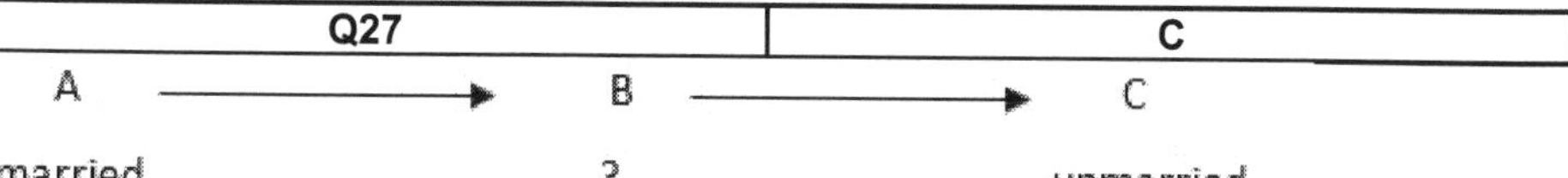

If Beth was married, a married person would be looking at a married person (A - B) and a married person would be looking at an unmarried person (B-C)
If Beth was unmarried, a married person would be looking at an unmarried person (A-B), and an unmarried person would be looking at a married person (B-C)
Therefore, the answer is C.

Q28	D

The above argument opposes the idea that children should witness harshness (we learn that they become vegetarian when faced '*so cruelly with this outcome*') and should be protected from this harm/witnessing cruelty. Only D acknowledges this conclusion, and so is correct.

Q29	E

Again, just like q26, if you find visualisation difficult, make a guess, and move onto the next question, only coming back to this question at the end if you have time. The only way you can solve this, if you find visualisation difficult, is to cut out the net and have a go folding it (this is a very helpful tip for practicing, though not so practical in the exam, due to time constraints). The answer option here is E.

Q30	D

The paragraph argues that wrinkles are an advantageous feature because they help us grip wet objects better and '*must have evolved because it gave humans a better grip underwater*' However it assumes that they gripping wet objects is advantageous, and assumes the reasons as to why certain characteristics evolve, so 1 and 3 are the assumptions. B is not an assumption, as without it, the conclusion still holds true.

Q31	A

These are the remaining numbers that fill the gaps: 3, 4, 7, 8, 11. The top row adds up to 14, the bottom to 22, and the right to 6. Therefore, the gaps on the top must add up to 15 (this is 11+4 or 8+7). The bottom gaps must add up to 7 (4+3). Therefore, the gaps at the bottom are 4 and 3, and the ones at the top are 8+7. The right gaps must add up to 23, and so are 11+8+4. So the bottom right gap is 4, and the top right is 8. Therefore, the person opposite 9 will be number 3.

Q32	B

80% of typical young people don't use cannabis, so in this sample it would be 8,000. If 1% of non-cannabis users develop psychosis, in this sample 8 would develop psychosis. Cannabis users are 41% more likely to develop psychosis than non-cannabis users, so 1.41% of cannabis users would do so in this sample. 1.41% of 2,000 is approximately 28. [Note 20 = 1%, and 41 is just over 2%, so the answer is B]

Q33	A

In that sample, 36 people develop psychosis. The probability of developing psychosis for non-cannabis users is x (who make up 80%), whereas in cannabis users it's 1.41x. (20%).
The probability that a person will get psychosis is: $(1.41x \times 0.2) + 0.8x$
The probability that a person will get psychosis from cannabis use is $(0.41 \times 0.2x)$
So the P(someone will get psychosis given they've used cannabis) = $[(1.41x \times 0.2) + 0.8x]$ / $(0.41 \times 0.2x)$ = approximately 0.08/1.1 = approximately 8%.

Q34	B

The passage suggests it is cannabis use that causes an increase in psychotic illness. B provides an alternative reason that explains why groups who may use cannabis have an increased risk of psychotic illness (that is not the fact that they use cannabis). A, C and D are not alternative reasons that could be the cause of this relationship.

Q35	C

A - this just provides more evidence to strengthen the correlation, as opposed to providing evidence to explain a causal link.
B - this weakens the link, suggesting that maybe ecstasy is the cause.
C - provides evidence to show that it is the cannabis causing the psychosis, as stronger cannabis results in more psychosis.
D and E are not relevant to proving the link between cannabis and psychosis.

2013 Section 2

Q1	H

This is another simple biology question which requires detailed knowledge of the specification material.
1 - both systems are involved in homeostasis (maintenance of constant internal environment).
2 - applies to both, since hormones are chemicals, and neurotransmitters (chemicals) are used in the nervous system at synapse.
3 - one of the parts of the central nervous system is the brain, and some hormones, such as ADH, are released from the pituitary gland, which is a part of the brain.

Q2	D

This question tests knowledge not currently on the BMAT specification.
A displacement reaction occurs when a more reactive element displaces a less reactive element from a solution of one of its salts. Learning the order of the reactivity series, and the properties of halogens helps greatly.
1 - Al is more reactive than Pb, so will displace it.
2 - this is a tricky one, here fluorine is in its ionic form, and therefore can't displace chlorine from KCl.
3 - Al is more reactive than Fe, so no displacement will occur.
4 - Zn is more reactive than Cu, so will displace it.

Q3	D

1 - is correct, as that is how microwaves cause damage.
2 - is correct, as X-rays are ionising radiation.
3 - incorrect, as this is not how IR causes damage. (IR causes burns and does not cause damage when it penetrates matter).

Q4	A

$$\frac{\mathbf{4.6 \times 10^7 + 14 \times 10^6}}{\mathbf{4.6 \times 10^7 - 4 \times 10^6}}$$

Because in the numerator and in the denominator, we are adding/subtracting values of different powers, we cannot simply add/subtract the terms. To be able to do that, we need to put everything in terms of 10^7.

$$\frac{4.6 \times 10^7 + 1.4 \times 10^7}{4.6 \times 10^7 - 0.4 \times 10^7} = \frac{6 \times 10^7}{4.2 \times 10^7} = \frac{6}{4.2} = \frac{60}{42} = \mathbf{\frac{10}{7}}$$

Q5	F

Carbohydrates break down into di/monosaccharides (in this reaction, there is no change in acidity/pH).
Proteins break down into amino acids (in this reaction, there is a decrease in acidity/pH as acids are formed).
Lipids break down into glycerol and 3x fatty acids (in this reaction, there is a decrease in acidity/pH, as acids are formed).
Therefore, only a breakdown of proteins (by proteases) or lipids by (lipases) would result in a decrease in the pH, so F is correct.

2013 Section 2

Q6	B

For this question it is necessary to know the effects of temperature, pressure, catalysts, and concentrations on the position of equilibrium.

- Increasing the temperature favours the endothermic change.
- Increasing the pressure favours the side of the equation producing the fewest molecules of gas.
- Increasing the concentration of reactants, shifts the position of equilibrium to the right (i.e. to the products).
- Using a catalyst does not affect the position of equilibrium.

Therefore, since the forward reaction is exothermic and there are fewer molecules of gas on the RHS, answer option B is correct.

Q7	H

P is an ammeter and measures current, whereas Q and R are voltmeters and measure voltage. When the switch is open, the current flows through the two resistors. When the switch is closed, the current flows through resistor Q and then bypasses resistor R. Therefore, no voltage will be measured in R, so the voltage in R decreases. Since there is now effectively only one resistor in the circuit, when the switch is closed, there is less resistance, and therefore there will be more current flowing for the same voltage (V=IR), so P increases. Also, we know that voltage splits in series between components. Since there is now only one component in the circuit when the switch is closed, the voltage of the cell will be the same voltage as R (as opposed to the voltage of the cell being double that of R when the switch was open, as the voltage had to be shared between the two resistors), so Q increases.

Q8	F

Step 1: divide both the numerator and the denominator by x^2

$$= 4 - \frac{(1-16x^2)}{2x(4x-1)}$$

Step 2: get 4 in terms of 2x(4x-1), so we can have one single fraction

$$= \frac{8x(4x-1)}{2x(4x-1)} - \frac{(1-16x^2)}{2x(4x-1)} = \frac{8x(4x-1) - (1-16x^2)}{2x(4x-1)} = \frac{8x(4x-1) + (16x^2 - 1)}{2x(4x-1)}$$

Step 3: Recognise that ($16x^2$ - 1) is a difference of two squares.

$$\frac{8x(4x-1) + (4x-1)(4x+1)}{2x(4x-1)}$$

Step 4: Divide by (4x-1), and then split the fraction into a whole number part and a fractional part.

$$\frac{8x + 4x + 1}{2x} = \frac{8x + 4x}{2x} + \frac{1}{2x} = 6 + \frac{1}{2x}$$

Q9	F

The sensory neuron is the longest (as it has to run from the receptors in the fingertip to the spinal cord), the relay neuron is the shortest (as it only runs inside the spinal cord), and the motor neuron is medium length (as it only runs from the spinal cord to the arm muscle).

Q10	B

For questions like this, first write out the balanced equation, so you can see the mole ratio between different compounds.
The equation is: $2Na + 2H_2O \rightarrow H_2 + 2NaOH$
1.15g of sodium is $\frac{1.15}{23}$= 0.05 moles of sodium.
The mole ratio between sodium and hydrogen is 2:1, so 0.025 moles of hydrogen are produced. Thus: 0.025 x 22.4 = 0.56dm^3 = 560cm^3

Q11	C

This question tests knowledge not currently on the BMAT specification.
Total Internal reflection occurs when the angle of incidence is greater than the critical angle <u>and</u> the light travels from a more dense to a less dense medium, since light only bends away from the normal in those circumstances.
In Diagram 1, angle of incidence < critical angle, so TIR does not occur, and the light leaves at P. In Diagram 2, light travels from a less dense to a more dense medium, so TIR does not occur, and the light gets refracted, going to S.

Q12	B

We recommend you do a quick sketch for these questions.

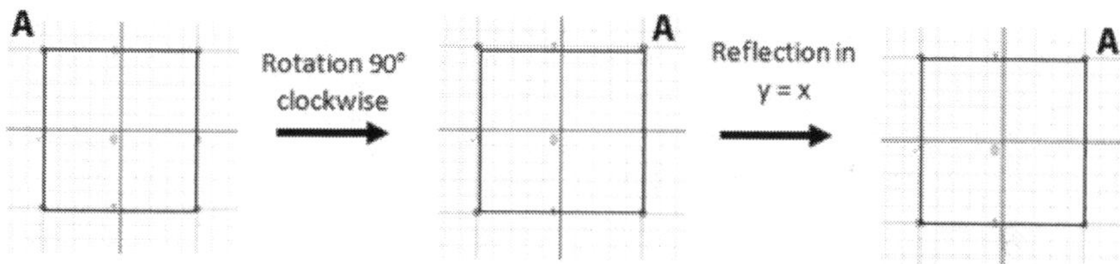

To get back to original conformation, all you need to do is reflect the third image in the y axis.

Q13	C

A - a ligase enzyme is needed to join the jellyfish DNA into the bacterial plasmid
B - a plasmid is needed for the exchange of DNA
C - a fluorescent protein is produced, it is not needed for the genetic engineering, as the implanted DNA is there to produce the protein
D - these enzymes are needed to remove the fluorescent 'gene' from the jellyfish DNA, and to cut the bacterial plasmid DNA

Q14	A

Again, work your way through the answer options until you find the correct answer. $MgCl_2$ consists of a magnesium ion (Mg^{2+}) and two chloride ions (Cl^-). The chloride ions both have the same electronic structure as argon, but magnesium has the same electronic structure as neon, so A is the correct answer. B-E all have the same electronic structures.

2013 Section 2

Q15	D

For this question, imagine X and Y were separate and work out the count rates for these substances after 24 hours as you would normally, and then add the two count rates at the end.
X has a half-life of 4.8 hours, therefore in 24 hours it will have 5 half-lives (24/4.8 = 5).
Therefore, 320 ----> 160 ------> 80-----> 40------->20 -----> 10 is the final count rate
Y has a half-life of 8 hours, therefore in 24 hours it will have 3 half-lives (24/8=3)
480---->240----->120------>60 is the final count rate
10+60 = 70 counts per minute = D

Q16	D

We know the following facts: $x \propto z^2$ and $y \propto 1/z^3$
In order to be able to equate the proportionality statements, we have to convert both z's to a common power (in this case we will use z^6 as 6 is the LCM of 3 and 2)
Therefore: $x^3 \propto z^6$ and $y^2 \propto 1/z^6$. Thus: $z^6 \propto x^3 \propto 1/y^2$ therefore D is correct.

Q17	A

This question tests knowledge not currently on the BMAT specification.
1 is correct because this is a possibility in somatic cell nuclear transfer (SCNT)
2 is incorrect because sperm cells are not involved in SNCT, as the male nucleus is transferred in vitro into the enucleated egg cell
3 is correct because this is a possibility with SCNT and the subsequent implantation of the embryo into the surrogate's uterus
4 The egg cells divide and not differentiate
5 is correct as this is a possibility in SCNT

Q18	E

n is the scientific convention to describe the number of moles.
n(HCl) = cv = (50/1000) x 0.50 = 0.025 moles of HCl
The molar ratio between HCl and NaOH is 1:1 (these are common questions, so it is best to learn the equation for this neutralisation reaction, or the fact that the ratio is 1:1). Therefore 0.025 moles of NaOH will get neutralised.
The maximum possible number of moles in a 1.20g sample of NaOH is (1.2/40) = 0.03 moles (as moles = mass/Mr).
Therefore, percentage purity is (0.025/0.03) x 100, which is (⅚) x 100 = E (83.3%)

Q19	D

For this question you need to use the equations $I = V/R$ and $P = I^2R$
The current is therefore, $I = \frac{V}{R1 + R2}$, and therefore power is $P = (\frac{V}{R1+R2})^2 R1 = \frac{V^2 R1}{(R1+R2)^2}$"

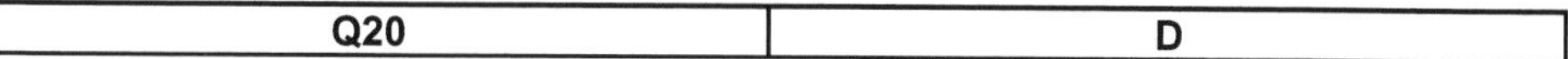

Q20	D

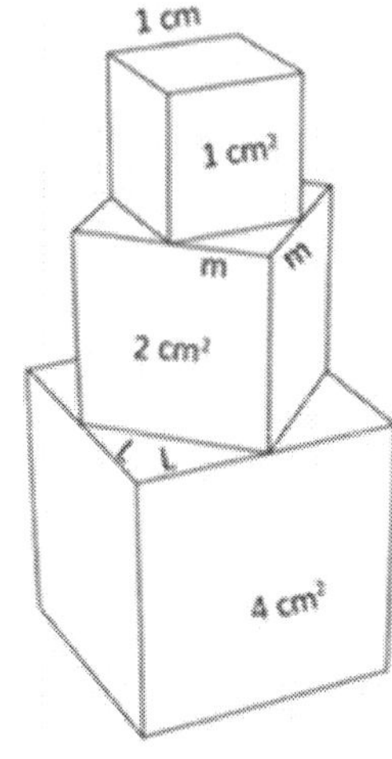

The small cube has 5 faces, so $5 \times 1cm^2 = 5cm^2$

On the top face of the middle cube, there are 4 triangles – let us call the length of the opposite and adjacent of each triangle m, and the hypotenuse is 1cm (as it is a side of the small cube). Using Pythag, $m = \frac{\sqrt{2}}{2}$ as $(1^2 = 2m^2)$.

Therefore, the area of each triangle = $\frac{1}{2} m^2$, and since there are 4 triangles, the area = $2m^2$. From before, $2m^2 = 2(\frac{\sqrt{2}}{2})^2 = 1cm^2$.

We know m is the midpoint of the edge of the middle cube, therefore the middle cube has side length of $2m = \sqrt{2}$. This time we only have 4 faces, so the area of the 4 faces = $4 \times 2 = 8cm^2$

We repeat this process for the large cube. The opposite and adjacent of the triangle (length marked L) is 1 cm (as $(\sqrt{2})^2 = 2L^2$ by Pythag). Therefore, the area of the 4 triangles is $2L^2 = 2cm^2$. The middle cube, therefore, has a length of 2L which is 2 cm and so the area of each face is $4cm^2$. 5 faces are shown so $5 \times 4 = 20cm^2$.

So total SA = $5cm^2 + 1cm^2 + 8cm^2 + 2cm^2 + 20cm^2 = 36cm^2$

Q21	E

This question tests knowledge not currently on the BMAT specification.
Every body cell has the entire genome (all the genes), so a liver cell will have the gene for amylase, so 1 is correct. Each body cell has 46 chromosomes, so a liver cell will have the sex chromosomes, so 2 is correct. Starch is not produced, nor stored in the liver so 3 is incorrect.

Q22	C

a = c so that the number of carbon atoms on both sides of the equation are equal. d = 2, so that the Chromium atoms are balanced. In order to balance the charge (there is 6+ on the RHS, and 2- on the LHS), b = 8. Therefore, e = 4 to balance the hydrogens.

Q23	D

A is correct; the equation needed here is $F = ma$. B is correct; the equation needed here is $V = IR$. C is correct; the equation needed here is $KE = \frac{1}{2} mv^2$
D is incorrect because wavelength and frequency are inversely proportional, whereas the graph shows a directly proportional relationship.
E is correct (the equation needed is $W = Fd$)

Q24	C

The only two combinations that will result in exactly two balls being the same colour are 1 red and 2 blue or 1 blue and 2 red.
P(1 red and 2 blue) = $\frac{2}{10} \times \frac{8}{9} \times \frac{7}{8} \times 3 = \frac{336}{720}$(we multiply by 3 because it could be RBB, BRB or BBR as the order we pick out the balls)
P (1 blue and 2 red) = = $\frac{2}{10} \times \frac{1}{9} \times \frac{8}{8} \times 3 = \frac{48}{720}$(we multiply by 3 because it could be BRR, RBR or RRB as the order we pick out the balls)
Total probability is $\frac{48}{720}+\frac{336}{720}=\frac{384}{720}=\frac{8}{15}$(we use the addition rule because it is 'OR' we either need 1 blue and 2 red or 2 blue and 1 red)

Q25	C

A Manx cat with a tail is tt and a Manx cat without a tail is Tt. Let us draw two Punnett squares for each of the crosses.

1. tt x Tt

	t	t
T	Tt (no tail)	Tt (no tail)
t	tt (tail)	tt (tail)

50% have no tail.

2. Tt x Tt

	T	t
T	TT (dead)	Tt (no tail)
t	Tt (no tail)	tt (tail)

75% have no tail, as dead organisms are not counted within a population.

Q26	B

We know that NO is a catalyst so must not be used up by the end of the reaction (i.e. for every 1NO used in the reaction, 1 NO must be produced). Reaction 3 followed by Reaction 6 is the only combination that would mean that the quantity of NO does not change. Also, this set of reactions produces only SO_3.

Q27	E

$KE = \frac{1}{2}mv^2 = 1800$. Therefore, the velocity is 30m/s.
$F = ma$, so current acceleration is $5\ m/s^2$
Rearrange the equation for acceleration giving v = u + at, so v after 2 seconds = 30 + 5(2) = 40m/s
Therefore final KE = 0.5 x 4 x (40 x 40) = 3200J.
We only want the extra KE though, so 3200-1800 = 1400J = E

2013 Section 3

To see the marking grid and mark bands that the BMAT examiners will use to mark your essays, please refer to the BMAT website.

"When you want to know how things really work, study them when they are coming apart." (*William Gibson*)

To see the question in full, please see:
https://www.admissionstesting.org/Images/164792-past-paper-2013-section-3.pdf

The statement suggests that the best way to understand the function of an object is to observe it when it is dismantled, disassembled, or dissected.

- When working with a piece of machinery or an object, by removing certain constituent parts and then observing the object functioning, one can determine the role of that constituent part by comparing the new functioning with normal functioning. This method is effective at working out the individual roles, functions and relative importances of the different parts in the object.
- The understanding of the human body that modern medicine is based on comes from dissections of the human body in the past, as through dissection we were able to better understand the roles of the different bodily structures.

- However, using the example above of the piece of machinery, simply identifying each part's individual role may not give the fullest understanding of the overall object's function. As Aristotle said '*The whole is greater than the sum of its parts*', and often it is the interaction between the constituent parts (which can only be seen when the object is functioning normal, and not when dismantled) that is key to understanding the functioning of an object, such as in the case of a living system like a plant.
- Dissection or dismantling is not possible for certain entities or objects, such as human behaviour and emotion which are difficult to break down and are better understood while the person is alive as opposed to when the brain is broken down on the dissection table.

- Dismantling or dissection has been helpful in the past to understand the workings of objects, such as human anatomy and clocks.
- However, Gibson's assertion may not be applicable for all objects due to their differing complexities.
- The more complex an object is, the more interactions there are between the constituent parts, and the less helpful dismantling may be to understand the intricacies of the object.
- Perhaps Gibson's assertion may hold more true for mechanical objects than biological systems.

2013 Section 3

'Good surgeons should be encouraged to take on tough cases, not just safe, routine ones. Publishing an individual surgeon's mortality rates may have the opposite effect.'
To see the question in full, please see:
https://www.admissionstesting.org/Images/164792-past-paper-2013-section-3.pdf

This statement means that publishing documents about doctors' success rates may decrease the quality of medical care provided, endanger patient safety and decrease the skills of surgeons as more competent surgeons would be drawn to the safer cases so that they have higher success rates.

- In the USA, within private practice, a doctor's reputation is very important and in order to safeguard their reputation, doctors may be more likely to take on safer, more routine cases, instead of tougher, more difficult ones to ensure they are high on the 'league table'.
- Publishing league tables/success rates could put undue extra pressure on surgeons, which could lead to worsened quality care, or more surgeons leaving the profession.
- Mortality rates are dependent on the type of surgery (for example a heart transplant will have a higher mortality rate than a corn excision), so mortality rates may not always be a good or fair representation of a surgeon's ability.

- Publication of mortality rates for each doctor could actually make medical practice safer, as it would allow for quicker identification of malpracticing doctors such as Dr Harold Shipman, or those who need more training.
- It could increase the standard of medical care provided, as publishing mortality rate tables may put pressure on surgeons to ensure that the surgery is done very carefully, with all safety measures put in place. It could make certain surgeons think twice about cutting corners in surgical procedures.
- It could also be used to improve surgical performance, as it could inspire/motivate doctors more to gain more training, so they can perform safer surgeries.
- A patient has autonomy to make an informed decision about whether they want a surgery; therefore, some people may say that a patient has every right to know about their surgeon's previous history/success rate.

- Regardless of league tables, surgeons should follow the Hippocratic Oath and relevant government guidance of good medical practice, to ensure they provide the best possible quality of care for their patients.
- Although publishing league tables may have a beneficial effect as discussed above, they will probably have more detrimental effects, such as putting too much pressure on surgeons. This could affect the decision of a surgeon to perform a surgery in the first place which could endanger patient safety and care. Fewer, riskier surgeries may take place, and although surgical mortality rates may decline, overall mortality rates would increase, as patients with more serious/complex ailments may not be able to get surgical interventions which could save their lives.
- Not publishing league tables may mean that doctors remain more confident and willing to take on riskier, tougher surgeries that may have higher mortality rates.

"Ignorance more frequently begets confidence than does knowledge: it is those who know little, and not those who know much, who so positively assert that this or that problem will never be solved by science." (*Charles Darwin*)
To see the question in full, please see:
https://www.admissionstesting.org/Images/164792-past-paper-2013-section-3.pdf

This statement argues that those who don't know much about a subject, in this case science are more confident about what they understand, because they either feel they know all there is to know about a subject, or they feel more confident because the level of study they are at is rather simplistic. With this confidence and limited knowledge, these sorts of people do not believe that certain problems can ever be solved by science. A person who knows more will better understand the complexities of the subject, and appreciate the vast amount of knowledge that they do not know, making them less confident in their total understanding of that subject, and believe more in being able to science to solve a problem.

The 2020 document; '*Our Plan to Rebuild: The UK Government's COVID-19 recovery strategy*' published by the UK government nicely sums up an example:

'*Now, with every week that passes,* ***we learn more about the virus and understand more about how to defeat it. But the more we learn, the more we realise how little the world yet understands about the true nature of the threat*** *- except that it is a shared one that we must all work together to defeat.*'

- A GCSE Chemistry student may feel they have a good grasp of what atoms are, and the basic Bohr model. An A Level Chemistry student would however know of different models of atoms, but may feel more uncertain that they understand the subject matter more clearly, as there are more complexities with the models of atomic structure, and similarly a degree student may know even more, but this would mean they are aware of far more exceptions, complexities and caveats.
- Members of the public who believe that coronavirus was caused by 5G are not very knowledgeable about biology and physics, yet so vocally assert that science will not be able to find solutions to coronavirus, without the destruction of 5G masts.

- Sometimes, people who have been studying a particular subject for a very long period of time, and are very knowledgeable in that area, may not be able to change their way of thinking, or may not be able to adapt to new technologies. A person who is less knowledgeable may be able to spot a different way, or offer a different view, as they may be able to take a step back and look at the bigger picture, which someone so engrossed in their work may be unable to do. This can be refreshing and highly productive for the research undertaken.

- The statement holds quite a lot of truth, as those who are less knowledgeable about a subject tend to be less open-minded about its possibilities. However, one must acknowledge that this is a generalisation, and cannot apply to everyone. There are examples, and may be more in the future, of ignorant people expanding our current shared scientific knowledge, by for example trialling new methods that those who are knowledgeable may have overlooked.

Authors' tip:

Using original, unique, or personal examples, such as the ones above, as well as up-to-date examples (such as COVID-19), make your essays stand out far more than generic, overused examples. However, make sure any examples you use are directly relevant to the question! A good way to prepare for the essay section is to read widely around medicine (this will help you for your medical interviews as well)!

Please remember there are many different ways to take questions like this. For example, you could argue that this statement is more about ignorant people being more vocal than those who are more knowledgeable, and that society often believes the 'ignorant', but this is now changing, with more sources of information available. What is important is that you follow your own line of understanding through to produce a clear and coherent argument.

Question 4 was written to widen access to the exam paper, as in the past, students hoping to study Veterinary Medicine would also have to take the BMAT. VetMed students no longer take the BMAT, and so in its current iteration (2017 onwards), there are none of these questions, so the authors have not included worked essays for these and recommend that you only attempt these after having attempted all the previous ones.

BMAT 2014

The BMAT website provides worked solutions for this paper, and therefore the authors have not included their own in this book.

Authors' tip:
Have a look at the examiners' comments for the essay responses - these are very helpful in explaining what the examiners are looking for in the high-level responses.

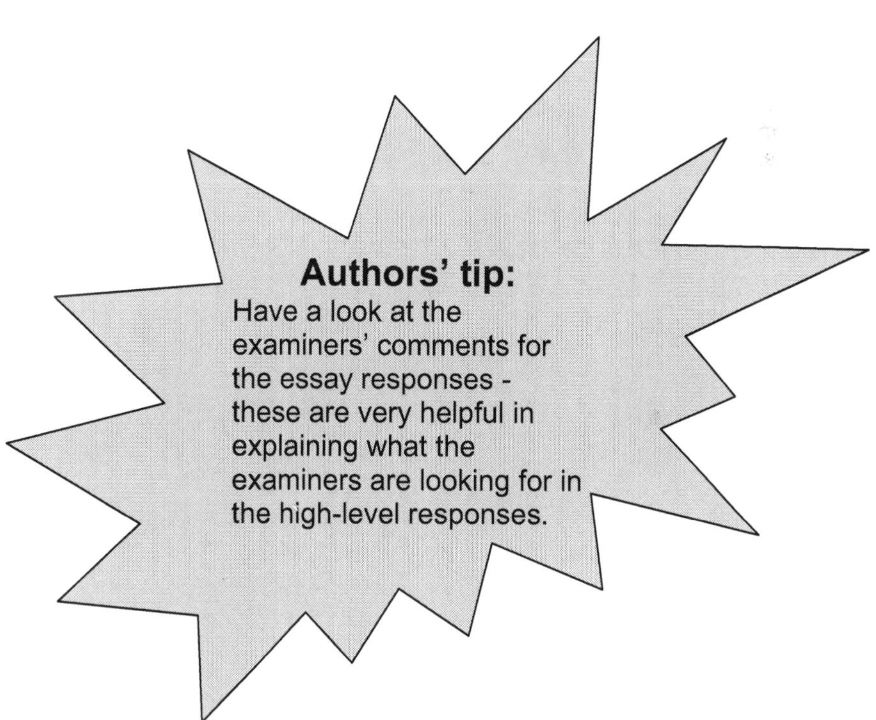

BMAT 2015

Section 1

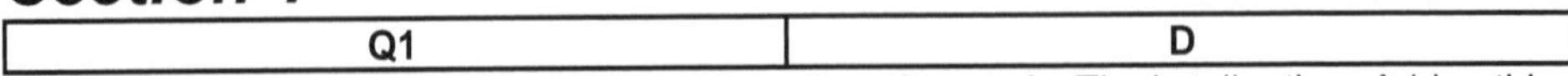

Q1	D

As Tim is shorter than Ruth, he is also shorter than Stuart. As Tim is taller than Adrian this means Adrian is therefore shorter than Ruth and Stuart. Already we can eliminate B, C and E. However, Margaret could be taller than Adrian or shorter than him because we do not know anything about her position other than the fact that she is shorter than Ruth and Stuart. This eliminates A leaving D.

Q2	E

A is incorrect, we don't have any comments on the immune systems of those from other countries. B is incorrect as this information is not in the passage, for all we know there could be lots of rich people with poor diets as well. C is incorrect because the only comment on the current generation of doctors is that they are unfamiliar with it. C implies they have heard of the disease i.e. they are familiar with it but they may not have appreciated the seriousness of it. D is incorrect because if anything, the figures would be underestimated given that some doctors do not consider the diagnosis. E is correct because the passage says ¾ of recorded infections were in people from deprived areas, thus implying that 1/4 of recorded infections were in people from relatively affluent areas which makes it more unlikely.

Q3	A

Notice the question says that '*at the last day of each month, the transport manager records the reading on the vans' meters*'. This means that the months we actually want are from the last day of August to the last day of November. Thus, we need to calculate the difference between the values for the November column and the August column and see which van has the largest figure. I have rounded to 3 significant figures to make calculations easier. The red van travels furthest. You can do a fair bit of this approximation in your head, such as easily eliminating Orange, Blue, Indigo and Violet just by looking at the numbers and this will cut down your calculation time.

	August	November	Difference
Red	68200	78900	10700
Orange	64400	73700	9300
Yellow	71300	81200	9900
Green	64800	75100	10300
Blue	74000	83400	9400
Indigo	68600	78200	9600
Violet	63100	72800	9700

Q4	A

A is correct because it gets at the heart of the flaw: the research has found a positive correlation between attractiveness of males and their success in a race but this alone is not sufficient for success because the research hasn't shown it to be causatory; only correlatory. B is incorrect because this argument only considers 1 sport, so can't comment on sporting excellence as a whole. C is wrong because it does not matter if these results aren't generalisable to all sports, that is why sports are considered separately. D is wrong because the argument makes no claim that cyclists are more attractive than other sportsmen as it gives no data or commentary on the attractiveness of males doing other sports. E is wrong because it is not the main flaw of this passage.

Q5	D

First, identify the top 3 competitors: these are 4, 10 and 13 when you count their better score qualifying. Subtract 50cm off of third place's score. This is 7.17-0.5 = 6.67. Going down the list from 1 to 15 (minus those we've already counted: 4, 10 and 13) we can see that 1, 6, 8, 9, 11, 12, and 15 will not qualify as their best score is below 6.67.
2, 3, 5, 7 and 14 will count. This is a total of 5. Adding on our 3 for 4, 10 and 13 gives us a total of 8 which is D.

Q6	C

The answer here is clear: '*to avert this disaster we need to develop worldwide seed banks with detailed catalogues...Farmers can then begin to trial crops*' hence C is correct.

Q7	C

Lay out the information given in the top paragraph about what each share was worth each day:
Monday: £1
Tuesday: £1.20
Wednesday: £x - we are using x as the question doesn't tell us what this is worth.
Thursday: £1.25x
Friday: £1
We know Helen bought 1000 shares on Monday, and if she sells them on Thursday and makes £350 this means 1.25x = £1350. Solving for x gives £1080 for 1000 shares. So, each share is worth £1.08 on Wednesday as this is when shares equal £x.
Having worked this out, we can see that on Tuesday £3000 worth of shares will equate to £3000/£1.20 shares which is 2500 shares. This will be worth 2500 x £1.08 on Wednesday which is £2700. As Paul initially bought £3000 worth of shares and then made £2700, he has a loss of £300.

Q8	B

We have no information on A as nothing is said about those who are released after half of their sentence has elapsed. B is correct because it is a mistake to send offenders to prison when they could be given a non-custodial sentence because the text clearly says at the end of the second paragraph that '*they are less likely to end up back in prison if the judge gives them a community service order rather than a prison sentence*'. C is wrong, this can't be asserted because for all we know young offenders may deserve their time in prison and the data doesn't comment on this. D cannot be inferred because the table in Study 1 only shows reoffending rates up to 9 years, and this has not hit 100%. E is wrong because this is not supported by the data in the passage at all.

Q9	D

As the data in the Study 1 table is cumulative, read across to 5 years and subtract the percentage for reoffending after 1 year from this giving 66% - 44% = 22%. 22% of the 50,000 participants is 11000.

Q10	A

A is correct because if the offenders with prison sentences don't normally have consideration for a non-custodial sentence like community service then they can't possibly have a chance to even try a non-custodial sentence. B is wrong as whether they are first-time offenders or not has no bearing on the matter as this isn't mentioned in the passage. C is wrong because if you had a prison sentence but most had already served a non-custodial sentence, then this would not explain why 55% of offenders released from a short prison sentence reoffended; because this should surely be lower if they had already gone through a non-custodial sentence. D is wrong because the third paragraph details how *'people who get a suspended sentence are 9% less likely to reoffend'* and this still doesn't explain the discrepancy in figures that the question asks for.

Q11	E

B, C and D can be eliminated because these are not supported by data in the passage at all. A is incorrect because if most of the offenders had received a prison sentence then the effect of restorative justice *'instead of being sent to prison'* as the question says, cannot be measured because the offenders would already have been to prison. E is correct because giving offenders community service orders *'reduces reoffending rates by 6%'* and subjecting them to restorative justice reduces reoffending according to government analysis by *'a more conservative 14%'*. 6% + 14% = 20%

Q12	D

Any possible score would be the sum of a combination of 9, 5 and 3 taking away a multiple of 2 if they finished after 30 minutes. The score of 22 for the Crosswords can be made up of a 9, 5, 5, 3. The Jigsaws' 21 can be made of 9, 9, 5, -2. The Rubiks' 24 can be made from 9, 5, 5, 5. The Tangrams' 25 can be made from 9, 9, 5 and 3. This leaves the Solitaires who's score can't be possible.

Q13	D

A is not correct because it uses strong language. It doesn't say some or a few, it simply assumes that all young football fans cannot distinguish from right and wrong; and in addition, the difference between right and wrong is incredibly broad whereas the footballer's crimes could be something very niche. B is wrong because this does not support the argument, there could be lots of people in high profile jobs and the argument states that people with high profile jobs should not be rehabilitated into society. C is wrong because we don't have any data on other sports; the argument doesn't even mention other sports. D is correct, the assumption is that the rights of the individual to rehabilitation is lesser than the risks of promoting less than ideal behaviour to young people in society. E is wrong because the argument doesn't ask anyone to accept the risks posed to their careers, it simply says there is no second chance for those with high profile jobs.

Q14	B

List the colours we need and the ratio of the sub-colours (if applicable) to make up their percentage as listed in the question.
Brown - 30% split R:B:Y in a 10%:10%:10% ratio
Red - 20%
Blue - 10%
Yellow - 10%
Orange - 10% split R:Y in a 5%:5% ratio
Purple - 10% split R:B in a 5%:5% ratio
Green 10% split in a B:Y 5%:5% ratio

Summing the total red percentage gives 10% + 20% + 5% + 5% = 40%
We know 20ml is left over from a 100ml bottle so 40% clearly equates to 80ml. This means 10% equates to 20ml.

The question asks for the remaining blue so we can work out how much blue is used and subtract this from 100ml.

The total blue % is 10% + 10% + 5% + 5% = 30% which is 60ml.
100-60 = 40ml left over.

Q15	A

The answer to this is quite clear in the argument: '*If we accept that it is ethical to test on primates rather than humans, such research could be done using primates*'. We already know that lesions can be created in primate brains so it may be possible to develop treatments for brain disorders hence why A is correct.

Q16	D

We know that there is a total of 16 girls (including Maisy) and 10 boys coming to a total of 26 pupils. Of the girls, 6 have sisters (we know this as if 3 have younger sisters, the younger sisters therefore have older sisters, so we need to double 3) and 2 have brothers. Of the boys, 4 have brothers (again we need to double 2 older ones with younger brothers with the same reasoning) and 2 have sisters. This leaves a total of 14 pupils accounted so 26 -14 = 12 which must be the pupils with no brothers or sisters.

Q17	A

B is incorrect because the argument only refers to research on women and makes no comparison to men at all. C is incorrect because the argument states that this blood test could provide a '*more accurate diagnosis*' but does not in doing so imply that a blood test is the only method of diagnosis. D is wrong because the research is concerned with diagnosis using a blood test, and therefore has no comment to pass on the efficacy of treatment at all. E is wrong because again, we have no reference to men and no reference to women themselves under-seeking medical help. By elimination we come to A which is also the most sensible because it confirms that you can't assert that a woman could start treatment earlier to reduce the risk of a further heart attack if essentially the same number of women are having heart attacks, it's just the distribution of old and recent attacks has become more pronounced.

2015 Section 1

Q18	E

42 spans = 42 x 8 = 336 points
36 beats = 36 x 5 = 180 points
This leaves a remainder of 204 points that were scored as tips as when you subtract the span and beat point totals from 720 you get 204. The pie chart is in terms of points, so we want the following ratio: Spans : Beats : Tipsin a 336 : 280 : 204 ratio so we want the spans to have the largest wedge. This immediately eliminates B, D and F. 336 is less than half of 720 so it's wedge will also be under half hence why E is correct because for A and C the span wedge is too large.

Q19	C

If 330ml is equal to 9 lumps, then 2000/330 is roughly equal to 6. 6 lots of 9 is 54 lumps.

Q20	C

Teenagers currently consume 150% of their recommended sugar amount as the second paragraph says, '*teenagers consume 50% more...than is currently recommended*'. 30% of this 150% is supplied by soft drinks; this is 45% of the total sugar intake as 30% x 150% = 45%. If as the question says, teenagers consume only a third of this with the new tax that means they only consume 15% of what is supplied by sugary drinks. So now the 30% contribution of sugary drinks of the new total amount consumed (x) can be expressed as below:
30% (x) = 15%. Solving for x gives 120%. This means the sugar intake is 20% greater than the recommended daily intake.

Q21	C

First, we need to work out what the 10% reduction in sales of sugary drinks would be 90% of 5.727 million litres which works out at 5 154300000. If there is a £20p tax per litre and there are 5.1543 million litres we need to essentially divide this figure by 5 to work out the total revenue from tax (as 20p x 5 = £1). This gives £1031 million.

Q22	A

A is the most sensible answer that highlights how if retailers reduce their purchase price, the sugary drinks would still be relatively cheap to buy so the tax would be rendered ineffective. B is wrong because food tax is not related to this. C D and E don't actually refer to sales tax or volume tax specifically, so they don't even provide anything related to what the question is asking.

Q23	E

One way to do this is to think about the 6 attractions and their location to the hotel in the centre. Radially we can see that the furthest attractions away are the Palace and the Tower so we can already eliminate the other shorter options and if you find this question challenges you now have a 50% of guessing the answer correctly if you are running out of time!
If not, it would be logical for the tourist to travel to the Courts first as this is the shortest distance away (60m) and from here the options are either going to the Palace or the Fountain; but there is no point going to the Palace because going there means a 90m walk to the Tower and then a 110m walk from the Tower to the Castle, which is very long. Whereas, going to the Fountain means going another 80m to the Arch and from there 90m to the Castle. This is shorter by 40m. The Castle-Tower distance and the Tower-Hotel (and Palace-Hotel distance incidentally) are the same so there is no point including them in the calculation.
So, to check we have picked a route adding to 530m:
Hotel to Courts: 60m. Courts to Fountain: 80m. Fountain to Arch: 80m. Arch to Castle: 90m. Castle to Tower 110m. Tower back to the hotel is 110m. The sum of this is 530m. So, the Palace is not visited.

Q24	B

1 and 2 are incorrect as reduction in sleep quality and duration doesn't directly weaker what is said in the passage, and 2 isn't related to sleep so these 2 taken together do not weaken the argument. 1 and 3 however do weaken the argument because lack of sleep is mentioned in 1 and 3 shows how this can cause lack of focus and poor memory which weakens the passage when it says that *'caffeine can boost the effectiveness of short-term memory'* by counteracting such a claim. 2 and 4 are incorrect because these 2 contradict each other, on the one hand caffeine withdrawal can cause headaches, and then moderate caffeine consumption has limited effects. 4 actually supports the argument, not weakens it! 3 and 5 are wrong as headaches and memory haven't been shown to have a connection in the argument so together these don't weaken the argument.

Q25	F

We can label the places as A to F from left to right for reference. We start with - 8 - - - - and then we are told that the passcode written as 3 2-digit numbers adds to 80. The only way of adding to get a multiple of 10 is to make 10 or 20 with the last digits of each 2-digit number i.e. D and F (as we can only use numbers 1-9 inclusive). However, we can't make 10 with the 8 because this would require 1 and 1 and we have to have 6 different numbers. This means we need to make 20-8=12 out of the remaining numbers. We could use 3 and 9 or 5 and 7. (4 and 8 aren't possible because we've already used an 8; and 6 and 6 aren't possible again because we need different numbers.)
We are then told that when written as 2 three-digit numbers the total is 800. This means that C and F must add again to make 0. Out of the options 3 9 5 and 7 our only option is for F to be 7. This is the only option that allows F and D to add to 12 (as D is 5) and it is also the only option where C and F (i.e. 3 and 7) can add to 10.

2015 Section 1

Q26	C

B can be eliminated because the argument does not make the assumption at all. D is also wrong because public health isn't mentioned anywhere in the argument. E is also wrong because it is extremely generic and not specific to the argument at all. This leaves us with A and D. A is wrong because it mentions a balanced diet, but there is no evidence that *'the tastes our grandparents enjoyed'* were indeed the tastes of a balanced diet. Hence C is correct by elimination because it is the assumption made when the passage says, *'now that this research has been discredited'*.

Q27	C

Set out the bounds:
Laptop computer: 55% to 65%
Mobile phone: 70% to 80%
Neither: 0% to 5%
Add the lower bounds and subtract 100%:
55% + 70% + 0% - 100% = 25%
65% + 80% + 5% -100% = 50%
Hence between 25% and 50% owned both a laptop and computer.

Q28	A

B, D and E can be eliminated because essentially, they don't really say anything relevant to the argument. This leaves A and C. C however actually wouldn't weaken the argument because the conclusion is that working hours need to be more flexible, but this isn't the same as changing shift patterns. A however gets to the heart of the problem; if melatonin follows people's behavioural patterns then employees shouldn't have flexible working hours because it is up to them to change their behavioural patterns as clearly these aren't caused by the hormone melatonin if A is true.

Q29	A

To work out the area that needs painting total the 4 walls and then take off the area of the door and the window. 2 of the walls have dimensions: 5m x 2.5m = 12.5m^2 each so 25m^2 total. This is the wider wall which will be painted in 1 colour. The other two walls have dimensions 4m x 2.5m = 10m^2 each so 20m^2 total. We have to take off the area of the door (2m x 1m = 2m^2) and the window opposite the door (1.5m x 2m = 3m^2) giving 15m^2 in the other colour.
For the wider walls painting in high quality would require 2 coats so 50m^2. This is equivalent to 4 pots of paint as 50/15 = 3.3... which has to be rounded up because you can't buy partial pots of paint. 4 pots of HQ paint costs £60. In the cheaper paint it would require 3 coats so 75m^2 which is equivalent to 5 pots of paint at £11 each. This comes to £55 which is cheaper than the HQ paint.
For the narrower walls painting in high quality requires 2 coats so 30m^2 which is equivalent to 2 pots of paint costing £30 in total. For them to be in low quality they require 3 coats so 45m^2. This is equivalent to 3 pots of lower quality paint which would cost £33. In this instance the HQ paint is actually cheaper.
Summing the 2 cheapest alternatives per colour gives £55 + £30 = £85.

Q30	D

A would weaken the argument as financial reward wouldn't carry sufficient motivation to incentivise the newly qualified doctors. B is wrong because although it could be true it doesn't strengthen the argument which is trying to get people to work in A&E, and not deter them. C is wrong because the argument's conclusion is about financial incentives not reducing the number of people using A&E services. D is correct because it is directly about the conclusion of the argument about financial incentives. E has no relevance to the conclusion of the argument.

Q31	B

We know the dies have 1 2 3 4 5 6 on them so they have to sum 21 spots each. The die that is shown must have the following pairs in order for no pair to add to 7.
3 must be opposite 1 to total 4.
5 must be opposite 6 to total 11.
4 must be opposite 2 to total 6.

This means the second die can't have these totals: 4, 6 or 11.

If we go down the answer list:
A: If 2 opposes 1 then the total for that pair is 3. 3 opposing 6 gives 9. 21 - 9 - 3 = 9 but we can't have two pairs adding to 9 as the question says they all have different totals.
B: 2 opposing 1 gives 3. 4 opposing 6 gives 10. This gives a remainder of 8 from 21 which is possible hence B is correct.
C: 4 opposing 1 gives 5. 2 opposing 6 gives 8. 21 - 8 - 5 = 8. But we can't have 2 8s.
D: 4 opposing 1 gives 5. 3 opposing 6 gives 9. 21 - 5 - 9 = 7 but we can't total 7 as in the question.
E: 5 opposing 1 gives 6. 2 opposing 6 gives 8. 21 - 6 - 8 = 7 but we can't total 7; nor can we have a total of 6 as this has been taken up by the other die.
F: 5 opposing 1 gives 6. 4 opposing 6 gives 10. 21 - 6 - 10 = 5 but we still can't have 6 as a total as this has been taken up by the other die as well.

Q32	G

1 is correct because just totalling the defendants convicted gives 4265 which is on average 98% of the total defendants as the prosecution success rate is about 98% averaged across all 3 years. If 4265 is 98% then 100% is over 4300 as it is 4352.
2 is correct because those acquitted would be the 2.1% that weren't prosecuted in 2012. 2.1% of 1552 is 32.6 which is over 30.
3 is correct because the total prison sentences imposed on individuals is 88 + 86 + 74 = 248. The suspended prison sentences total 538. If the suspended sentences made up ⅔ of all sentences then the individual sentences :suspended sentences is 1:2 to give the relevant fraction. We can see that 538 is clearly more than double 248 so 3 is also correct.

Q33	B

In England and Wales minus the North in 2013 the total was 1371-566 = 805. The trend in England and Wales was a decrease in 11.7% in convictions from 2012 to 2013. We are told in the North of England that convictions were at 531 in 2012. If they fell in line with the overall trends for England and Wales we need to calculate an 11.7% decrease of 531 which is the same as 88.3% of 531 which comes to 469 in 2013.
Summing 469 and 805 gives 1274.

Q34	C

1 is not correct, the inference cannot be supported, we only know how many convictions were in West Yorkshire in 2013, we have no 2012 information.
2 is incorrect because just like the above argument, we have no idea what the West Yorkshire numbers were in 2012 so we cannot comment on the change in convictions.
3 is correct because we are told 566 convictions were in the North out of 1371 as a whole. ⅖ of 1371 is 548 and 566 is clearly greater than 548.

Q35	B

weaken the view that northerners are less cruel to animals than southerners; essentially, we need to show that northerners are '*more cruel*'.
A won't do this because it actually supports a hypothesis presented in the reader's comments that more complaints could be because northerners are more concerned and hence aren't more cruel.
B is correct because an increase in proportion of convictions does show '*more cruelty*'.
C is incorrect because the fact that there are more animals in the North would justify more convictions because the convictions per animal could end up being relatively similar.
D is incorrect because it supports the reader and does not weaken their point.
E is incorrect because it doesn't even get to the core of the argument which is that there is a discrepancy between the North and South. This means the inference could be interpreted in the reader's favour which does not weaken their position.

Authors' tip

Make sure you read the question carefully - is it asking you to see which statement most weakens the conclusion, most strengthens the conclusion, or is it asking for a flaw or assumption.

2015 Section 2

Q1	E

The reflex arc is known to consist of:
Stimulus - receptor - sensory neuron - CNS (relay neurone across) - motor neuron - effector
Therefore, A is correct because this is the function of the sensory neuron. B is correct because a muscle is an effector and their cells do contract. C is correct because this is the function of a motor neuron. D is correct because relay neurons do this function. E is incorrect because the impulse goes across the CNS via a relay neuron, not from the brain to the relay neuron.

Q2	C

We know alkenes will decolourise bromine water due to the presence of a C=C bond and 1 is ethene so will decolourise bromine water. Don't get caught out for 2, although it has "propene" in the name, we know poly(alkenes) are in fact alkanes because the double bond is broken so that the repeating unit can be joined together. 3, if you draw it out, is 2-methylpropene and is an alkene so will decolourise bromine water. 4 is iodoethane which is an alkane so will not decolourise bromine water.

Q3	B

We know that black is the best absorber and emitter of infrared radiation so we can immediately eliminate all other answers but A and B. The better colour of clothes to keep a person warm in winter would be white because it will reflect heat back onto the person and won't emit heat well from the person as in winter. The amount of heat absorbed doesn't matter because it's Winter so it's unlikely to be warm outside.

Q4	B

If we draw a simple tree diagram to illustrate the probabilities, we can easily work out the probability of 2 black beads. Simply multiply down the black branches: ⅜ x 2/7 = 3/28 hence B is the correct answer.

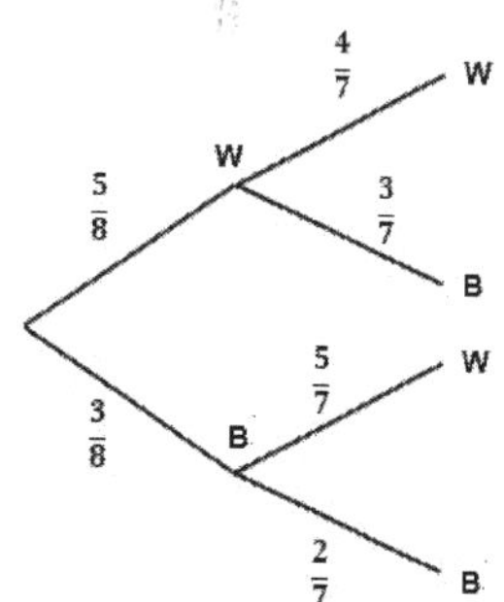

Authors' tip:

We recommend that you draw diagrams (such as tree diagrams) for probability questions to help make solving them easier

2015 Section 2

Q5	A

We know that in anaerobic respiration we take glucose and form lactic acid, with no oxygen used, no CO_2 formed, and no water formed. This is just a factual recall question.

Q6	A

To do this, we can just identify the change in energy from reactants to products, as shown on the diagram and reverse the sign of it to obtain the change in energy from products to reactants. So, reactants to products is a, so products to reactants is -a.

Q7	D

The power remains the same but because P = IV if current decreases I must increase to keep P the same so current increases.

Q8	E

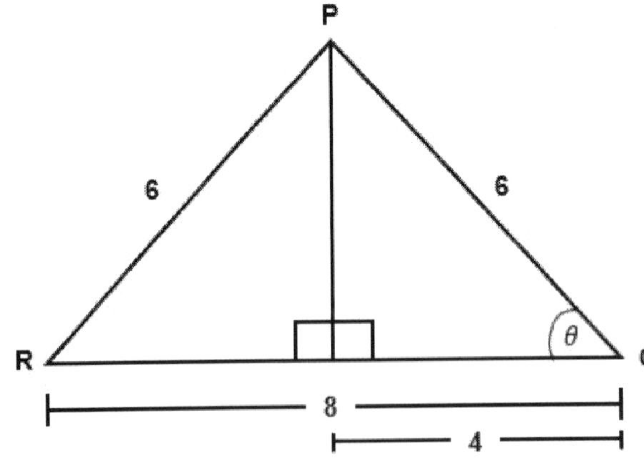

Using Pythagoras, we can work out the distance from P to the midpoint of RQ. as $a^2 + b^2 = c^2$ then $4^2 + b^2 = 6^2$ so $b = \sqrt{20}$

Working out tanθ =

opp/adj = $\sqrt{20}/4$

$= (\sqrt{5} \times \sqrt{4})/4 = 2\sqrt{5}/4$

We can cancel the 2

giving $\sqrt{5}/2$

Q9	D

The key here is to recognise that the white mouse must be homozygous recessive i.e. cc because all of its offspring are black. This means that mouse 1 (which we are told is homozygous in the question) must be homozygous dominant; meaning all of their offspring are Cc.

This means that Mouse 1 (genotype CC) crossed with Mouse 2 (genotype Cc) gives a Punnett square like the one on the right.

This gives a 100% black offspring, 50% homozygous dominant, 50% heterozygous hence why D is correct.

Mouse 2

Mouse 1	C	c
C	CC	Cc
C	CC	Cc

Q10	D

A is incorrect because the electrolysis will actually produce rubidium metal and H_2 gas because rubidium is more reactive than hydrogen. The melting point of the alkali metals decreases down the group as the ions get larger so the distance between the outer electrons and the positive nucleus gets larger thus reducing the attraction between the two. This means B is incorrect. C is incorrect because reactivity increases down the group as the outer electron is more easily lost, so rubidium will actually react faster with water than sodium. D is correct because alkali metals need to be stored in oil so they cannot be oxidised or react with water. E is incorrect because rubidium ions have a 1+ charge, whereas sulfate ions have a 2- charge. Thus, the formula would be Rb_2SO_4 not $RbSO_4$.

Q11	A

This questions tests knowledge not currently on the BMAT specification.
1 is correct because neutrons released can indeed go on to catalyse further fissions. 2 is incorrect, the half-life is the time taken for the radioactive nuclei in a sample to halve in number. 3 is incorrect, this is actually fusion not fission.

Q12	B

Simply substitute a positive whole number in for X. I will use 3. So, a = ⅜. B = 6/5 and c = 9/8. We can see that $a<c<b$ so B is correct. You may also try using other positive integers to check that G is not the case, but you will soon see that B holds.

Q13	B

The human will have less urine because it is a hot day so more water will be reabsorbed as the person will be sweating more. This increase in water reabsorption means the water mass in urine decreases. The urea mass remains the same because urea is still a toxic substance that needs to be removed from the body and it won't be absorbed.

Q14	C

A is incorrect, the general formula of a cycloalkane is C_nH_{2n}. B is incorrect because cycloalkanes do not contain a C=C double bond so they can't react with bromine water. C is correct, cycloalkanes are saturated because they don't contain any C=C bonds, only C-C single bonds. D is incorrect, complete combustion results in CO_2 and H_2O not H_2. E is incorrect, cycloalkanes are in a homologous series because each member differs by CH_2 and there are similar chemical properties. F is incorrect, this is a simple covalent structure.

Q15	A

You can work out net horizontal force as 10N to the right (50N-40N) and as F = ma then a = F/m = 10N/2kg = $5ms^{-2}$.
The net vertical force is 5N upwards and so the upwards acceleration is F/m = 5/2 = $2ms^{-2}$.

Q16	E

What you may find to be an easier way of answering this question is to make the denominator of the ratio the same to make calculation easier. By making the denominator 15 we have A:B:C as 15:10:12. Thus if C is £3000 then 12/37 is £3000. The total amount collected would be £3000/12 x 37 = £250 x 37 = £9250

2015 Section 2

Q17	H

Number 1 in the diagram is photosynthesis which requires neither type of stated enzyme. Number 2 corresponds to consumption which needs digestive enzymes. Number 3 is decomposition which needs digestive enzymes. Number 4 is respiration which needs respiratory enzymes.

Q18	C

A is incorrect as a catalyst speeds up the rate of reaction. B is incorrect because T is a gas so it being a powder i.e. in the solid state would not speed up the reaction. C is correct because a higher activation energy would actually make more of the backwards reaction take place as opposed to the forwards reaction because the forwards reaction is exothermic so applying a high activation energy would cause the reaction to counter the change by moving in the endothermic reaction to reduce the temperature/amount of energy. D is incorrect, again increasing temperature means more of the backwards reaction according to Le Chatelier's principle. E is incorrect because there is an equal number of moles on both sides of the reaction and they are all gaseous, so at a constant temperature the volume of gases on both sides will be exactly the same, so the gas volume will not change at all during the reaction.

Q19	G

Set up a full equation showing what goes on:
${}^{V}_{W}M - {}^{0}_{-1}\beta = N_X - {}^{4}_{2}\alpha = {}^{Y}Q$
As we can see this means X is equal to W - - 1 =W+1and Y is equal to V-4 hence why G is correct.

Q20	D

Set up an equation showing what is going on:
We want to show how the new mean (m-2) has been calculated. This will be the sum of the total score plus the other pupil who scored n divided by the total number of people. The sum of the total score is nm (i.e. the mean multiplied by the number of people taking the test) and adding n gives our numerator. The denominator is the new total number of people which is n+1.
(nm + n)/(n+1) = m-2
Rearranging this equation for n can be done as follows:
Multiply both sides by (n+1) giving nm + n = nm +m -2n -2
Collecting terms gives 3n = m-2
Dividing by 3 gives n = (m-2)/3 which is D.

Q21	A

1 is correct, bacteria have double helical DNA and white blood cells have double helical DNA. 2 is incorrect, whilst bacteria may possess a cell wall, human white blood cells do not because they are animal cells. 3 is incorrect, bacteria do not possess membrane-bound organelles, so they don’t have nuclei, their DNA is often in the form of plasmids and 1 long loop of DNA. 4 is correct, animal cells and therefore white blood cells have a cell membrane and bacteria possess a cell membrane as well.

Q22	C

The Cl^- ion has 18 electrons, the Cl^+ ion has 16 electrons, Ar has 18 electrons, K^+ has 18 electrons, Ca^+ has 19 electrons, K^- has 20 electrons. Hence C is correct.

Q23	D

The time from $20ms^{-1}$ to rest is double the reaction time (1.4s) plus 3.3s. So, the distance for the first 1.4 seconds will be speed x time for this portion which is $20ms^{-1}$ x 1.4s = 28m. Then the brakes are applied, and the car decelerates uniformly so the average speed is the (initial speed + final speed)/2 = $20ms^{-1}/2$ = $10ms^{-1}$. This means the distance = $10ms^{-1}$ x 3.3s = 33m. Adding the two distances gives 28m + 33m = 61m

Q24	D

Do the operations by finding a common denominator which is (2x-3)(2x+3).

This gives $\frac{(2x+3)^2 + (2x-3)^2 - 2(2x+3)(2x-3)}{(2x+3)(2x-3)}$

Expanding the brackets gives: $\frac{4x^2 + 12x + 9 + 4x^2 - 12x + 9 - 8x^2 + 18}{(2x+3)(2x-3)}$

Simplifying gives $\frac{36}{(2x-3)(2x+3)}$ which is D

Q25	G

We are told the male X:A ratio is 0.5:1 which can be expressed using integers as 1:2.
The X:A ratio for females is 1:1.
So going across the headings of the table from left to right:
We can see that XAA shows a 1:2 X:A ratio which expresses a male.
XYAA also shows a 1:2 X:A ratio which expresses a male.
XXAA shows a 1:1 X:A ratio which expressed a female.
XXYAA also shows a 1:1 X:A ratio which expresses a female.
XXYYAA also shows a 1:1 X:A ratio which expresses a female.

Q26	B

The reacting moles of methane = mass/Mr = 1.6/16 = 0.1moles
This means 0.2 moles of oxygen will react as methane: oxygen molar ratio is 1:2. So we can work out the mass of oxygen reacting and take this away from 8.00g of oxygen as we are told in the question is the initial excess mass.
The mass = Mr x moles = 32 x 0.2 = 6.4g.
8g-6.4g = 1.6g of unreacted oxygen.

Q27	D

F = ma so F = 4kg x $1.25ms^{-2}$ = 5N. Thus statement 1 is correct.
Wave Speed = frequency x wavelength = 4Hz x 1.25m = $5ms^{-1}$ so statement 2 is correct.
V = IR so V = 1.25A x 5Ω = 6.25V 6.25 V does not equal the 4V that is applied so this is incorrect.

2015 Section 3

To see the marking grid and mark bands that the BMAT examiners will use to mark your essays, please refer to the BMAT website.

"Computers are useless. They can only give you answers." (Pablo Picasso)

To see the question in full, please see: https://www.admissionstesting.org/Images/310869-specimen-bmat-2015-past-paper-section-3.pdf

Picasso may be referring to the ability of computers to offer a series of outputs for functional inputs and he may be highlighting the limitation of such an action: only the answer is supplied; the computer cannot come up with its own inputs or indeed its own set of functions. This is a human-made concept and not what a computer can do itself.

- Many people would disagree with this statement on the grounds of finding so many questions and thought-provoking statements on the internet for example, which is one of the applications present on many "computers" today. Indeed, Tim Berners-Lee who created the World Wide Web would probably be credited with making an accessible bank of information that sparks curiosity and challenges humans to come up with questions and intrigue. For example, digital artists can test the limit of their creativity using computers as a tool for expressing their artform. Much like Picasso except through the use of a different medium they would argue that the computer doesn't give an answer but rather a host of creative tools that provokes questions to which their artistry can supply a kind of answer through their artwork.
- Computers and technology also serve a variety of (arguably essential) functions in daily life, with examples including communication (on mobile phones, etc and through video-calling), navigation, online banking, business and commerce (many businesses operate online only presences, and computers are used for online shopping etc.). In medical fields, computers have revolutionised the quality of treatment provided, and helped improve care given, such as through showing HR and breathing rates on computer monitors, to organising patient data, and allowing the sharing of medical information between medical experts worldwide.

- Technology has current limits in the scope of what it can achieve today. For example all things need to obey the laws of nature in the universe, so we cannot (at least as far as hypothesising goes) construct a device that will travel faster than the speed of light, because this is a limit of the universe.
- Technology could be argued to be inequitable in its use and as such is limited because of how it can be manipulated by those who possess enough knowledge of computer science to control media and actions. You could use the example of censorship in China to illustrate this.
- Technology is also limited because those who are literate in its languages and well-educated in it are arguably a rather small number of people.
- Economically, technology is limited in its distribution; in lower income countries there is a limit to the scope of research and in the provision of technology; from material building technology to computer technology.

"That which can be asserted without evidence, can be dismissed without evidence." (Christopher Hitchens)
To see the question in full, please see: https://www.admissionstesting.org/Images/310869-specimen-bmat-2015-past-paper-section-3.pdf

Hitchens is arguing that the assertion of a statement, i.e. saying that something is the case, is utterly invalid if you cannot back it up with empirical data. He means that unless you have this evidence, your statement is void.

- Many rational philosophers would disagree strongly with Hitchens' claim. For example, take the assertion that a circle cannot be a square. This just is. We can't evidence such claims because they aren't up for testing empirically. They either obey the rational laws of logic or they do not and therefore many mathematicians would also agree that some assertions do not require evidence.
- Many religious people would also disagree such as those who do not need evidence for a God/deities in order to believe in them. It could be seen as offensive to propose the idea that evidence of an omnipotent, omniscient, omnibenevolent God (to use the Christian God) needs to justify His existence with evidence; and on a logical front these supernatural qualities could be seen as incompatible with the natural world we live in. Even if God tried to evidence himself, there is no telling that we as humans would be able to interpret such evidence correctly.

You may argue that Hitchens' line of argument is useful, but it is limited. It has use because it reminds us not to take assertions as gospel unless we see an evidence basis for these that we can judge and test as we please to attempt to validate such an assertion. This is important in our world of checks and balances because we need to test what people claim in order to consider it as somewhat useful. However, it does also fall short by the reasoning that we need evidence for absolutely everything. Take the assertion of "I love you". How are you supposed to evidence this in a way that is truly representative of the emotion you feel? There is an element of this evidencing that doesn't feel natural or organic to the concept of humanity.

2015 Section 3

'When treating an individual patient, a physician must also think of the wider society.'

To see the question in full, please see: https://www.admissionstesting.org/Images/310869-specimen-bmat-2015-past-paper-section-3.pdf

The reasoning of this statement is that it is vital that a doctor considers the balance of treating an individual patient and being constructive towards society well. This concept of balance could be applied to the allocation of resources, time and energy.
An example of when a physician should consider wider society is when treating a patient with a severely contagious disease, e.g. Ebola, doctors should also think about wider society by ensuring the patient is appropriately quarantined.

- A doctor should only consider the individual they are treating because that is how they can offer patient-centred care that is of the highest quality whilst facing minimal distractions from others so that their judgement is clear and suited to the situation of the patient. If this isn't the case, and a more paternalistic and less case-specific type of medicine is given then arguably this will not be helpful for each individual patient.
- In addition, by only considering the individual's clinical needs instead of society's view on what healthcare should be provided for a patient (such as if they were a smoker or an alcoholic and society at the time didn't wish to pay taxpayer money for people with arguably "self-inflicted diseases" to receive treatment) the quality of care given is unbiased and equal. It also renders the profession less discriminatory and upholds the value of care in all scenarios which is arguably a more preferable moral standpoint.
- A doctor's job is to treat the individual, so their main priority should be their patient. Therefore, the doctor should focus on the best and quickest method of treatment, instead of its potential impacts on society, fulfilling the ethical principle of beneficence as doctors should do all in their power (that is legal!) to help their patient.

In some cases, the wishes of an individual could conflict with those of wider society.

- A patient could want to refuse a full course of antibiotics when they have been prescribed, which is not in the interest of the wider population because failure to follow this advice generally leads to a rise in antibiotic resistance. This would be detrimental as when those with very serious infections needed treatment, the antibiotics would be ineffective.
- A patient can also be opposed to vaccination such as those who didn't wish for their children to have the MMR vaccine in the early 21st century at the time there was a paper alleging a link between the vaccine and the prevalence of autism (since shown to be incorrect). This reduces the chance of herd immunity for the population which means the most vulnerable in society will not be protected from measles, mumps or rubella.

Question 4 was written to widen access to the exam paper, as in the past, students hoping to study Veterinary Medicine would also have to take the BMAT. VetMed students no longer take the BMAT, and so in its current iteration (2017 onwards), there are none of these questions, so the authors have not included worked essays for these and recommend that you only attempt these after having attempted all the previous one.

BMAT 2016

Section 1

Q1	D

The most efficient way to answer this question is to first complete the table and then work out the probabilities.

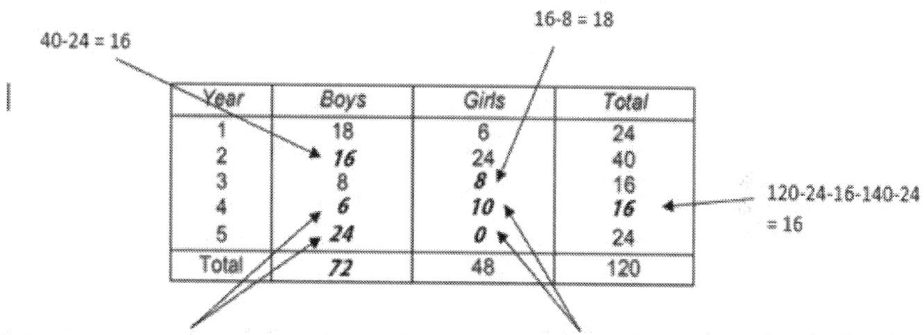

Year	Boys	Girls	Total
1	18	6	24
2	*16*	24	40
3	8	*8*	16
4	*6*	*10*	*16*
5	*24*	*0*	24
Total	*72*	48	120

P(Y4 student selected at random is a boy) = 6/16 = ⅜ = D

Q2	B

B is the correct answer as the text states that peat has also been burned releasing carbon dioxide, but only carbon dioxide from burnt plants can be taken back up '*as the plants regrow*'. Therefore, some CO_2 (from the peat) will remain in the atmosphere. A is wrong as we do not know about the rest of the world - they may have dramatically reduced their emissions. C is incorrect as the text does not mention anything about whether next year's forest fires (if they occur) and the CO_2 they emit. D is wrong for similar reasons to A - other factors may be bigger culprits when it comes to emitting carbon dioxide.

Q3	B

John's first stay: \$50 + \$50 + \$40 + \$40 + \$40 = \$220. [*hotel room*] + 5 x \$5 [car park] = \$245.
John's second stay: 8 x \$40 = \$320 [*hotel room*] + (\$25 + \$5) [*car park*] = \$350
\$350-\$245 = \$105

Q4	B

This passage concludes that there is an innate difference between non-musicians and musicians, and this is the flaw as it does not take into account that musical training (which musicians have over non-musicians) can improve one's ability to synchronise to slow tempo.

2016 Section 1

Q5	A

First work out the scale that each axis is using, and which axis refers to which test. The X axis is practical scores and the y axis is written because practical scores have a narrower distribution. The x axis increases in increments of 5, whereas the y axis increases in increments of 10.
Next, go through the students given in the answer option, and you will see there is no point to represent Con (there is no point at 10 on the x axis and 52 on the y axis).

Q6	D

The conclusion in this text can be identified as '*If justice is not to be out of reach of the majority of the ordinary people, the government must think again*', which is paraphrased by D. A is not correct, as not all claims are affected, only those of £200,000 or more, therefore '*justice*' for everyone is not affected. B is not correct as the text says the fees will be increased, not introduced, meaning that there have always been fees (so technically it has always been a saleable object). C is not correct because the statement is too general and E is incorrect because it is too general, whereas the text's last line is more specific. (i.e. fairness and prosperity cover more than simply a fair society and a prosperous economy)

Q7	D

For the figures to be correct, in 2014 Paul must be 49 and in 2015 Paul must be 50, so different bands will have to be used. (a clue for this is that they have provided two columns, and also the only way that you can earn more and pay less tax is if your tax rules are different).
2014: In the 20% tax bracket, the maximum tax payable is $5000 (0.2 x $25,000). Therefore, the other $600 of his tax must come from the 30% tax bracket, where $600 is 30%. Therefore, his income in this bracket is $2,000. So, his total income is $9,000 [untaxable] + $25,000 [$5,000 tax] + $2,000 [$600 tax] = $36,0000
2015: He earned $38,000 ($36,000 + $2,000)

Q8	C

We have to use the number of products sold in that quarter (which Fig 1 shows us) and then multiply the number by the cost of each unit (which Fig 3 shows us). Therefore, for April - June, 800 of product 1 are sold (so 8 x £1500 = £12,000), 800 of product 2 are sold (so 8 x £200 = £16,000) and 800 of product 3 are sold (so 8 x £1500 = £12,000). [remember: the price is per 100 units)
So, £12,000 + £16,000 + £12,000 = £40,000

Q9	D

Product 2 was released in March, therefore from Fig 1 we can see that 900 units were sold in March. The question that ⅔ of its sales in March, April and May had been in March, so 800 = ⅔. Therefore, sales in May and June are ⅓ which is 450 units. Therefore, in June 350 units were sold (800-450). Each unit costs £2,000 so 3.5 x £2,000 [prices are per 100 units] = £7,000.

Q10	D

In November and December 600 units were sold (Fig 1). The cost per 100 units is £4,000. In December, £6,000 was generated from sales of product 6, meaning that 150 units were sold in December (6,000/4,000 = 1.5, then x 100 = 150). Therefore, in November 600-150 = 450 units were sold.

Q11	E

Let us come up with a table to help us solve this - Product 5 has the highest monthly sales.

Product	Number of units sold	Months that it has been on sale	Number of units sold per month
1	3000	12	(3000/12) = 250
2	3200	10	(3200/10) = 320
3	2600	8	(2600/8) = 325
4	1200	6	(1200/6) = 200
5	1400	4	**(1400/4) = 350**
6	600	2	(600/2) = 300

Q12	D

21:23 in Bolandia means 21 minutes to 11pm, i.e. 20:39 in conventional time
23:04 in Bolandia means 23 minutes 4am, i.e. 03:37 in conventional time.
The difference between these two times is therefore 4 hours 58 minutes.

Q13	A

The passage concludes that children with rich parents have high IQs, because rich parents tend to have jobs which require high intelligence. It then goes on to say that the study didn't take into account parental profession, and that if children of high earners in sport were found to have lower IQs, the conclusion would be that IQ is genetically inherited from the parents. However, this argument assumes then that rich sportsmen aren't highly intelligent, which is paraphrased by A. B is not assumed by the argument as children's education level isn't mentioned. C is not assumed as the text says that it hadn't looked at professions. D is not relevant to the argument.

Q14	D

For these questions, the best approach is to work out how much money she has in each month.
January: $1300, February: $1100, March: $1300, April: $1300, May: $1700, June: $1500
July: $1100, August: $1300, Sept: $1200, Oct: $1500, Nov: $1400, Dec: $1400
Therefore, she has more than $1300 in 5 months.

2016 Section 1

Q15	B

B is correct as it says '*those elderly people who have lead a 'brain friendly' lifestyle when younger are thought to have created extra synapses*', and therefore this increase in synapses means after accounting for natural loss of synapses with ageing, these people will have more synapses than normal. A is incorrect as the loss of synapses in old age occurs to everyone. C is incorrect as it is not entirely relevant to the conclusion (we're arguing about brain friendly lifestyles as opposed to methods to study cognitive performance). D is incorrect as quality of life isn't mentioned or referred to in the text. E is incorrect as it is not a conclusion of the passage, and so isn't relevant.

Q16	A

Draw a diagram if it helps you to visualise each player and who sits on their left and right. To work out how many coins each person has at the end, look at who sits on their right and left, and see how many coins they gave to the person. From the diagram below, we can see that Alun has the least amount of coins.

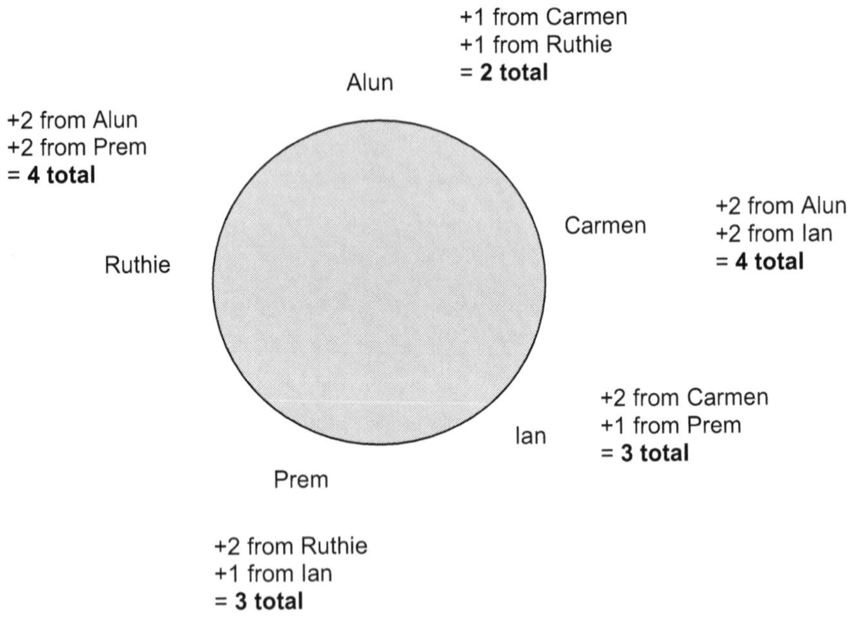

Q17	A

A is the only correct answer as it is the only one that would prevent over-prescription/use of this new antibiotic to prevent resistance, which is what the above argument is getting at. B, C and D may all be true but do not strengthen the argument as they are not relevant.

Q18	D

First work out the LTV. The person will have a £125,000 loan which is 83.3%, therefore mortgages 1 and 2 are not applicable to them. Let us work out how much it will cost for the first year for the remaining 3.
Mortgage 3: (0.05 x £125,000) = £6,250 [5% fixed] + £500 [fee] = £6750
Mortgage 4: (0.03 x £125,000) = £3,750 [2% + 1%] + £2000 [fee] = £5750
Mortgage 5: (0.04 x £125,000) = £5,000 [2% + 2%] + £1,000 [fee] = £6,000
Therefore, Mortgage 4 is the cheapest.

Q19	C

We have to use Texas' figures as a comparison. The number of Texan wells drilled in 2012 was approximately 40% of the 2005-11 figure (13,540 a/o to 33,753). Answer Option C is 40% of 2,694 [Oklahoma's number of wells drilled between 2005-11] and so is correct.

Q20	C

The amount of water used per well in Louisiana was (12,000 million gallons)/(2,327 + 139) ~ (12,000,000,000)/2500 = ~4,800,000 gallons per well.
The amount of water used per well in Utah was (590,000,000 gallons)/(1,336 + 765) ~ (600,000,000)/(2000) ~ 300,000 gallons per well
4,800,000 - 300,000 = 4,500,000 = C

Q21	E

1 - correct, since if 99.2% is 110,000 million gallons, then 0.8% is 880 million gallons. [see paragraph titled Chemicals used]. This paragraph also explains that the chemicals can also contaminate water supplies.
2 - incorrect, as 100,551,000/28 is 3,591,107 tonnes and not 36,000,000 tonnes.
3 - correct, as 26,000,000,000/200,000 = 130,000 gallons [see paragraph entitled water used, and the data for Colorado in the table].

Q22	H

1 is incorrect as consumption is not related to availability, as shown by the fact that Texas had the highest consumption yet being in a drought.
2 is incorrect as it does not explain how that technology development impacts the difference in water between the states.
3 is incorrect as like A consumption is not linked to availability, and also as shown on the table, water consumption per well varies.

Q23	D

D is correct as the square is inside both the triangles, with the right-angled triangles placed at such an angle to match the diagram. A is wrong as it is not possible to fit a square, B is incorrect because the two triangles will not fit, C is incorrect because the circle does not match the position of the circle of the middle triangle listed, E is incorrect because it is not possible to fit a square, as like A.

Q24	C

The argument claims that high impact walking is more effective in keeping weight down that conventional sports, because walking is a constant, uninterrupted activity, C is correct as it provides an alternative explanation for why sports players see a lower reduction in weight, which therefore weakens the argument that it is because sports tend to be more 'stop-start'. A is incorrect as age is irrelevant to the argument, B is incorrect as it does not focus on the crux of the argument, and D is irrelevant to the argument, as motivation is not discussed.

Q25	D

If there are 6 film showings (as each film is repeated twice, and there are 3 films), then there will be 5 intervals. Summing the film times, we get 117 + 109 + 119 = 345 minutes. We double this, since each film is shown twice, giving us 690 minutes of film, which is 11 hours and 30 minutes. The time gap between 10:15 and 22:45 is 12 hours and 30 minutes. Therefore, 12 hours and 30 minutes - 11 hours and 30 minutes = 60 minutes = total time of intervals. We know there are 5 intervals, so 60/5 = 12 minutes = the time of each interval.

Q26	B

The argument wrongly assumes that people become depressed and anxious after reading these books, whereas it could also be true that those who are depressed and anxious are more likely to read these books. This is paraphrased by B. A and D are irrelevant to the argument, C is incorrect as the text already notes this by saying that the people who read the books are '*more likely*' as opposed to being the only depressed/anxious people.

Q27	F

For this question, it is best to have a look at the table and pick a few select readings to calculate, as opposed to the whole table. To get the greatest difference in blood pressure, we know therefore that the systolic must be very high, and the diastolic must be very low. Looking at the table we can see that the lowest diastolic readings are at Mon pm (78) and at Thu pm (81), and the highest diastolic readings are at Sat pm and Tue am (163). Using these we get:
Mon pm: 145 - 78 = 67, Thu pm: 149 - 81 = 68, Sat pm: 165 - 99 = 66, Tue am: 163 - 96 = 67. Therefore, Thursday pm is correct, and the pulse then is 86.

Q28	D

The argument claims that cancer is more likely to be caused by extrinsic factors, and therefore people have some sort of control over this. The flaw in this logic is the assumption that people have some sort of control over the extrinsic factors, which is summarised by D. A is incorrect as the text does not assume this - it accepts that this study may not be definitive (*'If this study is to be believed'*). B is incorrect as the text states that only 75-90% of factors causing cancer are extrinsic, not all. C is incorrect as is not relevant to the argument.

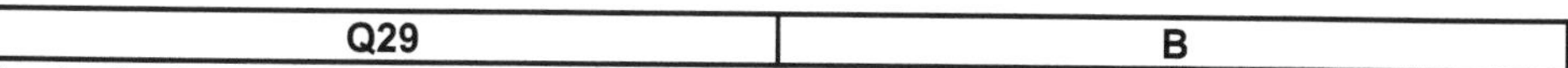

Q29	B

Again, for these kinds of questions, draw a diagram of what the question asks us. Remember that each subsequent time the string is folded, the number of strands doubles. From this we can see there are 7 marks between the two greens.

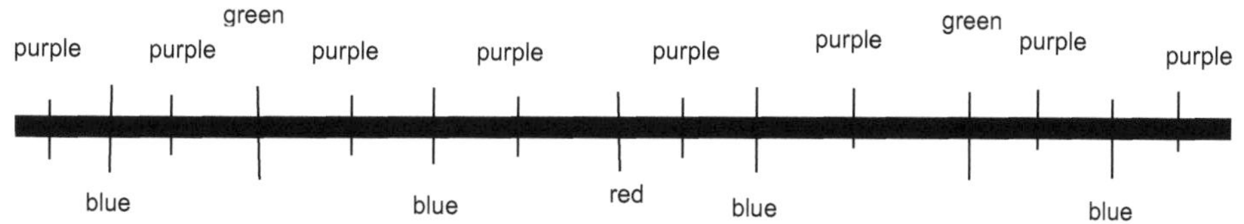

Q30	D

D is the answer here as the claims about the mind and the brain are not fully evidenced (*'if consciousness is just the result of the working of the brain'* - unwarranted claim). nor does the text prove that all machines are the same, or that the brain is like a normal machine.

Q31	D

For this question, let us work our way through the answer options. A - If the Argents scored 4 pales, they must have scored 2 fesses [total points score = 22]. The Sables would have scored 3 fesses and 3 pales [total points score = 27]. 27 is not one less than 22 so it cannot be A. Use this method for the other answer options, and you will see that D is the correct answer.

Q32	A

Imagine we had 100g of each oil (this would be a total of 200g in a 50:50 mixture). The table tells us that in 100g of oil, 10.0g of olive oil is polyunsaturated, and 65.7g of sunflower oil is polyunsaturated, so therefore in 200g of this mixture there is 75.7g of sunflower oil, which is roughly 37.9%.

Q33	A

The part of the text this question refers to is the end of the second paragraph. The text says that hunter-gatherers had a two-to-one ratio and is thus optimal. The assumption here is that hunter-gatherer diets are better for humans than modern ones, which is paraphrased by A.

Q34	B

This question requires using facts and figures from different parts of the data stimulus. A typical European consumes 143g of fat a day, 30% of which is from oil, therefore the grams of oil they consume a day is roughly 42g. Using the values in the table, in 100g of oil there is 0.6g of erucic acid which is 600mg. So, in 42g, there is (0.42 x 600) = 252mg of erucic acid. 252/500 ~ 50% which is closest to answer option B.

Q35	D

The table shows us that sunflower oil only contains omega-6, so all the omega-3 must come from the flaxseed oil. The ratio of omega 6:omega 3 in flaxseed oil is 0.2:1.
In 100g of flaxseed oil there is 53.3g of omega 3 and 12.7g of omega 6, but we need 106.6g of omega 6 in our mixture. Therefore (106.6 - 12.7) = 93.9g of omega 6 must come from sunflower oil. In 100g of sunflower oil there is 65.7g of omega 6, so roughly 150g of sunflower oil will be needed for 100g of flaxseed oil. Therefore, the proportion of flaxseed oil in the mixture is roughly 100/250 = 40% which is closest to answer option D (41%).

2016 Section 2

Q1	D

Vessel 1 is the vena cava because it has a larger internal lumen, and vessel 2 is the aorta because it has a smaller lumen. 3 is the renal vein because it attaches to the vena cava, and 4 is the renal artery because it comes off the aorta. 5 is the ureter. Urea is highest in the ureter, because the function of the kidney is to dispose of urea through the urine, so D is correct.

Q2	F

1 is incorrect because the element is in Group 3 (or 13), not 12, because of its 3 outer electrons. 2 and 3 are correct because the element would have a valency of 3+. 4 is correct since atomic number = number of protons = number of electrons = 2 + 8 + 3. 5 is incorrect because alkali metals only have 1 outer electron.

Q3	D

The mass of 250cm^3 of liquid and the scale is 170g, so the mass of one object is 470 - 170 = 300g. The volume of each object is (350-250)/2 = 50cm^3 as adding two objects increases the volume of the column of liquid from 250 to 350 cubic centimetres. Density is mass over volume, so the correct formula is 300/50 which is D.

Q4	A

A line that is parallel to another line will have the same gradient. Therefore to work out the gradient of the line between P and Q, we do $gradient = \frac{\Delta y}{\Delta x} = \frac{6}{9} = \frac{2}{3}$

The equation of a line is y = mx + c, where m is the gradient. Only line A has a gradient of $\frac{2}{3}$ so is correct.

Q5	B

W is a chromosome, X is a restriction enzyme, Y is also a restriction enzyme, and Z is DNA ligase, so B is correct.

Q6	E

A is correct as evaporating calcium carbonate will leave solid calcium carbonate.
B is correct, as fractional distillation is used to separate two liquids with different boiling points.
C is correct, as silicon dioxide is insoluble in water.
D is correct, as distillation is used to separate a solute from its solvent.
E is not correct, as ethanol is miscible in water, so a separating funnel can't be used.

Q7	D

1 - Isotopes have the same electronic configuration, and so have the same chemical properties.
2 - Isotopes have the same number of protons but different numbers of neutrons (if they had different numbers of protons, they would be different elements!)

3 - is incorrect as mass number ≠ number of neutrons.

Q8	B

75N is the total mass of N people. When J, K and L join, the total mass is 78(N + 3). J, K + L weigh together (3 x 90) = 270kg.
Therefore: 75N + 270 = 78(N+3), so 75N + 270 = 78N + 234, so 36 = 3N, so N = 12.

Q9	F

Statement 1 tells us that the enzymes must work in acidic conditions, which in the body are only found in the stomach. The pH of the mouth is neutral, and the pH of the pancreas and small intestine are alkaline, so F is the answer. Statement 2 tells us that it must be a protease (since proteins break down into amino acids). 3 does not help, as all these enzymes work at body temperature.

Q10	F

The mass number of an element is the top left number (the larger number). So, there are two nitrogens, 20 hydrogens (8 from $(NH_4)_2$ and 12 from $6H_2O$), 1 iron, 2 sulfurs, and 14 oxygens (8 from $(SO_4)_2$ and 6 from $6H_2O$). Therefore: the formula mass is:
(2 x 14) + (20 x 1) + (1 x 56) + (2 x 32) + (14 x 16) = 392.

Q11	B

Rotating the coil faster means the amplitude (more voltage is produced) and the frequency (more rotations per second) will increase, so B is the correct trace.

Q12	D

If the total diameter is 1.6cm = 16mm, and the thickness is 1mm, then the internal diameter is 16mm - 2(1mm) = 14mm. Area = $\pi r^2 = 7^2\pi = 49\pi\ mm^2$

Q13	B

Aerobic respiration in humans is: oxygen + glucose → carbon dioxide + water (+ATP)
Anaerobic respiration is: glucose → lactic acid (+ATP)
Glucose is the only molecule common to both reactions, so B is correct.

Q14	C

A is incorrect because hydrogen would be produced at the cathode since calcium is more reactive than hydrogen. B is incorrect because oxygen will be produced at the anode, not nitrate. C is correct. D is incorrect because aluminium is produced at the cathode, and oxygen at the anode. E is incorrect because sodium is produced at the cathode.

Q15	D

Microwaves are used in satellite communication, not UV so we can rule out E-H. The distance travelled is 90,000km or 90,000,000m. The speed of light is 300,000,000 m/s, so the time is distance/speed = 90/300 = 0.3s

Q16	C

Divide the quadrilateral into a right-angled triangle on the left with points P, Q and M (which is located on the line PS), and rectangle QRSM. MS = QR = 5cm, therefore PM = 11-5 = 6cm. Since tan is opposite over adjacent, $\frac{QM}{PM} = \frac{4}{3}$, therefore QM = 8cm = RS. Therefore, the rectangle's area = 8 x 5 = 40cm^2, and the triangles' are = ½ x 6 x 8 = 24cm^2, so the total area is 64cm^2

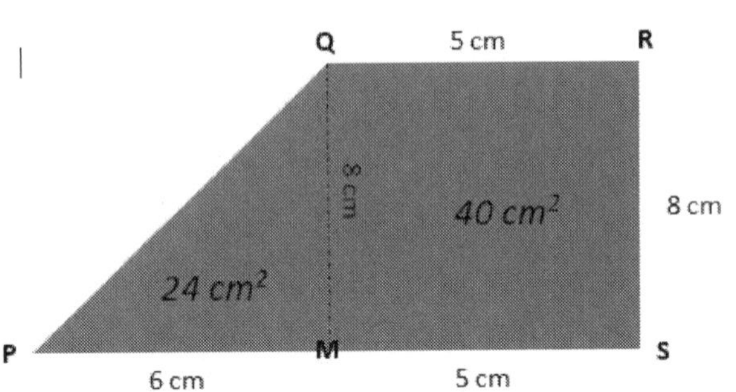

Q17	G

All 4 are correct, as a mutation in the gene changes the structure of the protein produced, which could have beneficial, negative or no effect, and could code for an enzyme, or another protein.

Q18	E

If it is a diprotic acid, then it means the mole ratio of NaOH : acid is 2:1. n(diprotic acid) = cv = 0.03 x 0.2 = 0.006 mol. So, 0.012 mol of NaOH is needed.
Volume = n/c = 0.012/0.1 = 0.12 dm^3 = 120 cm^3

Q19	D

We need this equation: Energy = current x voltage x time, so current = energy/(voltage x time), with time in seconds. I = 125/(500 x 0.01 seconds) = 25A. Note to convert milliseconds into seconds, divide by 1000.

Q20	C

$$\frac{e}{f} = \frac{a}{b} - \frac{c}{d}$$
$$\frac{e}{f} = \frac{ad - bc}{bd}$$
$$\frac{f}{e} = \frac{bd}{ad - bc}$$
$$f = \frac{bde}{ad - bc} = E$$

Q21	A

1 and 4 are the roles of mitosis. 2 is incorrect as mitosis causes growth of an organism, and not of an individual cell as that is to do with protein production, which is the same reason why 3 is incorrect.

Q22	B

$50cm^3$ of 2.0 $moldm^{-3}$ HCl has the same number of moles as $100cm^3$ of $1.0moldm^{-3}$. Therefore, the net amount of carbon dioxide produced will be the same, but since the concentration has doubled, the reaction will be quicker, so B is the answer.

Q23	E

Mass stays the same regardless of the planet. If something weighs 15N on Earth, it will have a mass of 1.5kg, ruling out A-C. The text tells us that on this new planet, it has a weight of 3.0N, and since GPE = mgh or w x h, the energy after 10m = 10 x 3 = 30J.

Q24	D

(9 + 3) = 12% of the population have just B antigens or both B and A antigens. The probability that a person has both A and B is 3%, so the P(someone has both A and B given that B was found) = 3/12 = ¼ = D.

Q25	H

Let us call the allele for black coat colour B and the allele for white coat colour b. We are looking for the maximum number of heterozygotes (Bb). Therefore, both the black coloured parents can be Bb, meaning all their offspring that are black would also be Bb. So we have 6 heterozygotes so far. The left cross would therefore be bb x Bb, and all of the offspring would be Bb, since they are black. The right cross would also be Bb x bb, so the two black offspring are Bb. So the number of heterozygotes = 6 + 4 + 2 = 12.

Q26	D

From the equation and the volumes, we can tell that Y is in excess. So $10cm^3$ of Y reacts with $20cm^3$ of X to form $20cm^3$ of Z. We also have $80cm^3$ of unreacted X in the final mixture, so the final volume = $20cm^3 + 80cm^3 = 100cm^3$.

Q27	C

360nm = ¾ of wavelength through air. So, wavelength through air = 480nm. Wavelength through glass = ⅔ of 480 ~ 320nm = C. NB: wavelength is proportional to speed, so we can use wavelength values instead of speed.

2016 Section 3

To see the marking grid and mark bands that the BMAT examiners will use to mark your essays, please refer to the BMAT website.

'You can resist an invading army; you cannot resist an idea whose time has come.' (Victor Hugo)

To see the question in full, please see:
https://www.admissionstesting.org/Images/378604-specimen-bmat-2016-past-paper-section-3.pdf

Authors' tip

Remember for the BMAT, you are not expected to explain the statement in its historical context or provide context about the author; nor are you rewarded for doing so!

The reasoning behind the statement is that forced change in a society can be resisted/won't be easily accepted, yet natural, passive change will be, and so is more powerful. Alternatively, it could mean that words/knowledge/ideas are far more impactful and powerful on changing society/societal opinion than violence.

- This can be because an 'invading army'/violence won't be accepted by the majority, and humans as a race will stand up to oppression/are not easily oppressed voluntarily without some form of lashing back (think of the slave revolts, numerous revolutions throughout the ages). Words and ideas, if accepted by society, are more powerful and can actually change society permanently, once people are convinced.(*'cannot [be] resisted'*) For example, during the Renaissance, scientific ideas came to the fore, and the foundations of scientific research started, and weren't able to be resisted by the Church (the powerful authority at the time). Society has changed, and since then, science has developed dramatically, and plays a major part in modern society.

- With sufficient force, anything can be suppressed, and there are many modern-day examples. In North Korea, the powerful dictatorship has suppressed any ideas of individual freedoms; anyone who fights back against the system is severely punished in 'internment'/concentration camps, such as Camp 14. This form of severe punishment twinned with a fear-mongering autocracy, has managed to successfully suppress any revolts for the past 60 years.
- No matter how good ideas are, force has the ability to oppress them, as humanity is afraid of injury to themselves or those that they love. Also, violent regimes have the ability to murder/remove those who are distributing these ideas, preventing propagation of these ideas in society, e.g. during the Nazi regime.

- The person/group of people who develop/propagate that idea. For example, many religious believers hold the ideas contained within their holy scripture to be very powerful as they have come from God, or other important religious figures.
- The number of people who support the idea: the more people who follow a trend/support an idea, the more powerful it becomes. For example, vegetarianism is becoming more powerful and popular and people are more likely to believe an idea that many other people do.
- The usefulness of an idea; more people are more likely to say the idea of building a computer is far more useful than an idea to throw a party in space.

'Science is not a follower of fashion nor of other social or cultural trends.'
To see the question in full, please see:
https://www.admissionstesting.org/Images/378604-specimen-bmat-2016-past-paper-section-3.pdf

The statement argues that scientific progress and development is independent of what is happening in society. It believes that there is no link between cultural or social phenomena and subsequent scientific advancement.
Some may argue that this is true since:

- Science deals only with truth, whereas cultural or social trends vary a lot (what is deemed correct in one time, is wrong at a different time in history).
- There have been examples where scientific thinking varies/contradicts the social trends of the time. For example, Darwin's theory of evolution greatly contradicted the religious ideas of creation.

- Science and scientists solve the problems that the world faces at a current time, and therefore do follow social/cultural trends. For example, a current 'social trend' is the increase in obesity and cardiovascular disease in the world, and so there is a lot of scientific research into cures and treatments for these sorts of problems.
- A current 'social trend' is dieting and weight-loss, and science has developed a lot in this field, to meet the demands of this trend.
- In the past the USA wanted to win the 'space race', and so scientific technologies were focused on space exploration. During the wars, scientific and technological effort and developments were focused on military technology,

Science can develop for the sake of science, for example some advancements in quantum physics do not seem to have much current use, nor seem to follow the desires of certain societal or cultural trends. It can also be seen to deviate from social or cultural trends. However, science is performed by humans, whose desires are impacted by current social and cultural trends, so inevitably, science will never be independent from these trends. Additionally, many may even define science as 'the field of study exploring new ideas, and searching for new information to solve world problems' meaning it is there to deal with social trends. In conclusion, science not always but mostly can be seen to follow ideas prevalent in society. Although science should not be used to follow trends that society perceives as wrong, it is necessary that science considers trends to ensure maintained global participation and interest.

2016 Section 3

'The option of taking strike action should not be available to doctors as they have a special duty of care to their patients.'
To see the question in full, please see:
https://www.admissionstesting.org/Images/378604-specimen-bmat-2016-past-paper-section-3.pdf

The statement argues that doctors should not be permitted to protest their working conditions or pay (by striking), since they have a responsibility to look after their patients.

- Proponents would argue that by striking and not being in the hospital/GP surgery, patient safety and care is compromised.
- Just because doctors are striking, patients are not going to stop requiring medical help. By not turning up to work and striking, doctors would be violating their principle of non-maleficence and would potentially be risking the lives of seriously ill patients, who may need urgent medical attention.

- Doctors are humans too and so are entitled to the same human/workers' rights as others, such as the right to strike (in the USA, for example, this is enshrined in the National Labor Relations Act). By denying medical professionals this basic right afforded to others, we would be discriminating unfairly against them, as well as breaking the law in some jurisdictions.
- Strike action is there to prevent employees being unfairly exploited, as it gives employees a voice to demand fair pay (e.g. the 2015 junior doctor strike) and safe and comfortable working conditions. Without the ability to strike, doctors could be at risk of wage-exploitation which could affect the doctors' mental health and consequently the patient care given to each patient. Content doctors make good doctors, and mean patient care is high.
- Other members of the emergency services, such as firefighters, have the right to strike, even though it can be argued that they too have a special duty of care to society, so on the grounds of equality, doctors too should be allowed to strike.

A doctor should try and provide the best quality of care to each patient, and has a duty of care to ensure that all patients receive the treatment and support that they need. This, however, shouldn't be at the expense of poor employment conditions for the doctor, as they have the right to work in comfortable, safe and appropriate environments, receiving a fair wage so they can live comfortably, Removing this right to strike against unfair conditions would not only be discriminatory but would negatively affect a doctor's wellbeing, and their ability to provide good quality patient care. This shows that while a doctor has a duty of care to all patients, this shouldn't supersede their right to fair employment. By treating doctors fairly, they will not have to make the difficult decision between patient care and their working conditions.

Question 4 was written to widen access to the exam paper, as in the past, students hoping to study Veterinary Medicine would also have to take the BMAT. VetMed students no longer take the BMAT, and so in its current iteration (2017 onwards), there are none of these questions, so the authors have not included worked essays for these and recommend that you only attempt these after having attempted all the previous ones.

BMAT 2017

Section 1

Q1	C

Pink: 60% split into 15% red : 45% white
Orange: 40% split 20% red : 20% yellow

Total yellow used is 20% which equates to 1500ml - 900ml = 600ml. Therefore 1% = 30ml. Total red used is 35% which is 30ml x 35 = 1050ml so red left over is 1500m l- 1050ml = 450ml

Q2	D

There is no evidence to suggest A is the case; there is no evidence about what worse outcomes are or that the antidepressants are the cause of the decline in mental health. B cannot be inferred as only data is mentioned, there is no mention of doctors at all. C is wrong because it's strong language of '*clearly not an effective solution*' is very generalising and the antidepressants may be very effective it just happens to be that more people have depression. D is correct because it refers directly to the data displayed and comments on the fact that there is little evidence to suggest mental health improving which is a statement informed by the figures.

Q3	D

Read the first line, we can eliminate Chestnuts because they have a budget of $900000 and Chestnuts is out of their budget. I have coloured the useful qualities in red for each house. We can now eliminate Bellavista and Everglade because they don't meet 4 wishes.

House	# of bed rooms	Garage	Garden	Distance to grocery store	Distance to sports	Cost	No. of wishes met
Acorns	5	double	large	2 km	8 km	825000	4
Bellavista	3	single	medium	2.5 km	4 km	810000	2
Dayview	4	double	medium	1 km	7 km	640000	4
Everglade	4	none	small	1.5 km	5 km	860000	3

Out of Acorns and Dayview we have to divide their cost by the number of bedrooms and find the cheaper one:
Acorns: 825000/5 = 165000
Dayview: 640000/4 = 160000. Therefore, the cheapest is Dayview.

Q4	A

A is correct because it tackles the argument's main problem with nuclear power which is the '*tens of thousands of tons of lethal, high-level radioactive waste*'. B is wrong because this would support the argument and not weaken it. C is wrong because wind itself will not weaken the argument as it has already suggested a mix of renewable energy sources simply mentioning wind as one of these. D is wrong because the argument has already pointed out that '*nuclear power may be less air-polluting*' but the argument has a problem with the waste not the reduction in CO_2.

2017 Section 1

Q5	D

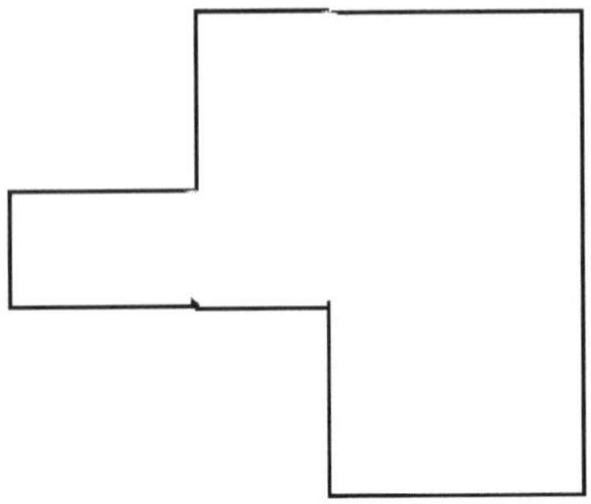

Some people may be able to do this simply by visualizing picking up each one of the shapes and trying to fit them to the piece of the puzzle. One way you may want to do this is by thinking about the shape that is created by a relief in 2D and finding the answer that matches this. By rotating this shape as necessary you can try and match it to A to E and you will see it only matches D in 2D pattern. Obviously as it's 2D it doesn't show the 3D dip that D has to account for the difference in height between the two protrusions on the puzzle piece, however it has clearly eliminated all the other options and left us with D.

Q6	C

A and D are incorrect because they are talking about other forms of cancer but the argument is only concerned with prostate cancer. B is incorrect because the argument does not allege all men can make major changes to diet and exercise it simply says by eating a healthy diet and taking regular exercise you can prevent the development of prostate cancer. C is correct because it directly refers to the conclusion of the argument and attacks the notion that "men can prevent the development of prostate cancer" because it allows room to consider other contributing factors to the development of prostate cancer.

Q7	B

We are told no girls chose swimming meaning if you add up the bars from swimming, 28 boys chose it. We are told no boys chose rounders, so that means 40 girls chose rounders. Adding up the bars for running shows 28 people chose running and the question tells us that there are an equal number of boys and girls who did so. So, there are 14 girls running and 14 boys running. Now adding up the total number of boys and girls so far gives 42 boys and 54 girls. This means of the 48 who do football the numbers need to be split so in total the number of boys and girls are equal. We can see that the total number of people will be 42 + 54 + 48 = 144 so there will be 72 each of boys and girls. Thus, there must be 30 boys playing football and 18 girls playing football; as for boys 42 (our previous total) + 30 = 72 and for girls 54 (our previous total) + 18 = 72.

Q8	C

The question asks for reconvictions per re-offender i.e. reconvictions/re-offenders and we know that the reconvictions is given by 1057.5 per 100. The re-offenders are given to us by the reconviction rate. Don't get confused by the re-offenders and reconviction appearing a lot; the information in the box is what tells you what each number represents and this is much clearer.
We want to do 1057.5 (reconviction frequency rate per 100) divided by 74% (reconviction rate) and since the frequency rate is per 100 we can essentially do 1057.5/74 = 14.3.

Q9	E

Statement 1 asks us to do 43% out of 55.2% and I obtained those figures looking at the reconviction rate column and reading across for the 1 year and 2 year values as the question asks. We need to know what the proportion of all offences over 2 years took place in the 1st year i.e. 43/55.2 = 0.779 which is 77.9% which is over 77%.

Statement 2 is wrong. The reconviction rate column is cumulative so to calculate the reoffences between year 2 and 3 we need to do 61.9% - 43% = 18.9%. This then needs to be calculated as a proportion of all re-offences in the 9 years (74% as read in the table) so 18.9/74 = 22.5%. This isn't even close to a third so 2 is wrong.

Statement 3 is correct because we need to calculate the reconviction frequency rate (which is 185.1 per 100) multiplied by the initial cohort of 42721 offenders. So, 1.1851 x 42721 = 79077 which is over 77000 reconvictions.

Q10	C

The information is found in the last paragraph of the passage: '*Offenders who received shorter sentences...committed 39 per cent of all offences that led to a conviction in the first year of the follow-up'*. Thus, we need to do 39% of what we actually worked out from Statement 3 of Question 9. 39% of 79077 = 30840 which rounds to C.
This is a prime example of needing to retain answers clearly from previous questions; don't waste time calculating this again because you have already done half the calculation.

Q11	G

1 is feasible, if you send re-offenders to prison then you reduce the number that are in the public who have the potential to reoffend hence why the reconviction rate could decline.
2 is feasible, the cohort is capped at the 42721 offenders in the study. Naturally following normal mortality rates some will inevitably die thus resulting in a decreased reconviction rate.
3 is feasible, offenders would be less likely to reoffend and hence be reconvicted if they were deterred by harsher sentences.

Q12	D

We can eliminate A because Gracie can only be played by 1 person as the question states. B is wrong because in Scene 1 Teddy and Guard 1 appear together and can't be played by the same person. C is wrong because again Guard 1 is played by whoever plays Rosie so another person can't play her as well. E is wrong because Sarah and Graham must be played by a female and a male respectively. F can be eliminated because whoever plays Rose already plays Guard 1 so she cannot play Guard 2 as well because both guards appear in Scene 1 and cannot be played by the same person at the same time. Hence D is correct.

Q13	B

A is wrong as the passage says the trace metals "*seemed to overlap*" with periods of living animals appearing but "*seemed*" is not the same as selenium HAVING to be the explanation; it is a possibility not a proof.
B is correct because it is a suggestion that matches the suggestive tone of the passage.
C is wrong because nowhere in the passage alleges the importance of selenium over any other trace element.
D is wrong because it says "*must*" whereas the passage says selenium dropping is correlated with marine life extinction not that it is causatory.

Q14	B

Draw up a table of the initial values for each party and how they change:

	Citrons	Jonquils	Saffrons
Beginning	80	126	34
	+47	+11	+18
	+10	+15	+33
	-11	-47	-10
	-18	-33	-15
End	108	72	60

So the pie chart can't contain any wedges of half or over a half as 108 < 0.5(240) so A, C and D are eliminated. E has 2 larger fairly equal wedges and 1 smaller one; but looking at our end figures we have 102, 72 and 60 and 72 and 60 are the 2 smaller ones and there is only 1 larger one so E can be eliminated leaving D.

Q15	A

The argument presented is that there are 2 possibilities for a scenario. 1 is shown to be incorrect leaving the other correct.
A does exactly that.
B does not refute the alternative so is incorrect.
C is incorrect because it doesn't refute one of the options.
D is incorrect because both alternatives of travelling by bus or taxi are still viable; you may just choose 1 out of preference; but the argument of the passage eliminates 1 possibility from existing so the reasoning isn't matched.

Q16	D

If each set of 4 numbers in the pin has to add to 19 then that means the sum of both pins is 38. This means the sum of all the 8 different digits is 38 and as from numbers 1-9 there is only 1 number that is excluded, we can try adding from 1-9 missing out 1 number each time to see which one sums to 38.
A Eliminating 1 : 2+3+4+5+6+7+8+9 = 44
B Eliminating 3: 1+2+4+5+6+7+8+9 = 42
C Eliminating 5: 1+2+3+4+6+7+8+9 = 40
D Eliminating 7: 1+2+3+4+5+6+8+9 = 38
E Eliminating 9: 1+2+3+4+5+6+7+8 = 36
Now, to save time here you obviously don't need to do all 5 calculations to see that the totals on the RHS are decreasing by 2 and you can save yourself working anything out by inferring that the answer will be D.

Q17	D

Nowhere in the argument does the author deny the fact that anyone can go through break-ups and mental breakdowns. The argument simply says it is wrong for a parent to knowingly subject their child star to this so statement 1 is wrong.
Statement 2 is wrong because the argument does not take the view that being adored as a child justifies or explains addictions or broken relationships. The argument does not seek to explain this notion; it just cites it as a bad consequence of being a child star.

Q18	B

If we subtract the cost of the relevant ingredients for pancakes alone, we can solve this question.

Ingredient	Flour	Eggs	Milk	Butter	Sugar	Lemon
Start	1000g	12	2500ml	600g	600g	5
Deduction for biscuits	-400g	0	0	-400g	-200g	0
Deduction for cake	-225g	-2	-250ml	-150g	-330g	0
Remaining	375g	10	2250ml	50g	70g	5

Going across our bottom row we need to find the limiting ingredient, which we can quickly see is butter. We only have 50g remaining and this is only enough to make 1 batch of 8 pancakes hence this is the answer.

Q19	B

A is incorrect as the information is only about genomics; widening the scope to other fields is essentially irrelevant.
B is correct because if the number of errors were overestimated by counting empty cells then that means there were less errors than the headline claims.
C is wrong because this would support the headline and not weaken it.
D is wrong because we aren't given any information as to whether these spreadsheets were made with new versions of Microsoft Excel.

Q20	B

1 is incorrect as although we know there were over 160 supplementary files with gene name errors (from the graph) we do not know the distribution of these files over all the papers being investigated so we cannot comment on this.
2 is correct because reading off the relevant graph shows in 2009 just under 50 files had gene name errors compared with over 100 in 2011.
3 is wrong because Nature published 23 papers affected whereas BMC Bioinformatics published 21 papers that were affected. If you were using the percentages in the left hand graph then you may disagree with this as Nature has 31% of papers with spreadsheet errors whereas BMC Bioinformatics has 14% but we don't know the total number of papers published, we only know the number of papers affected so we can't assert statement 3 from the information given.

Q21	D

The journals with a higher than average number of papers affected can be read off the graph on the top left-hand corner of the passage. They are Nature, Genes Dev, Genome Res, Genome Biol, Nature Genet, Nucleic Acids REs, and BMC Genomics. The corresponding number of papers affected can be read off the top right-hand table; and they come to 23, 55, 68, 63, 9, 67, 158 respectively. Summing this gives 443. 443/704 (704 being the total number of papers affected as shown on the top right-hand table) gives 63%.

Q22	C

We are told in the final paragraph that the '*number of genomics papers packaged with error-ridden spreadsheets increased by 20% a year over the period, far above the 10% annual growth rate'* so we can express this in a table.

Year	% of papers affected (increasing by 20% each year)	% of papers published compared to 100% in 2015 (increasing by 10% each year)	Is every genomics paper affected?
2015	80% - the question tells us this	100% - we are using 100% to make every calculation relevant to 2015 for ease	No
2016	96%	110%	No
2017	115.2%	121%	No
2018	138.24%	133.1%	Yes - the % papers affected exceeds the % papers published for the first time

Q23	E

It may be useful to assess what kind of puzzles we are looking for in the first place and we have 2 options per piece essentially.
For the left-hand piece, we know there have to be 2 "sticky-out bits" and 1 "inward bit" as shown.
For the right-hand piece there has to be 2 "sticky out bits" and 1 "inward bit" as well.
Remember, the bits in the middle (i.e. the part in the centre of the shading where we can't tell what the fitting together arrangement is) must be complementary so they have to be 1 of each: 1 "sticky out" and 1 "inward bit".
Overall, this means across the 2 pieces we need 5 "sticky out bits" and 3 "inward bits". We can therefore eliminate A, B, C, and D leaving our correct answer E.

Q24	E

E is the only answer that actually gets to the heart of the flaw; the argument has assumed the correlation of increasing life expectancy is caused by decreasing the number of children the average woman has when as E rightly points out; there could be other factors involved. A is not shown to be the case by the argument; B may be true but doesn't best express the flaw, C comments on infant mortality rates which have no effect on the lifespan of women and D is not relevant because multiple pregnancies aren't mentioned anywhere in the argument.

Q25	E

	Speed	Distance	Time
Route 1	30khm/h - we are told this in the question	X - we don't know this distance yet hence calling it x	x/30 - as time = distance/speed
Route 2	27km/h - the question tells us the average speed is reduced by 3 km/h	X+4 - the question tells us the distance increases by 4 km	1.25x/30 = x+4/27 We know that for the LHS of this equation the question tells us journey time increases by 25% which is the same as 1.25x/30 We also know that rearranging speed and distance using time = distance/speed gives us x+4/27

Now we just solve the equation for our new time to find x:
1.25x/30 = x+4/27
33.75x = 30x + 120
3.75x = 120
x = 32
The question asks for the new distance which is x + 4 = 36km

Q26	C

Be wary of statements containing strong language because often these will be wrong.
A is wrong because it claims the argument '*can be used to justify fully*' the resources spent on health checks when we can see that in the argument the '*researchers did not*' continue to monitor the health of the individuals so a full justification isn't appropriate to suggest.
B is wrong because some screening programmes can influence people's health related behaviours.
C is correct because the argument says the '*level of detection of risk factors COULD EQUATE to the prevention of over 2,000 heart attacks and strokes*' so like C says, it hasn't been proved conclusively.
D is wrong because this isn't actually directly related to the '*health checks*' conducted on individuals.
E is wrong because we cannot infer this from the information in the passage; it doesn't allude to other age groups at all.

Q27	B

You need not guess or trial and error your way to the answer; instead by using LCMs (lowest common multiples) we can come to the answer. The LCM of 400g, 200g, and 300g is 1200g. So 1200g of each seafood item will be bought.
1200g divided by 50g of each type of seafood comes to 24 plates.
To work out the cost of these work logically:
Prawns - 1200g/400g packets = 3 packets. We will pay for 2 and get 1 free.
Cockles, whelks, smoked salmon; 1200g/200g = 6 packets for each type so 18 packs altogether. We will pay for 12 and get 6 free.
Squid - 1200g/300g = 4 packets. We will pay for 3 and get 1 free.
Thus in total we are paying for 17 packets each costing £4.08 so in total costing £69.36.
This divided by 24 plates gives £2.89

Q28	E

Statement 1 is correct because the passage tells us that the aim is to *'lower levels of violence within these encounters'* by encouraging *'police officers to better regulate their own behaviour'*. Hence this implies that the level of force used by police in some interactions with the public exceeds that which is required by the situation.
Statement 2 is incorrect because the argument does not mention any sort of agreement between police departments around the world on what levels of force are appropriate; it simply asserts that police departments around the world should wear video cameras; not that the interpretation of the levels of force used as shown by the footage will be equal.
Statement 3 is correct because the last line of the argument: there is a *'clear warning from the start that everyone in an interaction is being filmed'* thus implying that when a bystander films everyone may not be aware that such filming is going on.

Q29	E

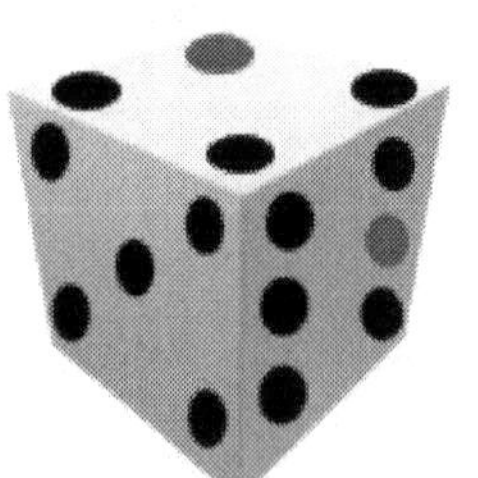

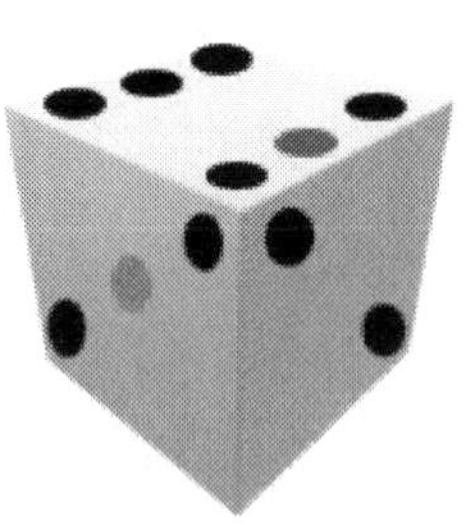

As we can see; the red dots have been added because they were missing from the dice. We also know that opposite sides must add to make 7. So what we can infer is that opposite the 4 on the left hand side is a 3 and opposite the 6 on both views is a 1. What we don't know yet is where the extra dot for the 3 goes because there are two 2s at the moment. We can tell from the orientation of the 6 relative to the 4 that the 4 on the right hand image must be the hidden face on the right (other hidden faces being to the left and the bottom). This means that the face that opposes the 4 is the 3 so we can infer that a spot is missing from the bottom left side of the dice in the RH diagram. This is shown in blue.

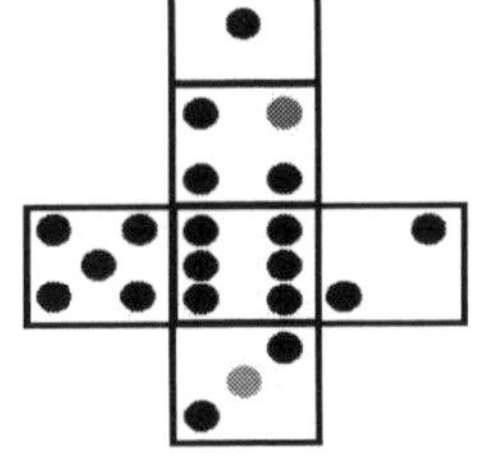

Making a net of this allows us to visualize how it will fold up in the orientation of the answer: E is the only cube that will produce this kind of net.

Q30	C

A is not true, the argument doesn't say this is the case it merely just exemplifies their definition of '*positive*' life traits but doesn't assert that that is true of everyone.
B is false because the argument says this is '*a beneficial use*' of the technology but does not say this should be the only point of study for fMRI technology so B is unfounded.
C is true because it harks back to the BMAT favourite of correlation not equalling causation. The argument's conclusion asserts something although there is only correlation in the evidence presented.
D is wrong because the argument does not ignore this; it simply says one would be '*more likely to exhibit 'negative' qualities'* but this inherently means that although less likely, those with weaker connectivity can still lead productive lives.

Q31	D

We can make 2 circles displaying the information shown:

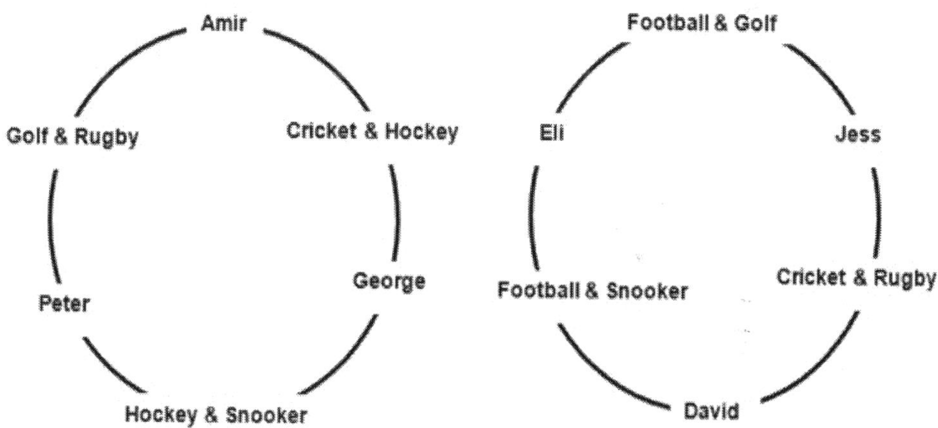

We know Jess shares 1 common interest with the people on either side of her so her options are either football and rugby, football and cricket, golf and rugby, or golf and cricket. Looking at the left-hand circle, the only option that matches is golf and rugby hence this is Jess and if we look at the person opposite this; it is George.

Q32	C

The fourth paragraph details the relevant parts to this question: there has been a '*long term loss of road space to bus lanes'* which would support Statement 1 and statement 2 is supported by the notion that road space has been lost which could happen if Statement 2 were to happen. Hence, as the question asks for what '*could*' account for this increase; both statements are correct.

2017 Section 1

Q33	E

We are told the most conservative estimate is '*£10 million each*' for '*the six Underground strikes in 2015*' from the Centre for Economics and Business Research. Thus, this comes to £60 million. The cost of congestion to London's GVA in 2015 is '*an astonishing £5.5 billion a year*'. So, 5.5 billion/60million = 5500/60 = 550/6 = 91.667 which rounds to 92.

Q34	C

Statement 1 is not supported by the passage; although the last paragraph seems to indicate that car ownership has declined and that road congestion in the capital has not been resolved; this could be because car ownership may have reduced but other factors caused the congestion to remain high.
Statement 2 is incorrect because 2% of people travelled by bike in 2014 and creating bike lanes doesn't appear to help the problem according to the passage.
Statement 3 is correct because we know that certain methods of public transport including buses or taxis are detailed in paragraph 3 have experienced decline, due to the deterring factors of '*slower speeds and worse reliability*'.

Q35	B

A is incorrect, we do not know that the additional buses will have the effect of making more congestion and thus reducing London's GVA because the 300 buses could be replacing a much higher number of cars for example.
B is correct; London's GVA is made of the value added to the economy and this will be from profitable retail areas, and if they are in the congestion charge zone less people will be entering these areas so there will be less spending here thus a smaller contribution to the economy.
C is wrong because qualification as mini cabs just means that congestion is still there so GVA will still decrease.
D is wrong because the length of traffic delay being the same would seem to indicate the damage to the GVA would be the same, not increased hence why it is wrong.

2017 Section 2

Q1	A

P is the gallbladder which secretes bile.
Q is the stomach which releases proteases and has a high H^+ concentration because this corresponds to its acidity as it has a lower pH value.
R is the pancreas and secretes insulin, protease, lipase and amylase.

Q2	E

We know oxidation takes place at the anode (from OIL RIG - oxidation is loss of electrons) and already we can eliminate B C and D because these show reduction equations taking place at the anode which we know to be incorrect. Out of A and E we know Copper will preferentially discharge its Cu^{2+} ion over the sulphate group due to the sulphate group's stability hence why the answer is E.

Q3	A

Statement 1 is incorrect; on the EM spectrum microwaves have a longer wavelength than visible light.
Statement 2 is incorrect; all EM waves travel at the same peed in a vacuum.
Statement 3 is wrong; Gamma rays have the shortest wavelength and the highest frequency.
Statement 4 is also wrong; X-rays are used, not radio waves.

Q4	F

$$(\sqrt{5} - 2)^2 = (\sqrt{5})^2 - 4\sqrt{5} + 4 = 5 - 4\sqrt{5} + 4 = 9 - 4\sqrt{5}$$

Just expand the initial set of brackets as you would any other quadratic.

Q5	G

SCID is when an enzyme cannot be made, and all enzymes are made of protein. We know that proteins are coded by DNA so a change in the DNA will change the amino acid sequence and hence the protein product it codes for.
An allelic change changes the DNA hence could change the protein.
The amino acid order could change how the protein folds so could change the protein product.
A change in the bases in the gene could change the protein.
The shape of the active site could change the function of the enzyme because as we know the active site is specific to a substrate and a change in the active site means a n enzyme-substrate complex cannot be formed hence the enzyme can't carry out its function.

2017 Section 2

Q6	D

1 contains 18 neutrons and 18 electrons.
2 contains 20 neutrons and 18 electrons.
3 contains 22 neutrons and 18 electrons.
4 contains 20 neutrons and 18 electrons.
5 contains 20 neutrons and 20 electrons.
Hence D is correct.
To work these out you need to remember your atomic structure; the neutron number is given by the mass number minus the atomic number. The electron number is equal to the number of protons as well as the charge on the species i.e. a proton number 20 and a charge of -2 gives 22 electrons as -2 indicates a gain of 2 electrons as electrons are negatively charged.

Q7	F

This question tests knowledge not currently on the BMAT specification
1 is correct; at higher temperature water molecules have more kinetic energy and can overcome the intermolecular forces between them to change state from a liquid to a gas.
2 is incorrect; if the air is still then the evaporated water i.e. the water vapour above the puddle remains there creating a high concentration there thus reducing the concentration gradient for evaporation.
3 is correct; with a large surface area more water molecules can gain energy from the sunlight and thus evaporate.

Q8	A

The probability we want from this tree is that for which 2 people suffered from migraines. This means we have to multiply down the branches so 5/20 x 4/19 = 1/19 hence why A is correct.

$^{4}/_{19}$ Migraines
$^{5}/_{20}$ Migraines
$^{15}/_{19}$ No Migraines
$^{5}/_{19}$ Migraines
$^{15}/_{20}$ No Migraines
$^{14}/_{19}$ No Migraines

Q9	E

It is important to read that the partially permeable membrane allows both glucose and water to pass through it.
In experiment 1 there is only distilled water so only water will move. This means we can eliminate A and B.
In experiment 2 the 10% glucose solution is the same within the tubing and on the outside. But, although there may be no net movement the water and glucose are both still moving through the partially permeable membrane.
In experiment 3 the glucose will be moving from in the tubing outwards, and the water will be moving from out the tubing inwards hence it belongs in both columns.
In experiment 4 the glucose this time will be moving into the tubing and the water will be moving out of the tubing so it also belongs in both columns.
E fits with all of these.

Q10	C

Statement 1 is incorrect firstly because it seems to insinuate that all the particles have less energy however if gaseous products are still being formed then they clearly have more energy than the solid metal ribbon.
Statement is correct because as the HCl concentration decreases so does the rate of reaction because there is a lower frequency of successful collisions between reacting particles hence why less H_2 gas is evolved.
Statement 3 is incorrect; the activation energy is fixed; it doesn't change so long as the temperature remains the same.

Q11	C

1 is incorrect; we know in a series circuit current remains the same; so, if the resistance is different across the resistors then this means the voltage has to be different across the 2. We can eliminate therefore A and B.
2 is correct; call the resistance across R_1 x and the resistance across R_2 2x. As V = IR we can arrange for I as it remains the same so I = V/R. Subbing in our numbers and equating shows us that for R_1 I = $\frac{V_1}{x} = \frac{V_2}{2x}$ and if this is to be the case we can cancel the x on the bottom and multiply up the 2 showing $2V_1 = V_2$. This eliminates F, G and H.
3 is wrong because of the former reasoning.
4 is correct because we know current remains the same across a series circuit.
5 and 6 therefore are incorrect because of the same reasoning.

Q12	F

As triangle PQT and RSP are similar this means that we can set up an equation of lengths to solve for the length PT firstly which we can add to TS (which we know to be 1.8cm) to solve. We can do this by saying that the relationship between PT and PS is the same as that of QT to RS. The bigger length is 5 times the other length.
So 1.8 + x = 5x
Solving this gives x = 0.45 so the length PS must be 0.45 + 1.8 = 2.25cm

Q13	E

The gamete nucleus contained the haploid number of chromosomes which is 27 as all gamete cells contain half the genetic information of all other body cells.
Statement 2 is correct as embryonic cells need to contain embryonic stem cells so that they can differentiate into all of the types of cell needed in a lamb. 3 is incorrect; the gametes were produced by meiosis.

Q14	E

There is no disproportionation in 1, Fe is oxidised, Cu^{2+} is reduced and Cl^- are spectators.
In 2 Cu^+ in Cu_2O is reduced to Cu and also oxidised to Cu^{2+} in CuO.
In 3 Cl_2 is reduced to Cl^- in HCl and oxidised to Cl^+ in HOCl.
In 4 there is no disproportionation, all ions remain the same.
In 5 the Hg^+ is reduced to Hg and oxidised to Hg^{2+}.

Q15	F

The first stage of fission is a neutron hitting the Uranium-238 so we can actually already eliminate A, B, C, and D. Now the overall change is from $^{238}_{92}U$ to $^{239}_{94}Pu$ so we need to write an equation for our neutron absorption so we can work out what decay occurs as a result to get from Uranium to Plutonium.

$^{238}_{92}U + ^{1}_{0}n = ^{239}_{92}U$

We now need to gain 2 protons, which will only happen by emitting 2 Beta particles, as when they release electrons, they convert a neutron into a proton in the process. The other alternative, i.e. answer E would not work; emission of 2 alpha particles would decrease our atomic mass by 8 and our atomic number by 4 which does not take us to the correct end product.

Q16	A

First rearrange the expression for M. This gives M $=\frac{gR^2}{G}$

Substitute in the numbers given in the question:

$$\frac{10 \times (6 \times 10^6)^2}{7 \times 10^{-11}} = \frac{10 \times 36 \times 10^{12}}{7 \times 10^{-11}} = \frac{36 \times 10^{13}}{7 \times 10^{-11}} = \frac{36}{7} \times 10^{24}$$

What may catch you out are the rules for indices; with brackets you multiply the powers and with fractions like $10^{13}/10^{-11}$ subtract the indices (i.e. 13- -11 = 24)
36/7 is approximately 5 hence the answer is A.

Q17	G

1 is not true; capillaries are where glucose and oxygen diffuse into muscle cells; not arteries.
2 is true, arteries carry blood at high pressure.
3 is correct; the walls of arterials have a muscle layer to contract or relax to regulate blood pressure.

Q18	C

As propanoic acid is monoprotic it will dissociate to form its anion and H^+ and we know that when we have a metal carbonate + acid we form a metal salt, CO_2 and H_2O so we can eliminate A for forming the wrong products.
Because Mg will form a 2+ ion and the anion of propanoic acid has a 1- charge we need 2 propanoic acid anions for every 1 Mg. This eliminates B and actually D and E because the correct anion has formula $CH_3CH_2COO^-$ whereas in D this has not got enough H atoms and in E there are no H atoms in the anion.
This leaves C which is balanced, forms the correct products and shows the acid: carbonate in a 2:1 ratio as we would expect for a monoprotic acid and a M^{2+} ion.

Q19	E

It is important to read that the microphone is placed next to the sound source because this means the distances, we use have to be doubled to account for the wave hitting the wall and returning.
For the wave that hits the wall 2m away; speed = distance/time = 4/t
For the wave hitting the wall 8m away; speed = distance/time = 16/t+0.01
The speed is the same so equating these gives 4/t = 16/t+0.01
Multiplying up gives 4t + 0.04 = 16t and taking the t's over gives 12t = 0.04 so t = 0.04/12 = 4/1200 = 1/300.
Thus, the speed can be found by substituting this time into one of the equations above; for ease I'll pick the first one. Speed = 4 divided by 1/300 = 1200m/s

Q20	E

The common denominator here will be 2x(x-1) and then we simply add as we would normally with fractions:

$$\mathbf{1/2x + 1/x - 1 - 1/x = x - 1 + 2x - 2(x-1)/2x(x-1)}$$
$$\mathbf{= x - 1 + 2x - 2x + 2/2x(x-1) = x + 1/2x(x-1)}$$

Q21	D

We know that having no freckles indicates a homozygous recessive individual. We can tell this is the case because 7 and 8 were both born to 5 and 6 who have freckles, and therefore having freckles cannot be a recessive trait. The only way for two freckled individuals to have recessive children without freckles is if they themselves are heterozygous (5 and 6). So the probability that the next child of 5 and 6 has freckles can be worked out from a Punnett square of 2 heterozygous individuals:

	Y	y
Y	YY	Yy
y	Yy	yy

We can see that the probability is therefore 0.75 which eliminates all the answers apart from C and D.
If 5 is heterozygous this means that as 2 has to be homozygous recessive (as they have no freckles) 1 must be heterozygous. This is because 1 and 2 have been able to have 4 who is recessive, and this is the only way for such an offspring to be formed. Thus the probability that the next child of 1 and 2 will have freckles can be shown by the Punnett square:

	Y	y
y	Yy	yy
y	Yy	yy

We can see this probability is 0.5 so D is correct.

Q22	B

We first need to work out the moles of $CuSO_4.5H_2O$ which = mass/Mr

$$= \frac{10g}{64 + 32 + 4(16) + 5(18)}$$ = 10/250 = 0.04 moles.

Concentration = moles/volume = 0.04moles/0.1dm^{-3} (N.B 100cm^{-3} has been converted to dm^{-3} as this is the unit of concentration all of the answers are in).
This comes to 4/10 = 0.4moldm^{-3}

2017 Section 2

Q23	F

Newton's third Law requires that if an object exerts a force on the second object; the second object will exert an equal and opposite force on the primary object. This only fits with F.

Q24	C

We can work out the area of the quarter circle first; this will be $1/4\pi(6)^2 = 9\pi$
We need to find the length of the base of the triangle using Pythagoras, so we know that $a^2 + 6^2 = 9^2$ and so this means $a^2 = 81 - 36 = 45$ so $a = \sqrt{45}$
The area of the triangle is equal to ½ x base x height = $\frac{1}{2} \times \sqrt{45} \times 6 = 3\sqrt{45} = 3\sqrt{9}\sqrt{5}$ $= 3 \times 3 \times \sqrt{5} = 9\sqrt{5}$
Summing the two individual areas gives $9\pi + 9\sqrt{5}$ which is C.

Q25	G

The general maxim we can work out from the information given is below:
Inactive gene = paler = warmer
Active gene = darker = cooler
Statement 1 is wrong because the gene changes activity depending on the temperature so the enzyme formed isn't denatured when it is warmer because it wouldn't have been coded for in the first place.
Statement 2 is correct; we know that a darker coat colour matches with a cooler temperature from the information in the question.
Statement 3 is correct; we know the gene is either inactive or active and that this activity depends on the temperature of the environment hence both these facets are correct.

Q26	B

We can write equations for what happens here (it is important to note that regardless of the equation the molar ratio of sodium to hydrogen is the same in both cases)
Either: $2Na + H_2O = Na_2O + H_2$
Or: $2Na + H_2O = 2NaOH + H_2$
So $Na:H_2$ is 2:1 either way.
The moles of sodium reacting = mass/Mr = 0.23/23 = 0.01 moles
Thus the moles of H_2 produced is 0.005 moles using our ratio.
We know 1 mole of any gas at room temperature and pressure is $24dm^3$ so 0.005 moles of hydrogen gas would be $24dm^3/200 = 0.12dm^3$

Q27	C

We know that because the line plotted is straight we can say that it can be represented by y = Bx (we don't need a +c here because it is actually 0 as nothing can have KE without velocity). N.B I have changed the gradient function from an m which it normally is to a B to avoid confusion as this question has deliberately put 2 different m's together when they represent something different to confuse you). We are told y = KE (as it's on this axis) and that x is v^2. So this means $KE = Bv^2$ as represented on the graph.
We already know though that $KE = \frac{1}{2} mv^2$ (from our knowledge of physics) so that means B (the gradient function) = ½ m (m here standing for mass) = ½ (2.5) = 1.25

2017 Section 3

To see the marking grid and mark bands that the BMAT examiners will use to mark your essays, please refer to the BMAT website.

'He who has never learned to obey cannot be a good commander'. (*Aristotle*)

Explain what you understand by this statement.

- You may think that this statement highlights the importance of what good leadership is in that in order to be able to lead effectively one needs to be able to sympathise with the team-players and those to whom tasks are delegated. This could be for the benefit of efficiency and good teamwork as a leader must understand the working capacity of their team and ensure that delegation is fair and even.
- You could argue that learning to obey provides one with critical skills of resilience and reliability that are also equally important qualities in a leader. For example, becoming a leader in an academic field generally only happens after years of learning and guidance under the tutelage of experts. This builds up an affinity for the field itself resulting in a source of inspiration for new research and it also means that there are good working relationships forged in the field that could really aid future research.
- If a commander or leader has learned to obey or follow it also gives experience of obeying under different types of leadership; and you could argue that leaders or commanders need to have a wide range of experiences under different leadership so that they know what works well in different scenarios. This means their arsenal of leadership tools is wide and ready for when and if a situation requires adaptation and quick thinking whilst still maintaining the best outcome possible. For example, a military leader may build up good intuition for decision-making only after years serving as a soldier and a strategist building up experience and learning discipline.

Argue to the contrary.

- Arguably a good commander/leader needs to be someone who can come up with innovative and new ideas unblemished by someone else's ideas. If, for example, all one has ever known is to obey the ideas of another without challenging these notions and presenting debate; how is there scope for innovation and change? In creative fields generally this is how new ideas come about.
- You could relate this back to medicine in the sense of medical research today. If scientists didn't question the information presented to them; or what they had been taught because all they knew was to obey whoever was more senior to them how expedient would that be for scientific discovery? Ideas need to be challenged and plenty of commanders/leaders would argue that they don't simply want to be obeyed; they want peer-review at most stages of investigation to encourage good research.

2017 Section 3

To what extent do you agree that someone cannot be a good leader without learning how to follow?

You may wish to comment on how this statement relates to medicine if you want to exemplify how broadly speaking one does need to learn how to follow in order to become a good leader. The natural progression within the progression of medicine has this inherent to it.

Alternatively, it really does depend on your personal views; you need to work out to what degree you think being a good leader depends on learning how to follow. You may wish to reflect on your own experiences of being a team-player and contrast those with leadership and your progression to leadership as commenting on your own experiences are unique and will be much easier for you to express.

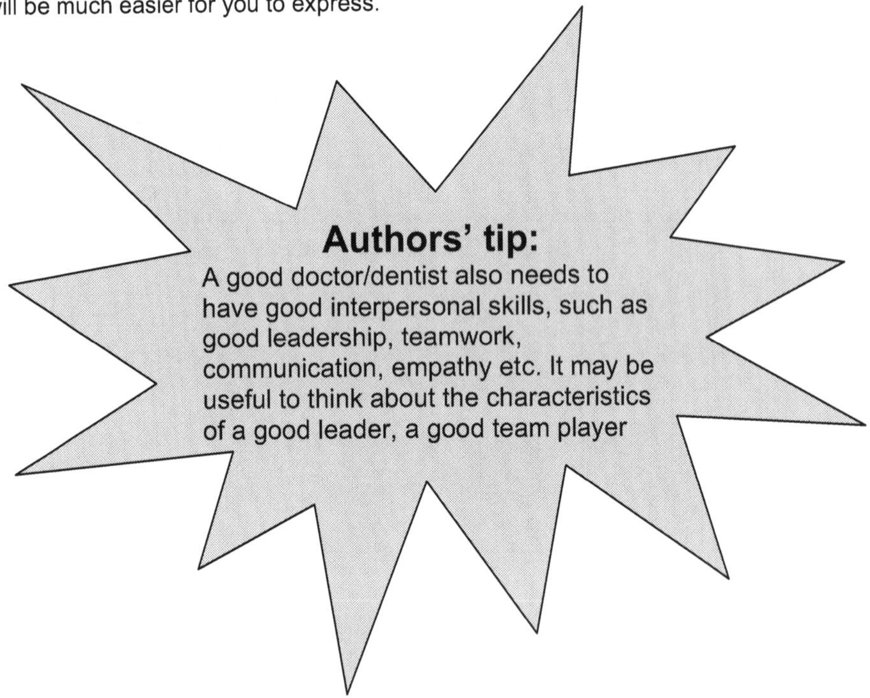

'The only moral obligation a scientist has is to reveal the truth.'

What is the reasoning behind this statement?

- This statement makes a rather sweeping claim that morality for a scientist is to reveal "truth" potentially because that is the only value they ascribe to discovery of new scientific knowledge. The reasoning may be to deter scientists from being caught up in sponsorship or distortion of evidence and statistics for political or economic gain. This way if their only moral obligation is to reveal the truth then there is so much transparency that facts arguably can't be distorted and that true knowledge (potentially akin to Platonic ideals) can be sourced.
- This question may also be hinting at the use of the scientific method as a means of ensuring that only the truth is presented by ensuring fair testing and repeat readings. Hence the statement may be indicating that scientists carry out truth revelation which is in line with scientific methods that are peer reviewed and empirically verifiable.

Present an argument to the contrary.

- Supporting and manufacturing a drug with higher prices that may only be patented to make money as opposed to help people is arguably the moral obligation of the big American company Turing Pharmaceuticals which charged much higher prices for some drugs in the USA that were much more readily available elsewhere in the world. This is an example of moral obligation that is self-serving and money-making as opposed to truth discovered. (maybe you could counter later and say this wasn't the fault of the scientists but of the company CEOs instead)
- The discovery of truth shouldn't be the only moral obligation, it should also be what to do with the truth when it has been discovered. For example, should it be widely known how to make an atomic bomb? Should information that can be used to the detriment of society be revealed or should a scientist's moral obligation be to also assess how information is released and in what capacity this can take place?

To what extent do you agree that the only moral duty a scientist has is to reveal the truth?

- With regards to the point that I made above, maybe you might like to take the line that it is not the moral duty of a scientist to arbitrate the distribution of knowledge; but that that job lies with politicians or advisors. If you think this then a scientist does have a single moral duty to reveal the truth because in many ways this is the domain of their profession; just like the domain of teachers is to teach.
- However you may argue that that is too narrow-minded, and that scientists have a moral obligation to do a whole lot more than simply discover "the truth" in that they must teach; innovate; manage and budget research. They must be able to interpret results and pursue "the truth" in an ethical and sustainable manner. These are all moral obligations that our society would deem appropriate to follow therefore you may disagree with the narrow parameters of the question.

2017 Section 3

'The healthcare profession is wrong to treat ageing as if it were a disease.'

What do you understand by this statement?

This statement is getting at ageing being an irreversible and natural process that most people go through normally. Ageing ought to be accepted as a part of life. This differs from the notion of treating it as a disease which implies that it is acquired, has detrimental effects and thus requires intervention. The statement instead seeks to accept and embrace the inevitable concept of ageing as opposed to trying to "go against Mother Nature" as it were.

Argue that it is not wrong to treat the effects of ageing as if they were a disease.

- Ageing can be debilitating and can massively reduce quality of life if it isn't treated in some cases as if it was a disease. Take dementia for example. This can be a very emotionally painful and difficult disease not only for the patient experiencing the disease but also their family and carers. The difficulty of experiencing arguably dehumanising symptoms of memory loss and loss of motility and self-awareness is upsetting. If dementia was left untreated some could argue that this is morally unethical because we have the means of staging some interventions with current medical research; but to decide to not treat diseases like this despite having the means could be considered cruel.
- In addition, the defining factor of humans like many other living organisms is that they are mortal. Surely if we have the means of trying to eliminate the negative effects of ageing that include wear and tear and reduced higher cerebral functions we can promote QALYs (Quality Adjusted Life Years) which will improve the life experience of many people.
- It is also worth noting that ageing itself may not be the root cause of disease but that it is ageing in conjunction with other acquired diseases during life that can be dangerous and life-threatening. As this can be the case then surely we should absolutely treat the effects of ageing as if they were a disease because to fail to do so shows a failure to recognise the acceleration ageing provides to the decline of health.

To what extent do you agree with the statement?

- You might like to consider the fact that ageing (like with many things) varies from person to person. What would be the implications of not treating ageing as if it were a disease? If genetics plays a part in the process of ageing (i.e. how early it starts and how it progresses) then is it not unfair to simply condemn some people to their biology when we have the means to help them?
- Alternatively, you could disagree with the point above on the grounds that our genetic constitution is what makes us all different and that the treatment of ageing would disproportionately affect some people and leave others disadvantaged which is unequal. In addition, some people would argue that intervening with nature is unethical and "playing God" when we ought to be following the natural progression of our lives.
- Arguably, the medicalisation of ageing could give rise to lots more problems such as several global ageing populations that means the allocation of resources is heavily towards the end of life care as opposed to an even distribution among the population demographic thus disadvantaging a large number of people.

BMAT 2018

Section 1

Q1	B

If the path is 3.2 km long, and there are seats at each end and every 400m in between, there will be 9 seats. Therefore, there will be 18 bins next to each seat. Between the 9 seats, there will be 8 gaps, each of 400m. Therefore, between any two seats there will be 3 litter bins (see diagram), therefore between the seats there will be 8 x 3 = 24 bins. So, 24 + 18 = 42 = total number of bins.

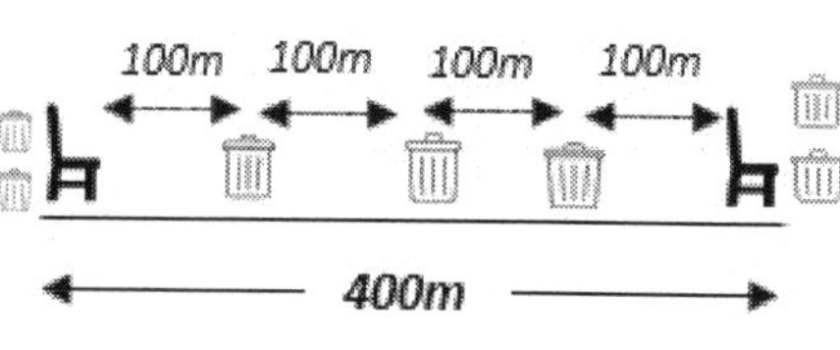

Q2	B

B is correct as those with MV combination (thereby having one variant of V) have died from vCJD, and therefore don't have resistance. A is incorrect as the passage does not discuss the VV variant, C can't be assumed from the text as we don't know if all those with the MM combination who ate beef had vCJD or did not have it (although we do know that some of those with MM got vCJD), and D is incorrect as we don't know what percentage of the population eats beef, or are susceptible etc.

Q3	D

The best way to work out this question is to quickly work out the time in the office for each person

Phil: 10:00 - 11:03 (63 mins) + 11:42 - 12:00 (18 mins) = 81 minutes
Quentin: 11:23 - 11:46 (23 mins) + 11:55 - 12:00 (5 mins) = 28 minutes
Rob: 10:00 - 10:17 (17 mins) + 10:26 - 11:00 (34 mins) + 11:38 - 12:00 (22 mins) = 73 mins
Sanna: 10:00 - 10:10 (10 mins) + 10:16 - 11:50 (104 mins) = 114 minutes
Theresa: 10:00 - 10:02 (2 mins) + 10:42 - 12:00 (78 mins) = 80 minutes
So Sanna is in the office for the longest time between 10:00 and 12:00.

Q4	C

The evidence in this text is based purely on an anecdote - that is the experience of the author's child. The author goes on to generalise this to every child and every nursery, which is the flaw of this argument, which is paraphrased by C.

Q5	D

The pie chart shows that the two largest segments are equal in size (the left and the right), and so are the smallest (at the top; black and white). The 5th category is equal to the sum of the two smallest categories. Now look at the table, and you will see that only Dolly fits this pattern.

Q6	C

The passage talks about the negative impacts of social media on democracy, with the conclusion being in the last line - *'Social media has become a vehicle for spreading untruths and has thereby undermined democracy'*. C paraphrases this, and so is the answer. A is wrong as the passage does not suggest censorship, B is wrong as the passage does not make a conclusion about whether the benefits outweigh the negatives or vice versa, D is wrong as no definition of democracy is provided or implied and E is not relevant to the passage, as it talks about the effects of social media on democracy, and not about the nature of protest.

Q7	D

Let us first work out the order of the lift:
From 11, it will go to floor 15 (12 seconds of travelling time), and it will wait there for 9 seconds. From 15, it will go to 24 (27 seconds of travelling time), and it will wait there for 9 seconds. From 24 it will go to 6 (54 seconds of travelling time), and it will wait there for 9 seconds. From 6 it will go to 4 (6 seconds of travelling time), at which point the person gets off.
So, 12+9+27+9+54+9+6 = 126.

Q8	B

For this question we need to look at table two and work out the ratio of women to men doing unpaid work. To save time, glance at the table and see which categories have the highest relative difference, and then work out the ratios for them.
26 to 35: 34.60/17.47 = ~2:1
36 to 45: 33.26/20.87 = ~1.6:1
Therefore, the answer is B. Note if you are unable to quickly ascertain the relative difference between the categories, it may be easier to work all of them out.

Q9	B

1 - 4.66/2.42 is less than 2, so 1 is incorrect.
2 - Again have a quick glance down the table to see the relative difference between female and male unpaid hours, and then work out the ratio for a few of the categories with the highest relative difference. (simply divide the female values by the male values, and we are looking for the highest value). Childcare: 4.67/1.89 = 2.47:1, Laundry: 2.40/0.39 = 6.15:1, therefore we can see that 2 is correct.

Q10	C

A, B and D are all plausible explanations. C is not, since using public transport still counts as 'non-leisure travel', and therefore that explanation holds no weight.

Q11	C

The data says that the total value of unpaid work is £1000 billion. Using the totals in table 1 we can then use this equation to work out the answer:

$$\frac{25.54}{25.54 + 15.99} \times £1000\, billion = 614.97\, billion = C$$

Q12	C

Let's see which customers need a refund, these are 3, 4, 9 and 10. Customer 4 needs a $4 refund, and 3, 9 and 10 all need a $6 refund. So, the company needs to pay $4 + $6 + $6 + $6 = $22.

Q13	D

The main argument of this passage is that '*rugby enables players to channel aggression in a positive, controlled way*' and so '*a ban...must not be implemented*'. 1 strengthens the argument, as it implies that there would be no other way for school children to channel their aggression in a controlled manner, so they would channel that aggression in other, more violent ways, thereby strengthening the idea that a ban shouldn't be implemented. 2 strengthens the argument because it strengthens the fact that such sports that channel aggression in a positive way are needed, since that aggression cannot be avoided. 3 contradicts the argument presented in the passage, and actually weakens the argument.

Q14	F

Let us see who is mentioned the greatest number of times, and then proceed from there. Roger is mentioned by 3 of the people. If we assume he is in the team, then Qayla, Phillip and Trista can't be in the team (as no one correctly named both people). We then see that Roger says it is Qayla and Sam, and Trista says it is Ursula and Sam. If Sam is the team player, then Trista must be wrong for both names (as P, Q, R and S would have all named one person correctly), however this is not possible as Trista also names Sam. Therefore, Roger must be totally wrong, and Trista must have correctly named Ursula. Therefore, Roger and Ursula are in the team.

Q15	A

1 can be concluded as the text states that the Right promotes the '*prosperity of business*' and that newspapers are owned by a '*few businessmen*'. Therefore, we can conclude that the Right promotes the interests of these businessmen/newspaper owners.
2 cannot be concluded as we don't get any data from the text about percentages of newspapers who are aligned to the right or the left.

Q16	A

This question is quite difficult to work out algebraically. Let us assign a value to the smaller container, e.g. 6 litres. Using the slow pump, it will take 30 seconds to fill half of the container. We then switch to the fast pump, which will take 15 seconds to fill it up. So, 45 seconds is taken in total.
Now, let us imagine the big container. It will use the fast pump for 30 seconds (since the small container took this long with the slow pump to get to halfway), meaning it will pump out 6 litres. After 30 seconds, we switch to the slow pump for 15 seconds, which will pump out 1.5 litres in this time. So, the volume of the big container is 7.5 litres, when the small one is 6 litres. Therefore, the larger container is 25% bigger than the smaller one.

Q17	A

First summarise the argument: If his location remains secret, the level of risk can be managed, but if his location is revealed, the level of risk can't be managed.
Put this in terms of x and y: If x is true, then y is true. If x is not true, then y isn't true.
This is the logical flaw that the argument has committed, which is the same as what A commits.

Q18	E

This is a difficult and long question, if you are unable to answer the question within the first 1 minute, make a guess, move on and come back to it at the end if you have time.
Let us work out the possible combinations that we can have: we have 4 red skittles, 4 yellow ones, and only six spaces to fill. The combinations are therefore: 3r + 3y, 4r + 2y and 2r + 4y.
The first potential combination: 3 red and 3 yellow
There are 6 places where the first 3 red skittle can go, 5 places where the second red skittle can go and 4 places where the third red skittle can go. There are 3 places where the first yellow skittle can go, 2 places for the second, and 1 for the third yellow. So, there are 6 x 5 x 4 x 3 x 2 x 1 total ways that the skittles can be arranged for this combination.
However for the red skittles and the yellow skittles we do not care which red one goes where, so we divide our overall total by 36 (as there are 3 x 2 x 1 ways to arrange 3 red skittles in 3 spaces, and 3 x 2 x 1 ways to arrange 3 yellow skittles in 3 spaces).
So: $\frac{6\times5\times4\times3\times2\times1}{3\times2\times1\times3\times2\times1} = 20\ arrangements.$
The second potential combination: 4 red and 2 yellow
There are 6 places to put the 1st red, 5 for the 2nd red, 4 for the 3rd red, and 3 for the 4th red. There are 2 places for the first yellow, and 1 place for the second yellow. We again don't care about which red goes where, or which yellow goes where, so similarly to the first combination we do:
$\frac{6\times5\times4\times3\times2\times1}{4\times3\times2\times1\times2\times1} = 15\ arrangements.$ The third combination is the same but 4 yellows instead of 4 reds, so again we will also have 15 arrangements.
20 + 15 + 15 = 50 total arrangements.

Q19	A

We need to work out the ratio of fatal crashes : onboard fatalities. Again, glance along the table and look for the largest relative difference and work out the ratios for those phases only to save time. We want the phase with the highest onboard fatalities per crash.
Take off and initial climb: 20/30 = 1:1.5
Cruise: 8/16 = 1:2
Therefore, A is the correct answer.

Q20	C

The exposure from the end of cruise to landing = 11 + 12 + 3 + 1 = 27%
27% of a 1.5 hour flight = 0.27 x 90 = 24 minutes.

Q21	D

A is incorrect as there were similar proportions of crashes due to pilot error in the 60s and the 70s.
B is incorrect as although the absolute value for mechanical failure in the 2010s is the lowest, the number of total crashes has also reduced. Both the total number of crashes and the number of crashes due to mechanical failure have reduced proportionally, therefore it is not proportionally lower in the 2010s.
C is incorrect as in fact it has increased proportionally over the years (the number of crashes due to weather has decreased at a slower rate than the total number of crashes).
D is correct because compared with the 1970s and 1990s where there was roughly the same total number of crashes, in the 1960s, there were far fewer crashes due to sabotage (12 as opposed to 25 and 19).
E is incorrect as both the absolute values and the proportion have decreased not increased.

Q22	C

The final paragraph says that 2015 was the safest year, when figures for sabotage is not included, which therefore means it assumes that sabotage is not a factor to be considered when determining air safety, so C is correct. E is very similar but incorrect, as it is too broad and does not link sabotage with safety of air travel.

Q23	B

The first digit can be called x, and the third digit y.
So, my pin is: x, x+1, y, y+1.
$x + (y+1) = (x+1)y$
So $x + y + 1 = xy + y$, so $x + 1 = xy$
x + 1 is the second digit, which is equal to multiplying the first and third digits together. This can only occur if the first digit is 1 to satisfy this rule and the rules given in the question - for example if x was 4, then x+1 would be 5, but there is no way you can multiply 4 by any other integer (the 3rd digit) to make 5 . Therefore, the second digit is 2, the third digit is 2 and the 4th digit is 3.

Q24	C

The evidence upon which this argument is based comes from only one study in one particular location; however, the text's final line generalises this to a much larger scale. The flaw is therefore that the text assumes that everywhere will be similar to Canberra, which is summarised by C. A is incorrect as this is not assumed by the text as the argument is the effect of domestic cats on wildlife, and not on the reasons for keeping pets, B is incorrect as the text states that it is the cats who are killing the invasive species and D is incorrect as it is not entirely relevant to the argument.

Q25	B

Assume that one of the charities receives $100 from Simone (this will allow us to see the minimum that STARS could get, as we are limiting the pot of money the most). Therefore, we have $100 for the remaining 4 charities, so on average each one will receive $25. To see the least amount of money STARS could get, we need to 'give' the most amount possible to the other charities, whilst following the rules. So, the other charities could get $23, $24 and $26, meaning STARS would get a minimum of $27.

Q26	D

The main crux of the argument is that more women should breastfeed their children as it has health benefits for the child and is more beneficial than bottle feeding. D is correct as it would represent another strength of breastfeeding and would strengthen the text's argument to get more women to breastfeed. A does not strengthen the argument as the argument doesn't mention specifically targeting certain groups based on education level. B doesn't strengthen the argument, as it provides reasons why women would bottle-feed, and not methods to increase breastfeeding. C doesn't strengthen the argument as limiting promotion of bottle-feeding, doesn't mean breastfeeding is or will be promoted instead.

Q27	A

The least possible cost is attained by paying for the cheapest pizzas and getting the most expensive ones for free. In total, the group wants seven pizzas so we will use one buy four get one free deal, and one buy one get one half price deal.
I's pizza is $5, K's is $6 and J and L's are $8. M's is $12, N's is $9 and O's is $10.
Therefore, since M's is the most expensive that will be the free one.
The buy four get one free deal's cost = $5 + $6 + $8 + $8 = $27
The buy one get one half price = $9 + ½ x $10 = $14
$27 + $14 = $41.

Q28	D

The main conclusions of the paragraph are that routine health checks do not always improve health or reduce mortality, and these health checks may not reach those that need it the most, and suggests at the end that we shouldn't discount '*targeted screening programmes in geographical areas where levels of disease are more prevalent*'. Therefore, D is the statement that can be drawn from the conclusion.

Q29	C

The die on the left is the one from 2-7 as if it was the dice from 0-5, 3 and 2 cannot be on adjacent sides. Therefore, the die on the right is the 0-5 one.
Dice A and D must belong to the die with 2 - 7 on their faces due to the presence of six spots. A can be ruled out as 6 + 3 cannot be adjacent as they must be opposite each other to add up to 9. Dice D can be ruled out as if we reposition the die on the left to have two on the top in the same orientation as in D, we should have a 3 on the left and not 6, so we can rule out D.
B must be the die from 2-7 as the faces with 3 and 2 are adjacent. However, it can be ruled out because looking at the die on the left, we can see that the face with 4 dots is in the same position as the face with 5 dots.
E is the dice from 0-5 as the 4 and 5 sides are adjacent. It is incorrect, however, because if we rotate the die on the right to match the positions of the 4 and the 5 as in E, we will see that 2 spots should be on the top, not 3 dots.
Therefore, C is correct. It is the die from 0-5 as it has a face with one dot. Rotating the left die to C's orientation, you will see that this is in fact compatible, as the side to the left of the 5 in C must be 4 and the side underneath the 5 must be two (which is shown by the right die).

Q30	D

The conclusion of this argument is that more biofuels should be used and less fossil fuels should be used, despite the damage to food security and biodiversity by planting more biofuel crops. 1 does not explain how longer growing seasons and climate change will affect biofuel crops. 2 states that if waste products can be used, then we do not need to convert the land used for food crops into land to produce biofuels. However, this does not weaken the conclusion of the argument, as the conclusion is simply that we must transition from fossil fuels to biofuels.

Q31	A

For simplicity's sake let us call research, r and design, d. From the second paragraph we know that construction = d -2 and evaluation is d-11.

48 = r + d + d - 2 + d - 11 = r + 3d - 13

61 = 3d + r

Now let us use the answer options given, to test whether they would work in this equation. Only A or C can work as 61 - r must be a multiple of 3, as d has to be a whole number.

If the answer was A, r = 13, d = 16, c = 14 and e = 5; this cannot be correct as it does not satisfy the fact that the smallest difference is 2.

Therefore, the answer is C.

Q32	D

Conditionally indispensable amino acids are those that '*can be made by our body under many circumstances, but under others cannot be made…*' (paragraph 1). In paragraph 2, we learn that cysteine and tyrosine can be converted from amino acids, but only in certain circumstances when other molecules are present, and so are conditionally indispensable.

Q33	B

Table 1 suggests that 0.8 x 70 x 4 = 224mg of tryptophan should be consumed

Table 2 suggests that 70 x 5 = 350mg of tryptophan should be consumed.

350 - 224 = 126mg

Q34	A

In 560g breastmilk for newborns there is 0.025 x 560g = 14g of protein

In 700g breastmilk for 8-week olds there is 0.01 x 700 = 7g of protein

There is therefore double the amount of protein in new-born milk, so double the amount of isoleucine, so the ratio is 2:1

Q35	B

21 x 19/44 = 9.07 mg = 9mg

2018 Section 2

Q1	H

Pancreatic juices contain amylase (a type of carbohydrase that breaks down starch), lipase (break down fat) and protease (break down protein), and so all 3 will be needed in the medication, given the fact that CF prevents secretion of pancreatic juice.

Q2	C

Q has an atomic number of 12, so its electronic configuration is 2,8,2. Therefore it is an alkali earth metal (group 2) with 2 electrons in its outer shell. Z has an atomic number of 9 so its electronic configuration is 2,7. Therefore it is a halogen (group 7) with 7 electrons in its outer shell. Therefore, one molecule of Q must react with 2 molecules of Z to ensure all atoms have full outer shells, so the formula is QZ_2. A halogen is a non-metal, and an alkali earth metal is a metal, so the bonding is ionic.

Q3	E

1 is incorrect because the speed of light is the same for all colours of light.
2 is correct because red light has a longer wavelength (and smaller frequency) than green light.
3 is incorrect because EM waves travel slower in denser media, and water is more dense than a vacuum.
4 is correct, because blue light has a greater frequency (and shorter wavelength) than red light.

Q4	B

Step 1: Divide the numbers so: $\frac{48m^5p}{40m^2p^3} = \frac{6m^5p}{5m^2p^3}$
Step 2: Divide the m's and p's (remember the laws of indices - division of powers means subtraction): $\frac{6m^5p}{5m^2p^3} = \frac{6m^3p}{5p^3} = \frac{6m^3}{5p^2}$
Step 3: Use the law that $\frac{1}{p^x} = p^{-x}$, to give $6m^3p^{-2}$

Q5	A

This question assumes knowledge not currently on the BMAT specification.
Denitrification is the conversion of nitrates to nitrogen gas in anaerobic conditions by microbes in the soil, and in root nodules of certain plants, so 1 is correct.

Q6	C

1 is incorrect because covalent bonds are not broken during evaporation/boiling or reformed during condensation. These changes in matter are due to breaking/reforming of intermolecular forces.
2 is correct because particles are closer in the liquid phase than in the gas phase.
3 is incorrect because boiling/evaporation needs heat/energy from the surroundings to occur, so is endothermic.

Q7	E

This is a two part question, which requires recall of two different equations.

$$speed = frequency \times wavelength = 50 \times 0.4 = 20m/s$$
$$time = distance/speed = 100/20 = 5\ seconds$$

Q8	C

We want to see the probability of picking a 50p coin and a 20p coin. This can occur in two combinations - 50p first then 20p or 20p first then 50p

P(50p first the 20p) = $\frac{2}{7} \times \frac{5}{6} = \frac{10}{42} = \frac{5}{21}$

P (20p first then 50p) = $\frac{5}{7} \times \frac{2}{6} = \frac{10}{42} = \frac{5}{21}$

$$\frac{5}{21} + \frac{5}{21} = \frac{10}{21}$$

Q9	B

The type of division is mitosis since the products of meiosis (gametes) cannot then undergo divisions themselves to produce more gametes. Therefore 2 and 4 are incorrect. 1 is correct because mitosis produces genetically identical cells, and 3 is correct for the same reason.

Q10	C

A is incorrect because iron ions are positively charged, and so would need to gain electrons to become Fe.

B is incorrect because each oxide ion has a charge of -2.

C is correct because CO gets oxidised, while Fe_2O_3 gets reduced. The definition of an oxidising agent is a substance in a redox reaction that oxidises another substance, and itself gets reduced - Fe_2O_3 fulfils this definition.

D is incorrect because ΔH is negative, meaning the reaction is exothermic.

E is incorrect as carbon is not involved in an electrolysis reaction, and iron is less reactive than carbon, and therefore can be extracted by heating with carbon compounds.

Q11	E

This question tests your understanding of scalar and vector quantities, and this question asks you to identify the vector quantities. Velocity and momentum are the only vectors, so E is correct.

Q12	F

Call the width of the rectangle x and the length 3x (since the ratio is 3:1). Therefore, we know that 3x + x + 3x + x = 8x = 24cm, so x = 3cm. Therefore, the area of the rectangle is 3 x 9 = 27cm2. To find the area of the shaded bit, we need to subtract the area of the rectangle from the area of the circle.

We can work out the diameter of the circle, as this is the diagonal of the rectangle. Using Pythagoras, we know the diameter is therefore $\sqrt{3^2 + 9^2} = \sqrt{90}$. Therefore the area of the circle = $\pi r^2 = \pi(\frac{\sqrt{90}}{2})^2 = \frac{90\pi}{4} = \frac{45\pi}{2}$

Shaded area = area of circle - area of rectangle = $\frac{45\pi}{2} - 27$ = F.

2018 Section 2

Q13	H

1 is found in skin tissue, 2 is a part of blood tissue and 3 is found in muscle tissue. Therefore, H is correct.

Q14	B

The 5 peaks on this MS are split into two groups (2 at a lower m/z value, and 3 at higher values). If we call the peaks in the group of 2 A and B, we can see that these peaks represent the isotopes of Element X. That is because when X appears as X_2, there can be 3 possible masses/peaks (A+A, A+B, B+B). Therefore, the answer is B = 2.

Q15	E

$GPE = mgh = 200 \times 10 \times 1.8 = 3600J.$

$$GPE = KE \text{ and } KE = 0.5mv^2$$

Therefore, $3600 = 0.5 \times 200 \times v^2, so\ v^2 = 3600/100 = 36, so\ v = 6.0m/s$

Q16	B

Looking at the details of the pattern that they have given us, we know that the difference between the rth and the $(r+1)^{th}$ triangular number = r+1.

Therefore $\mathbf{126 = (r+1) + (r+2) + (r+3) = 3r + 6}$

$$\mathbf{120 = 3r, so\ r = 40}$$

Q17	F

Pulling the rubber diaphragm down is equivalent to the diaphragm contracting and flattening (2). The diaphragm contracting causes the volume of the thorax to increase (3), and therefore, the pressure in the thorax will decrease (6), so air will rush in.

Q18	E

During addition polymerisation, the double bond breaks allowing the monomers to join together to form one long polymer. The monomer shown tells us that a CH_3 group and a H atom are attached to each carbon atom. Therefore, E is the correct option. D is incorrect as the middle 2 carbons lack a CH_3 group, as does C. B is incorrect as only 1 out of the 2 carbons in the repeating unit has a CH_3 whereas both should have one, whereas A is incorrect as it lacks any CH_3 groups.

Q19	B

The maximum current will occur when the resistance is the least and the least current will occur when the resistance is greatest. I = V/R

Maximum current = $\frac{6}{10+2} = 0.5A$

Minimum current = $\frac{6}{10+20} = 0.2A$

0.5 - 0.2 = 0.3 so B is the correct answer.

Q20	A

The total mass must be greater than 200g (20 x 10), but less than 210g (20 x 10.5)

The total mass of the first 16 sweets = 16 x 9.5 = 152g.

Therefore, the mass of 4x must be between (200 - 152) $\leq 4x <$ (210-52)

$48 \leq 4x < 58$ so $12 \leq 4x < 14.5$. The reason it is ≤ is because the mean mass of the sweets must be greater than 200g, and not equal to it

Q21	A

If the cell is unable to respire, that means there will be a build-up of glucose in the cell. Therefore, water molecules will move into the cell as there will be a higher solute concentration inside the cell than outside. Glucose molecules will not move, as there is a higher concentration of glucose inside the cell than outside.

Q22	C

In 105g of compound, 57g are F and (105-57) = 48g are O.
Therefore, there are 57/19 = 3 moles of F and 48/16 = 3 moles of oxygen. The O:F mole ratio is therefore 1:1, so the empirical formula is OF.
The Mr of OF is double its empirical formula mass so the formula is O_2F_2.

Q23	B

The difference in mass number is 24, and the difference in atomic number is 8. Emission of an alpha particle causes a decrease of 4 in the mass number, and a decrease of 2 in the atomic number. Emission of a beta particle doesn't change the mass number but increases the atomic number by 1. As the mass number decreased by 24, 6 alpha particles must have been emitted. Therefore, the atomic number should have decreased by 12. However, it has only decreased by 8, so 4 beta particles must also have been emitted.

Q24	B

$$\frac{x}{x-1}-\frac{x^2+3}{x^2+2x-3}=\frac{x}{x-1}-\frac{x^2+3}{(x-1)(x+3)}=\frac{x(x+3)}{(x-1)(x+3)}-\frac{x^2+3}{(x-1)(x+3)}$$
$$=\frac{x^2+3x-(x^2+3)}{(x-1)(x+3)}=\frac{3x-3}{(x-1)(x+3)}$$
$$=\frac{3(x-1)}{(x-1)(x+3)}=\frac{3}{(x+3)}$$

Q25	C

The dominant allele (brown body) is B, and the recessive allele (black body) is b.
So we cross Bb x Bb.
The genotypes we can get are BB, Bb, Bb and bb. There are 3 possible genotypes. There are only two phenotypes (brown body [BB, Bb] and black body [bb]). So, the ratio is 3:2.

Q26	C

$\boldsymbol{Energy\ change} = \boldsymbol{\Sigma(bonds\ broken)} - \boldsymbol{\Sigma(bonds\ made)}$and the equation is:

$$3F_2 + X \rightarrow XF_6$$

$-330 = [(3 \times F-F)] - [(6 \times X-F)]$, so, $330 + (3 \times 158) = [(6 \times X-F)]$
Therefore, $[(6 \times X-F)] = 804kJ/mol, so\ X-F = 134kJ/mol$

Q27	E

If the ratio has changed to $100:10^{15}$then we need to work out how many half-lives will cause the decrease from 1000 atoms to 100 atoms. After 1 half-life, 500 atoms will remain, after 2, 250 will remain, after 3, 125 will remain, and after 4, 62.5 will remain. So approximately 3.5 half-lives are needed.
$3.5 \times 6000 = 21{,}000$which is closest to answer option E.

2018 Section 3

To see the marking grid and mark bands that the BMAT examiners will use to mark your essays, please refer to the BMAT website.

'Liberty consists in doing what one desires.' (*John Stuart Mill*)

Explain the reasoning behind the statement.

Liberty means the state of being free from restrictions, and the statement means that true liberty/freedom means that one can do anything that they please. The reasoning behind this is that if someone truly is thought of being free, or having liberty, they therefore should be able to do anything that they want.

Present a counterargument.

- Liberty does not mean doing what one desires, if this means harming others either physically or verbally. Mill also presents a harm principle whereby you are free to do what you please as long as it doesn't cause harm to others. Many countries therefore give their citizens liberty but punish those who use their 'freedom' to hurt others (for example by depriving them of their liberty through custodial sentences in prison).
- You might like to consider using Mill's harm principle as a means of critiquing his own statement, he clearly doesn't mean "liberty consists in doing what one desires", he means "liberty consists in doing what one desires, so long as this does not cause harm."

Authors' tip:

You are not expected to know about Mill's harm principle, but we have included it as an example of wider reading or knowledge that you probably possess in other ways. If you know something unique this is an opportunity to show off your knowledge; but please stick to answering the question and only include it if it is relevant.

To what extent do you agree that freedom is doing what you want?

- Freedom is doing what you want, but there should be limits on how far we can exercise it, and what society can or cannot do to limit it.
- Everyone has freedom, and for the most part this does equate to the ability to do what you want. However, freedom shouldn't include the liberty to cause harm to others, and there should be consequences for those who decide to use their 'freedom' to cause harm upon others.
- But who decides what consists of 'harm'? It is subjective, and as such the arbitration of these judgements will not be consistent.

'Rosalind Franklin said that science gives only a partial explanation of life.'

Explain what you understand is meant by her statement.

The statement means that science can only explain certain ambits of life, and that some aspects of life and their explanations lie outside the remit of what science can do and will ever be able to do.

Reasons for her statement could include: (this could be included here or in the conclusion)

- It is the role of religion and ethics to try to answer certain philosophical questions about life (meaning and purpose), for example 'Why are we here?', 'What is our purpose?', 'How should we behave with others', which is outside the remit of science, which deals with form and function - science would not be able to provide answers to some kinds of questions
- There is a lot that science can still not explain at this moment in time, for example complex space phenomena. As such, for certain ideas (termed theories), science can only give partial explanations at the moment (for example, science has not been able to prove definitely how the universe formed).

Argue to the contrary that science can give a complete explanation of life.

- The scientific method deals with the physical and function, which for many is a complete explanation to life. Many people are not religious and may not seek answers to certain philosophical questions about religion or God, for example, and may feel satisfied that science allows them to understand life fully.
- Science is constantly advancing and improving - just because science can't explain something now, it doesn't mean that science will never be able to. For example, if you had asked someone in the Middle Ages whether science would ever be able to explain the surface of the moon, they may not have believed you.

To what extent do you agree with Franklin's statement?

- Science can explain a lot about the world, but may not be able to answer everything for everyone - many people say science deals with the What? And How (function and form), whereas religion deals with the deep, Why? Questions (meaning and purpose).
- Essentially, the validity of the statement depends on personal views. It is good for you to explain this in your conclusion (as opposed to solely presenting your personal view). If a person wants a more functional explanation, science provides those answers, if one wants a more purpose-driven answer, religion and philosophy may hold those truths, and the majority want both kinds of answers, so for them science alone won't suffice.

Authors' tip:

For more information about the debate between religion and science (or the limitations of science), have a look at BBC GCSE Religious Studies Bitesize.

2018 Section 3

'In the age of modern healthcare, every time a patient dies after a routine operation or procedure, it's a case of medical error.'

Explain the reasoning behind this statement.

The reasoning behind the statement is because medical technology has become so advanced, and that because there exists numerous safeguards and checklists, the only way for a patient to die during an operation would be because of medical error.

Argue that there can be reasons other than medical error behind such deaths.

- A patient may have multiple comorbidities, which means that even a simple surgery can become very complex and carry a lot of risk. Therefore, in such situations, if the patient were to die, it may not be down to medical error.
- A patient may not be completely truthful when declaring any other conditions, they may have, or allergies, or may not have stuck to preoperative guidelines suggested by the doctor to enable the surgery to have the best chance of success. Therefore, in such cases, even if the doctor performed the surgery to the best of their abilities, and there was a mistake, in this circumstance it could not be assigned to medical error. Similarly, some patients may not know they are allergic to certain medication or anaesthesia, and may have allergic reactions on the operating table, which could cause death which could be argued to not fall under the remit of medical error.
- If you have defined medical error as an error committed by the medical professionals, you could say that administrative errors may be the cause instead. For example, in rare circumstances, the manufacturer of the drugs/anaesthesia used in the operation may have mislabelled the name and/or concentration of a substance on the bottle, or there may have been problems with the manufacturing process, resulting in impurities added, all of which could cause death on the operating table.
- Technology could also be the source of error; for example, in developing countries, there may be a power cut during an operation, which could lead to machinery supporting a patient to fail, which could result in the patient losing their life.

To what extent do you agree with the statement?

While modern healthcare and advanced technology has reduced the probability of death on the operating table, and increased the safety of many routine operations, it is not correct to say therefore that it is the only source of medical error. Each patient is different, and may present different comorbidities, or may not always tell the full truth in all circumstances, which could lead to unexpected consequences on the operating table. Perhaps, what is more important than saying all causes of error must be medical error, is to identify the source of error when something goes wrong, and reflect on it and see what can be put in place to make sure that the mistake doesn't happen again.

BMAT 2019

Section 1

Q1	C

If last year's total cost was $330 then we can take away the $50 booking fee and appreciate that the remaining $280 was split in a 3:2 ratio of basic cost: taxes. This means the actual cost of basic cost : taxes was $168:$112. I have displayed this information in a table along with how each cost changed. Summing the final row gives our answer.

	Basic Cost	Taxes	Booking Fee	Total
Cost last year	$168	$112	$50	$330
Change	Increased by 20%	Increased by 10%	Halved	
Cost this year	$201.60	$123.20	$25	$349.80

Q2	C

The main premise of the argument is that with the rise of the *'internet-connected smartphone' there is a worry about parents shifting their 'attention away from the young children around them'*. The argument wants us to focus on maintaining existing relationships "*face-to face'* in the real world, not via the internet.
A is irrelevant to the conclusion as the size of families isn't mentioned anywhere.
B is wrong because it would actually weaken the argument as it claims this "*face to face*" interaction can be done via the internet which is what the argument claims cannot happen sufficiently.
C is correct, it highlights the "*rise of the internet-connected smartphone*" and the problem that this has on society which is exactly what the argument does.
D is incorrect, like B that could be seen to weaken the argument as if robots could interact with humans like other humans this undermines the premise of the argument.

Q3	C

This is relatively straightforward, reading through each requirement allows us to eliminate our answers. The car needs to be picked up from the hotel at the beginning of the holiday, this eliminates Ashla. All cars can be dropped off at the airport so we can't eliminate further here. The car has to have a sunroof and air con so we can eliminate Bezza, Dega, and Fire as they do not contain both of these features. The car can't be above 1600cc but neither Cronal or Elox are above 1600cc so we can't eliminate further here. The car cannot cost more than $160 per day for 7 days of hire, so reading down the relevant column we can see that Elox costs $180 for 7-day hire whereas Cronal costs $150. Hence Cronal is the answer.

Q4	B

A is not true, the argument is centred around attacking the idea and has expanded heavily upon this subject so A can't be true. The people who came up with the idea are being "*attacked*" but so are the ideas.
B is correct; if the people who would have bought online now buy from physical stores instead then the number of sales across both types remains about the same. This means that companies will sell the same number of products and hence their profits will not go down. This best expresses the flaw in the argument.
C is wrong; it says that the "*economy will suffer ONLY if sales fall*". The argument does not say that the economy will only suffer if sales fall; nowhere in the argument does it narrow the possibility of the economy suffering down to this cause.
D is wrong because it seems odd to suggest that taxation wouldn't be the cause of decreased sales. Hence, although it could seem plausible it doesn't best characterise the flaw.

Q5	B

This question requires some visualisation. It may be a little tricky to understand but there is an alternative way to answer this question if visualisation doesn't come naturally to you. Look at the nets and identify what the faces are that we need to be concerned with: they are the ones with the arrows as this is the discriminatory factor between the nets. Now, in relation to the bottom face of the cuboid we can see that the ends of the arrows closest to the bottom face will be 1 arrowhead and 1 tail.
If we now go through A to D and look at the relation of the arrows to the bottom face on the nets we can see that A will fulfil having 1 arrow head and end closest to the bottom face; as will C and D. The only one that will not is B; it has 2 arrow ends instead. Hence B cannot possibly be correct as it can't be rotated or moved to produce the above configuration at all.

Q6	C

Statements A and B are both incorrect; the argument doesn't say it is "*impossible*" to measure the true value of a product; nor does it say there is "*no such thing*" as true value. Instead it says the value is "*hard to quantify*" which implies it exists and could be possible.
Statement C is correct; the passage states that the market price as a means of judging value "*is starting to break down with new technologies*" implying that we need to find alternatives.
Statement D is incorrect; the judgement that "*there are more serious costs to consider than merely financial ones*" isn't propagated by the passage at all. The passage simply suggests other costs but doesn't pass judgement on whether they are more serious.

Q7	E

This is rather straightforward; the question asks us to calculate the probability that a child actually has the disease given that they tested positive. So we need to calculate $\frac{true\ positive}{all\ positive\ test\ results} = \frac{72}{164}$ which is answer E.

Q8	E

A is not correct; at the end of the paragraph concerned with there being more men in senior roles (the second paragraph) the passage states '*discriminatory behaviour by employers might be partly responsible*'. This is not evidence of discrimination; it is evidence that suggests discrimination may be partly resposible.
B is wrong because the beginning of the third paragraph states otherwise: '*this did not mean that two thirds of the gap must be attributable to pay discrimination*'.
will provide greater evidence of discrimination'; the use of strong language with '*will*' is a red flag here.
D is wrong because as we saw earlier '*discriminatory behaviour by employers might be partly responsible*' and this disagrees with the notion that there is no evidence for the gender pay gap being partly the result of discrimination.
E is correct because this summarises the findings of the gender pay gap investigations; there may be discrimination and the extent isn't known.

Q9	D

If the gender pay gap in 2017 was 9.1% and the average weekly earnings were £550 per week we know that men would earn 9.1%/2 more than the average, and women would earn 9.1%/2 less than the average.
So, 9.1%/2 = 4.55% so a 4.55% decrease comes to 95.45% of £550 which comes to £524.98 which rounds to D.

Q10	H

If 1 and 3 were true, this would mean that women would have greater hourly earnings than men which we know is not true as they passage says they have less.
For 2 if women have shorter tenures, they will earn less than men so this is consistent with the passage.
For 4, if the logic of the statement is that a sorter tenure leads to greater income and that men have a shorter tenure in their jobs, this is correct as men having greater average earnings is consistent with the passage.

Q11	E

Immediately from looking at the figures we can see that women's earnings must have risen more than men's (the men's rise being 75% as stated in the question) in order to reduce the gender pay gap from 17.4% in 1997 to 9.4% in 2016. Hence, we can eliminate A, B and C.
We can tabulate the data to reflect the changes over time:

	Men	**Women**
1997 ***(gap was 17.4%)***	x	17.4% less than x which comes to 82.6% of x or $0.826x$
Change	Increase of 75%	We can now work out the percentage increase in women's earnings: $\frac{difference}{original} = \frac{1.5855x - 0.826x}{0.826x} = 92\%$
2016 ***(gap was 9.4%)***	$1.75x$	9.4% less than $1.75x$ = 90.6% of $1.75x$ = $1.5855x$

Q12	C

We know that the crossing takes 2 hours 30 mins and that the ferries need at least 1 hour to load and unload. This comes to 3 and a half hours. The closet difference between departure times from X and Y to the turnaround time is 3 hours 45 mins (e.g. 00:00 departure from X and a 03:45 departure from Y). We can see that by numbering the ferries departing from X from 1 to 5 only 5 ferries are needed as by the time 07:30 rolls around at X; ferry 1 has already made it back and is ready to travel again.
The table has been included in full as well; but as soon as you understand that 5 different ferries are needed before 1 can go again you have answered the question so do not feel as though you need to write corresponding numbers down the whole table! I have just included it for clarity.

Departures from X	Departures from Y
00:00 (1)	00:45 (4) - this will be the 4 from the previous day
01:30 (2)	02:15 (5) - this will be the 5 from the previous day
03:00 (3)	03:45 (1)
04:30 (4)	05:15 (2)
06:00 (5)	06:45 (3)
07:30 (1)	08:15 (4)
09:00 (2)	09:45 (5)
10:30 (3)	11:15 (1)
12:00 (4)	12:45 (2)
13:30 (5)	14:15 (3)
15:00 (1)	15:45 (4)
16:30 (2)	17:15 (5)
18:00 (3)	18:45 (1)
19:30 (4)	20:15 (2) - when this gets back to X it stays there until it departs at 01:30 the next day
21:00 (5)	21:45 (3) - when this gets back to X it stays there until it departs at 3:00 the next day
22:30 (1) - this ferry remains at X until departure at 00:00 the next day	23:15 (4) - this stays at Y for the 00:45 departure

Q13	B

The main conclusion of the passage is that the longer one spends drinking a coffee (which is dictated by coffee culture) the more expensive coffee is. This is exemplified with case studies from Greece, the UK and Italy.
A is wrong, *'the most significant cost is staff wages, though in fact that's not the key difference'* so this cannot be the main conclusion of the argument.
B is correct; it summarises the conclusion well.
C is wrong, although the information may be correct this is not the MAIN conclusion of the argument.
D is wrong, again although the information is correct this isn't the MAIN conclusion of the argument.
Although the difference may seem irritating, do remember the question asks for the MAIN conclusion meaning you may find it helpful to try and find the main conclusion before looking at the answers so you already have an idea of what you are looking for.

Q14	C

We can quickly eliminate Tuesday as we can see that there is already a very small pie wedge on the chart that can only be Tuesday. We can also eliminate Monday and Friday on the grounds that there are 80 and 70 sales respectively on these days and this is the closest interval between any 2 days; corresponding to the darkest pie wedge and the lightest pie wedge. There are no 2 other days that would be represented by these wedges in any case.
This leaves us with Wednesday and Thursday.
If Wednesday was removed, total sales would be 300 and the split would be 80:30:120:70. This is plausible as an option so far.
If Thursday was removed, total sales would be 280 and the split would be:
80:30:100:70. This can't be though; because taking the 70/280 portion we would expect a pie wedge that was exactly a quarter large; however, the pie in the diagram does not contain a quarter wedge. Hence, we can eliminate Thursday leaving Wednesday.

Q15	C

A is incorrect as the passage states indefinite hyperbolic numbers give a "*sense of size*" but this doesn't imply that they encourage exaggeration or rhetoric.
B is incorrect; nowhere in the passage is it suggested that indefinite hyperbolic numbers are misunderstood by native speakers.
C is correct; the statement rightly says that indefinite hyperbolic numbers are more *'rule-based than might be apparent at first sight'* referring to the *'language models that underpin the terms'*. This is a good summary of the conclusion of the passage.
D is incorrect; the passage does not make the inference at all that the language models are used unusually.

Q16	A

All those tested can be calculated easily by adding the top row: 50 + 50 + 200 + 150 = 450
Those who could read the bottom line are:
28% of 50 = 14
32% of 50 = 16
12% of 200 = 24
18% of 150 = 27
Totalling these gives 81.
Thus, the percentage of all those tested who can read the bottom line is 81/450 x 100 = 18% hence A is correct.

Q17	D

A, B and C all contain strong language that should be a red flag for you when you read through them.
A is wrong because the argument states that there can't be '*reliable evaluation of judgements'* but this does not make drawing conclusions impossible.
B is wrong because the argument does not assume this at all.
C is wrong because again the passage states there '*can be no reliable evaluations of judgements'* during the war so C cannot be true.
D is correct because it is a conditional statement that reflects the uncertainty and the unreliability of past events.

Q18	D

If Jasper's book bag capacity is 5 and the question asks what day he doesn't need to visit his locker at break time then we need to find the day where Jasper needs 5 books or less for the lessons until lunch (i.e. the first 3 lessons of the day).
On Monday he needs 3 for maths, 1 for English and 2 for history totalling 6.
On Tuesday he needs 1 for music, 2 for science and 3 for geography totalling 6.
On Wednesday he needs 3 for maths, 2 for history and 2 for science totalling 7.
On Thursday he needs 1 for music, 1 for English and 3 for maths totalling 5.
On Friday he needs 1 for art, 3 for geography and 2 for science totalling 6.
Hence Thursday is correct as this is the only day where his bag book capacity isn't exceeded by lunchtime.

Q19	D

Reading off the table, the Mirror average daily sales in 2018 were 583192.
From Figure 1 we can see that from 1992 to 2018 the Mirror had an 80% decrease in average daily sales. This means that the average daily sales in 2018 (583192) correspond to 20% of the average daily sales in 1992.
Hence the average daily sales in 1992 are equal to 5 x 583192 = 2915960 which is approximately 2.9 million.

Q20	C

Rounding to the nearest decimal place we can see the relationship over the years with time and average daily sales of the Mirror.

1995	2000	2005	2010	2015
-	2.3 million	1.7 million	1.2 million	0.9 million

Line 1 cannot be right as the drop from 2010 to 2015 as shown on the line compared to 2005-2010 is much steeper but the figures tell us that the drop should be steeper from 2005-2010 than 2010-2015 as there is a 0.5 million drop compared with a 0.3 million drop respectively.
Line 2 is wrong because the sales never increase as line 2 suggests they do.
Line 3 is correct because the intervals between the lines are equal and match the drop in numbers from our table above.
Line 4 is wrong because the drop from 2005-2010 and 2010-2015 line 4 suggests that the drop is consistent whereas the figures tell us that there is a 0.5 million drop then a 0.3 million drop; and these obviously aren't equal in magnitude.
Line 5 is wrong because there is no plateau in the figures at all; line 5 suggests the sales remained the same in 2000 and 2005 which we know is not the case.

Q21	D

The argument expressed in the second and third paragraphs is that newspapers have enormous ability to influence public opinion. We want to weaken this argument.
D is the only statement that does this because it directly attacks the notion of influence as it suggests the public just buy what they are already thinking and not that the newspaper has guided them to change their opinion.

Q22	B

Between 2017 and 2018 the combined sales of all papers fell from 6008137 to 5381969 which is a drop of 626168. The percentage decrease is therefore 626168/6008137 which is 10.4% and hence not between 11% and 12%. An easier way to do this maths is to consider that between 11% and 12% is roughly equal to 1/9 so if you calculate 1/9 of 6008137 you can see this comes to 667571 which is definitely bigger than 626168 hence the statement cannot be correct.
Statement 2 is correct. The total sales of the 5 pro-Leave newspapers (Mail, Star, Sun, Telegraph and Express) is 1589471 + 470369 + 1787096 + 472033 + 408700 = 4726969
Hence the percentage these newspapers accounted for out of total sales is
$\frac{4726969}{6303371} \times 100$ = 74.99% which is more than 70%.

Q23	D

We know that the numbers for the second diagram down on the question could either be 2, 3, or 7 as these are the only numbers that can form the pattern shown. Then we are told after the first 4 is scored there is no change in the pattern. This means we know the score was originally - - 3 and then went to - - 7 (as this is the only way you can add 4 with the digits 2/3/7).
Then we are told that after the first 6 was scored the pattern changed; this time with the middle number of the pattern changing. This tells us something, we know 7+6=13 so the score has to be - - 3; but the middle number has changed from either 2/3/7 to a number that could be 8/9/0 as shown by the pattern. Now, as the middle number will only have increased by 1 (as the score has only increased by 13) sp the only possibility is that 7 went to 8 as these are consecutive. So, the score now is -83. We are told it doesn't change for the next 4 and 6, and this makes sense. -87 and -97 will look the same on the pattern. However, on the next 6 we know that 97+6=103 so the first digit will increase by 1 and will be -03. As it started at 2/3/7 and still doesn't change pattern we know the first digit has gone from a 2 to a 3. So, the score is 303.

Q24	B

The passage states, '*it provides a good example of convergent evolution*' and '*to demonstrate that this is an example of convergent evolution*'. The majority of the passage is concerned with exemplifying convergent evolution in cuckoos, cowbirds and honeyguides hence why B is correct.

Q25	E

1 is incorrectly Nicola could have bought 8 Venus bars which would've come to £2.40.
2 is incorrect; again, by buying 8 Venus bars Nicola has not bought a single Flaky bar.
3 is incorrect again as Nicola could have bought 8 Venus bars.
4 is incorrect; Nicola could have 2 of each type of bar; 2 x 30p + 2 x 40p + 2 x 50p = £2.40.
Hence E is correct.

Q26	C

1 is incorrect; although swimming has had a relatively high number of new work records over the past few decades the passage does not allude to this continuing into the future.
2 is incorrect; the passage does not allude to this at all; it only focuses on technological developments but does not pass the judgement that as a result natural ability no longer matters that much in racing.
3 is correct; the passage is focussed around exemplifying the technological advancements in swimming that can shave off times from races such as '*swimsuits that create less resistance*'.

Q27	D

This is a long and difficult question so to save time come back to it at the end if you can. We can ignore the final 2 columns of the table, because no combination with these would give us the minimum amount possible (nor anything that is in the answers).
The Times has to be included and we need 2 printed newspapers a week. It would be sensible to recognise that as you go down the table the prices increase for both printed and digital copies. Hence, if we have to include the Times we want to include Dispatch and Express as well to come to our 3 newspapers per week as these are the 2 other cheapest newspapers.
The cost of 1 printed newspaper per week for a year for each of the 3 newspapers is as follows:
Dispatch: 52 x £1 = £52
Express: 52 x £0.80 = £41.60
Times: 52 x £1.50 = £78
The cost of the tablets is £30 and £20 respectively for Dispatch and Express. We can infer then that the Times shouldn't be bought for online and tablet use because £60 alone is more than the cost for Dispatch and Express together!
Thus, the Times will be printed and we know this will cost £78.
We need 1 other printed copy, so the next cheapest is the Express which cost us £41.60. Thus, we can now pick the online and tablet option for the 3rd newspaper as it will be cheaper and we have fulfilled the requirements of the question so we will pick Dispatch's subscription for £30.

The final combination is summarised below:
A printed Times copy once a week = 52 x £1.50 = £78
A printed Express copy (as it is the cheapest) = £0.80 x 52 = £41.60
Dispatch online and tablet: £30
Adding these gives £149.60 which is D.

Q28	E

1 is correct as it is a flaw in the reasoning as the passage states '*following the state's recent legalisation of marijuana, the rates of murder and of violent crime overall increased*' which perfectly summarises the assumption that the rise in crime was caused by the legalisation as opposed to something else.
2 is wrong, the problems associated with other substances that are already legal is not the focus of the passage; the beginning of the passage states that the subject is '*legalising previously illegal substances*'.
3 is correct. The passage states '*for evidence of such effects, we need only look to Colorado in the USA*' and this immediately narrows the focus of the claim to one area so 3 rightly points out that Colorado as 1 place is not representative enough to conclude that drug legalisation has negative effects.

2019 Section 1

Q29	A

It is important here to read the question, '*which of the statements, taken independently, COULD be true?*'. This means we need to consider each in turn and find a scenario where they could be true.
Well, for 1 It could be that 30% only use the climbing wall, 10% use the climbing wall and swim, and 60% only swim. This is a possibility that fits with statement 1 as well as the information in the question.
For 2, it is entirely plausible that all of the members either swim, climb or do both because in 1 we have seen that this was possible.
For 3, at least half of those who climb comes to at least 20%. If 70% of the members use the swimming pool, this leaves 30% of members who don't swim and hence the 20% who climb but never swim < 30% who never swim so this is entirely possible.

Q30	C

We cannot infer A from the passage; we just know women are using self-help baby books.
B is wrong because the passage doesn't state that this is the case at all.
C is correct; the passage states, '*most of the mothers in the study had used routine-led baby manuals that advise others to implement routines of feeding and sleeping, implying that such routines are easy to establish*'. This implies that some of the mothers experienced difficulty establishing these routines for their babies.
D is incorrect; we do not know that this is the case; although there seems to be a correlation with depressive symptoms, this is one facet of harm and the good that these books bring is not known either, so comments like this cannot be inferred from the information given to us.

Q31	F

The largest amount you could sell shares for would be if you buy them on the day they are worth the least (day 5) and sell them on the day they are worth the most (day 7 or 8). So if £6000 worth are bought on day 5, this equate to £6000/£0.15 = 40,000 shares. Selling these shares for £0.30 each on day 7 or 8 makes £0.30 x 40,000 = £12,000.
The smallest amount you could sell shares for would be if you buy them on the interval with the largest drop: this could be from Day 2 to Day 5 or day 8 to day 10. However, we will make less money in the first case (hence why we will look at this interval) because the share price is lower all-round on this interval.
So, buying £6000 worth of shares on day 2 gives £6000/£0.25 = 24,000 shares. Selling these on day 5 for £0.15 each gives £0.15 x 24,000 = £3600.
So, the difference between the largest and smallest amounts you could sell the shares for is: £12,000 - £3600 = £8400 hence F is correct.

Q32	C

Reading off the graph we can see that the lowest risk of dementia corresponds to the smallest hazard ratio, and this is at approximately 0.6; and the corresponding alcohol units consumed per week is 6.

Q33	A

B is incorrect; the study defines the region where the hazard of developing dementia increases as over 14 units of alcohol a week, not 40.
C is wrong, the study has already said that it is investigating how the risk of dementia varies with drinking and not drinking in middle age, so it doesn't need to consider other health risks.
D is wrong, the study has stated clearly that '*we don't know about their drinking habits earlier in adulthood, and it is possible that this may contribute to their later life dementia risk*'. Hence they haven't assumed this, they have just pointed out the limitation of their own study.
E is wrong, the study doesn't assume this is the case, it just comments on the risk of developing dementia.
A is correct; the conclusion of the passage is in the first sentence as the question points out, but this conclusion has been drawn from a study done on 10308 civil servants. This has not taken into account other occupations, hence there has been an assumption that the relationship between alcohol and dementia risk doesn't vary with occupation in order to make the conclusion the author has.

Q34	B

Drinking 3 glasses of wine a day means per week 21 glasses are drunk. As 7 glasses = 14 units this means 21 glasses is 42 units. Reading the hazard score for 42 units of alcohol from the graph gives us a hazard score of 1.5.
We know from the ratio given in the passage that:
$hazard\ score = \frac{proportion\ of\ participants\ consuming\ 42\ units\ per\ week\ who\ go\ on\ to\ develop\ dementia}{proportion\ of\ participants\ consuming\ 14\ units\ per\ week\ who\ go\ on\ to\ develop\ dementia}$ and we want to find the numerator because that is what the question asks for.
The question also tells us that 40% of the study cohort (i.e. 40% of 10308 = 4123.2) consumed 14 units of alcohol a week and of them 80 went on to develop dementia. This tells us that the denominator is 80/4123.2 x 100 = 1.94%
Solving for the numerator gives:

$$1.5 = \frac{proportion\ of\ participants\ consuming\ 42\ units\ per\ week\ who\ go\ on\ to\ develop\ dementia}{1.94\%}$$

So the numerator = 2.91% which rounds to 3%.

Q35	C

The question wants to undermine the claim of the passage; so we need something that would support the notion that drinking in mid-life causes the same risk of developing dementia as heavy drinking.

A is wrong, it would actually support the claim of the report as the abstainers (i.e. those who don't drink in mid-life) would become heavy drinkers later on in life which would carry a greater risk of developing dementia.

B is wrong, it doesn't undermine the claim made because it just shows that heavy drinking can lead to development of health problems (which could include dementia) but the abstinence that follows doesn't negate the damage done in terms of increasing the risk of developing dementia.

C is correct; it undermines the claim because where the claim argues that heavy drinking increases the risk of developing dementia, C states that this claim can't be made, because people were more likely to die from alcohol-related causes before they had the chance to develop dementia so this measurement is not really possible. If many of the heavy drinkers were to die before being able to develop dementia, then this would push up the proportion of the population with dementia who abstained from alcohol in mid-life, and therefore the figures would be misleading, and so would undermine the claim.

D is wrong, it does not actually say what the effect of '*mentally astute*' people controlling their drinking consumption in mid-life is on the risk of dementia in later life.

2019 Section 2

Q1	E

W is a section on a chromosome as shown by the picture; and a section on a chromosome is known as a gene. We can eliminate A, B, C and D alone from this.
X is a restriction enzyme because the diagram shows the enzyme cutting the gene from the chromosome and again cutting the DNA on the plasmid and these cutting games are called restriction enzymes.
Y is a plasmid which is the circular piece of DNA into which our sample DNA is inserted. Y cannot be a bacterium because the gene must be inserted into the coding region of the bacterium which is the plasmid.
Z is ligase because this is the enzyme that essentially "sticks" the sticky ends of the gene in the same DNA to the plasmid DNA.

Q2	C

$CaCO_3$ is a fairly insoluble base. This means in order to be removed we need to add acid as this will allow us to do the following reaction:
metal carbonate + acid = metal salt + CO_2 + H_2O
This is a neutralisation reaction so the cleaning solution must be acidic in order to react with a base, so Statement 1 is correct.
Statement 2 is wrong, as we can see from the word equation the only gas produced is CO_2 not H_2.
Statement 3 is wrong as well because this is a neutralisation reaction so the pH of the reacting solution (which we know is acidic to begin with so must have a low pH) must end at around 7 (pH neutral). This is an increase in pH not a decrease.
Statement 4 is correct, $CaCO_3$ as we know from the question isn't very soluble as '*it can't be removed with water alone*' and the point of a cleaner is to dissolve the offending substance on the surface so it can be wiped away. This means the salt produced will be more soluble than $CaCO_3$.

Q3	B

We can calculate the resultant force of the cyclist using F = ma where F = 50kg x 4.0ms^{-2} = 200N (we are given the mass and acceleration figures in the question).
Taking the direction of acceleration as positive we know that the Resultant force (right across the paper) = 600N (the forward force produced by the cyclist and the bicycle) - the resistive forces against the cyclist and bicycle (300N + air resistance).
Hence 200N = 600N - (300N + air resistance)
So 200N = 600N - 300N - air resistance
So air resistance = 600N - 300N - 200N = 100N hence B is correct.

Q4	B

The equation in the question tells us:

$$p + q = 3(p - q)$$

Expanding and collecting like terms gives the following:

$$p + q = 3p - 3q$$
$$4q = 2p$$
$$2q = p$$

We can then substitute the p in the equation the question asks us to solve:

$\frac{pq}{p^2 + q^2} = \frac{2q(q)}{(2q)^2 + q^2} = \frac{2q^2}{5q^2} = \frac{2}{5}$ hence the answer is B.

2019 Section 2

Q5	A

We know that shading represents passive processes therefore areas of no shading (i.e. all of 1) must be active. This means that 1 has to always be active as everything in its section is active. This also means 2 and 3 must be passive because they don't overlap with the non-shaded section. By looking down the column for 1, we can eliminate C, D, and E for being passive.
Going down column 2 we can eliminate D, E, and F for being active.
Going down column 3 we can eliminate B, C, E, and G for being active.
This only leaves A.

Q6	D

We can actually eliminate C straight away because neither of the electrodes are a copper rod and the question tells us the electroplating requires a copper rod.
Looking at the cathode column first, we know reduction (gain of electrons) goes on here. As we want to electroplate a copper rod with silver the reduction equation at the anode must therefore be $Ag^+ + e^- = Ag$ so we can already eliminate B, C and E as reduction at the cathode must be taking place on a copper rod.
But we need to obtain the Ag^+ from somewhere so at the anode where oxidation takes place the equation must be $Ag = Ag^+ + e^-$. This means that the anode must be a silver rod that is oxidised. Hence, we can eliminate B, C, E and F.
This leaves A and D. Looking at the electrolyte, we have copper nitrate versus silver nitrate. The electrolyte is the aqueous solution of the ions that are travelling and we know that Ag^+ will need to be travelling here hence why the answer is D.

Q7	C

We know density = mass/volume
We can calculate mass from the difference of the masses from the electronic balance. Hence 950g - 750g = 200g
We can calculate volume from the displacement caused when object X is placed into the measuring cylinder. The displacement is the reading from diagram 2 - reading from diagram 1. This comes to $500cm^3 - 375cm^3 = 125cm^3$ hence density = $200g/125cm^3$ which is $1.6gcm^{-3}$.

Q8	E

We can first write all terms in full by expanding the standard form:

$$\sqrt{\frac{600+400}{0.012+0.004}} = \sqrt{\frac{640}{0.016}}$$

Then we can rewrite the numerator and denominator as square numbers (as this is convenient to square root) and we can do so by writing them back in standard form:

$$\sqrt{\frac{64\times10^{1}}{19\times10^{-3}}} = \frac{8\times10^{1/2}}{4\times10^{-3/2}} = 2\times10^{1/2--3/2} = 2\times10^{2} = 200$$

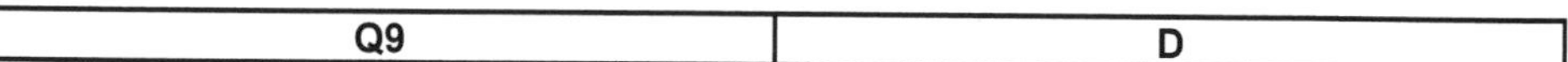

Q9	D

Statement 1 is incorrect because the graph shows that the rate of respiration of the lizard decreases as temperature decreases and this is a direct proportional relationship; not an inverse one.
Statement 2 is incorrect; there is no proof the lizard is only respiring aerobically; anaerobic respiration in lizards produces lactic acid which isn't being measured here so for all we know some anaerobic respiration could be taking place.
Statement 3 is correct because as we know from chemistry, the test for the presence of CO_2 is a white precipitate forming when CO_2 is bubbled through limewater.

Q10	H

Statement 1 is correct; the reactivity of the Group 1 metals increases as you go down the group because the outer electrons are less strongly attracted electrostatically to the positive nucleus and thus are easier to lose.
Statement 2 is correct because all groups are named so because they have the same number of outer electrons in their highest energy level.
Statement 3 is also correct; we know oxidation is the loss of electrons and as you go down the group (as mentioned above) the outer electrons are further away from the nucleus and thus experience weaker electrostatic forces of attraction so the electrons are more easily lost.
This is a relatively straightforward recall question, so you just need to remember what you have already learnt from your science notes.

Q11	C

The smaller sphere will have a positive charge because if the electrons have flowed from the sphere to the earth as they are repelled by the large sphere (as we are told in the question) this leaves a positive charge on the sphere itself because electrons are negatively charged.
The larger sphere is still negatively charged as shown in the diagram so there must be fewer protons than electrons as this produces a negative charge.

Q12	H

The gradient can be expressed by the following formula where we can input the coordinates of M and N:
$\frac{y2-y1}{x2-x1}=\frac{2-(3p-1)}{1-p-6}=\frac{2-3p+1}{1-p-6}=\frac{3-3p}{-p-5}=-3$(as we are told in the question)
Solving for p gives the following:

$$3p+15 = 3-3p$$
$$6p = -12$$
$$p = -2$$

If we substitute our p value into the coordinates (using M as an example here) we find that M becomes (6,-7) and can be represented by$y = mx + c$ as $-7 = -3(6) + r$
So r = 11

Q13	H

Amino acids, cellulose and lipids all contain carbon firstly and secondly are all consumed by a wide range of animals including humans. They can all be used as forms of respiratory substrates so are all involved in producing CO_2, they can all be eaten and digested by animals and when animals decay the carbon can remain in fossils. Essentially, there are so many ways each of these 3 molecules are involved with the carbon cycle.

2019 Section 2

Q14	A

The first thing to see from the graph is that Y has a faster rate of reaction than X as its curve is steeper initially. However, Y produces ⅘ of the product that X does as observed by counting how many squares up on the y axis product is produced (measured as total volume of oxygen gas).
The second thing to do is to work out how many moles of hydrogen peroxide are used for experiment X. moles = volume x concentration = 50 x 10^{-3} x 0.1 = 0.005 moles.
Thus, if curve Y produces ⅘ of the product it follows that the amount of hydrogen peroxide used initially is ⅘ of that for X, hence ⅘ of 0.005 = 0.004 moles.
Working from A to E, we can calculate the number of moles of hydrogen peroxide and see which one matches 0.004 moles that we know would produce the graph shown.
A produces 0.004 moles, hence is correct. B produces 0.005 moles. C produces 0.005 moles. D produces 0.002 moles. E produces 0.005 moles.
Looking at the table, we would expect the manganese (VI) oxide to be a powder because the increased surface area would increase the rate of reaction hence why A is correct.

Q15	F

A is incorrect, it is transverse waves that travel at the same speed (only in a vacuum); longitudinal waves can travel at different speeds.
B is wrong, longitudinal waves cause vibrations that are parallel to the direction of energy transfer.
C is wrong, sound waves are longitudinal.
D is wrong, longitudinal waves could travel faster than transverse ones if the conditions were correct.
E is incorrect; although all EM waves are transverse this doesn't mean all transverse waves are EM.
F is correct; ultrasonic waves are a type of sound wave and are therefore longitudinal.
G is wrong, ultraviolet waves are a type of EM wave so are transverse.
H is wrong, X-rays are EM waves so can travel in a vacuum.
This question is purely testing factual recall so make sure to revise physics knowledge thoroughly.

Q16	D

We know 1 side of the rectangle is $(7-\sqrt{5})$ so we can call the other side x. If the rectangle area is 66cm^2 this means $x = \frac{66}{7-\sqrt{5}}$(as the area of a rectangle is the product of the 2 different side lengths) but we will rationalise this fraction first to eliminate a surd from the denominator by multiplying the fraction by $\frac{7+\sqrt{5}}{7+\sqrt{5}}$:
$\frac{66}{7-\sqrt{5}} \times \frac{7+\sqrt{5}}{7+\sqrt{5}} = \frac{66(7+\sqrt{5})}{49-5} = \frac{66(7+\sqrt{5})}{44}$ and at this point we can see that 66 and 44 will cancel to 3/2 so we end up with:
$\frac{3(7+\sqrt{5})}{2} = x$
The perimeter will be expressed by $2x + 2(7-\sqrt{5})$ so substituting our x in gives:
$\frac{2\times 3(7+\sqrt{5})}{2} + 14 - 2\sqrt{5} = 3(7+\sqrt{5}) + 14 - 2\sqrt{5} = 35 + \sqrt{5}$ hence D is the answer.

Q17	D

If the pea plant is heterozygous for seed colour it must have the genotype Yy so we can already eliminate 3 and 5 as these don't contain any alleles.
If the pea plant is homozygous for seed shape it must be either RR or rr so we can eliminate 1, 3 and 6 for being heterozygous.
This leaves 2, 4 and 7 as possibilities hence D is correct.

Q18	E

We can work out the moles of MnO_4^- ions reacting using the information in the question; moles = concentration x volume = 0.05 x 10 x 10^{-3} (we have converted the cm^3 to dm^3 as all the answers use these units) = 0.0005 moles.
As the ratio of reacting moles of MnO_4^- : Fe^{2+} is 1:5 this means the reacting moles of Fe^{2+} is 5 times that of MnO_4^- which comes to 5 x 0.0005 = 0.0025 moles.
Thus the concentration of Fe^{2+} = moles/volume = 0.0025/25 x 10^{-3} (we are told this volume in the question; I have again converted it to dm^3).
It may be helpful to convert the numerator into standard form:
$\frac{25 \times 10^{-4}}{25 \times 10^{-3}} = 1 \times 10^{-1}$ hence why E is correct.

Q19	A

The question tells us that the initial EM radiation was in the form of gamma-rays and that now, we are in the microwave region of the spectrum. This means the wavelength of the radiation waves has increased and the frequency of the waves has decreased.
You should be able to work this out from your knowledge of how wavelength and frequency trends change across the EM spectrum. This means statement 1 and 2 are incorrect. 3 is incorrect regardless of the question because wavelength and frequency are always inversely proportional and not directly proportional.

2019 Section 2

Q20	E

We can represent this information in a tree diagram. To work out the probability that the bus

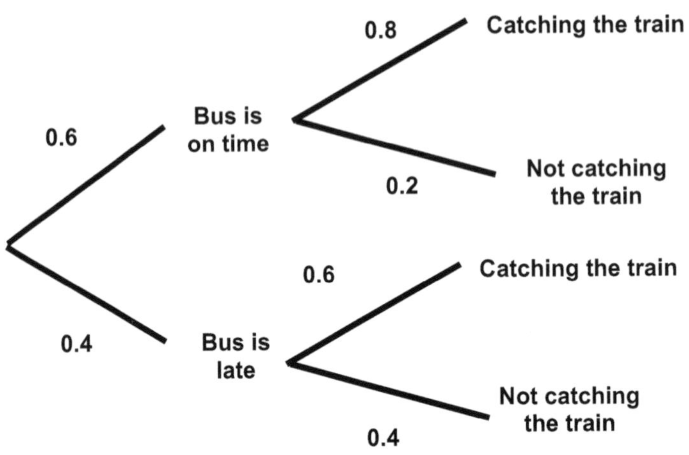

was on time given that Sylvie catches the train.

This means we are working out: $\frac{P(bus\ was\ on\ time\ and\ Sylvie\ caught\ the\ train)}{P(Sylvie\ caught\ the\ train)}$

P(Sylvie caught the train) is the multiple of going along the branches ending in Sylvie catching the train: 0.6(0.8) + 0.4(0.6) = 0.72

P(bus was on time and Sylvie caught the train) = 0.6(0.8) = 0.48

0.48/0.72 = 2/3

Q21	B

Statement 1 is correct; 500 base pairs will code for a maximum of 166 amino acids. We know that 3 base pairs can code for 1 amino acid and 500/3 to the nearest whole number is 166.

Statement 2 is wrong; a mature red blood cell has no nucleus therefore contains no chromosomes.

Statement 3 is wrong because adenine is complementary to thymine (not guanine as the question implies) so the number of A bases = the number of T bases and A doesn't necessarily equal G.

Q22	D

We can eliminate A and C on the grounds that these are not straight-chain alkanes as they have the wrong formula. The general formula of an alkane is C_nH_{2n+2} which A and C do not correspond to.

We also know that molar gas volumes mean that 1 mole of any gas at a given temperature takes up the same volume. As 105cm^3 of CO_2 is produced relative to 35cm^3 of the alkane we can see that CO_2 is produced in a 3:1 ratio to the alkane being combusted (as 105/35 = 3). This means that for every 1 alkane molecule combusted, 3 CO_2 molecules are formed. This implies that the alkane must have a multiple of 3 number of carbons in it, so the only options could be C and D but C has been eliminated already hence why D is the answer.

Q23	A

Momentum = mass x velocity which is 400kg x $15ms^{-1}$ as we are told in the question per nozzle. This comes to 6000 kg ms^{-1} so we can eliminate all options other than A and B.
The force ejected by each nozzle can be worked out using F = ma.
The mass we are told is 400kg per nozzle.
The acceleration can be worked out as a = v-u/t = 15-0/12 = 15/12 = 1.25 ms^{-2}
This means F = 400(1.25) = 500N. Remember though, we just worked out the force of 1 nozzle, but the jet pack has 2 nozzles, so we need to double our answer giving 1000N.

Q24	H

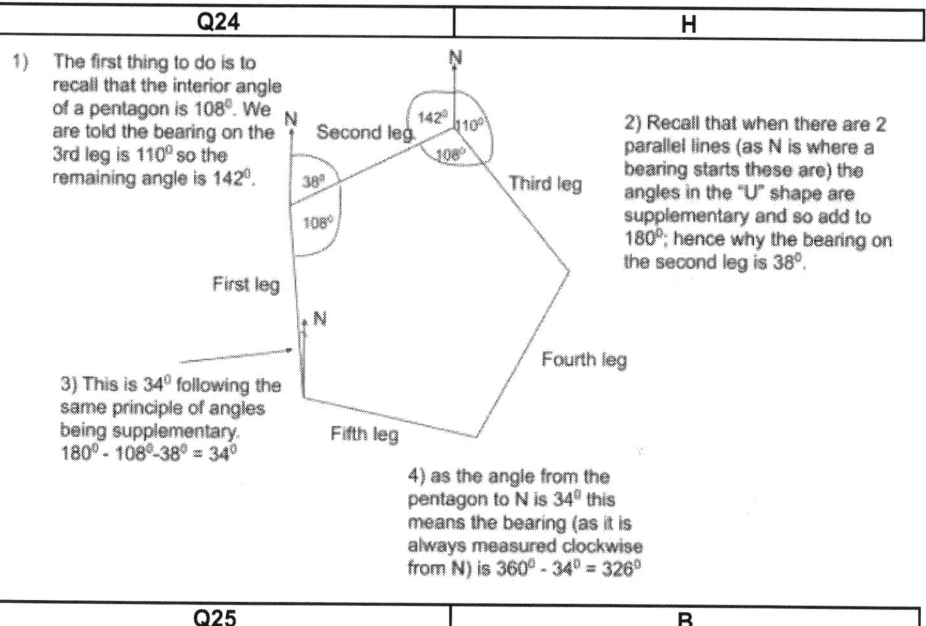

Q25	B

If large protein is present in urine this means there has been a problem with ultrafiltration in the kidney because only very small molecules of water, salts, urea, amino acids, and glucose are supposed to be ultrafiltrated. Hence statement 1 is the only correct statement because damage to cell membranes between the blood vessels and the Bowman's capsule means that larger proteins could pass through the damaged membrane and enter the filtrate. It is the only statement relevant to problems with ultrafiltration.

Statement 2 is wrong because problems with active transport and selective reabsorption are to do with the small molecules mentioned earlier not with proteins; if there were these problems there wouldn't be large proteins in urine, there may be an imbalance of salts and urea instead.

Statement 3 is incorrect because it is concerned with the concentration of the urine based on how much water is reabsorbed and is not to do with the presence of protein in urine.

Q26	E

The options for how diborane can be made as are follows:
$^{10}B^{10}BH_6$ giving Mr 26. The probability is 20% x 20% = 0.2 x 0.2 = 0.04
$^{10}B^{11}BH_6$ and $^{11}B^{10}BH_6$ each giving Mr 27. The probability is 2 lots of 20% x 80% = 2 x 0.2 x 0.8 = 0.32
$^{11}B^{11}BH_6$ giving Mr 28. The probability of this one is 80% x 80% = 0.8 x 0.8 = 0.64.
So the ratio of Mrs of 26:27:28 in terms of their probability is as follows:
4:32:64 which simplifies to 1:8:16 so E is correct.

Q27	B

Recall the equation relating voltage to the number of turns on coils in a transformer:
$\frac{Vs}{Vp}=\frac{Ns}{Np}$ Inputting the information in the question and solving for the voltage in the secondary coil (the output voltage) gives:
$\frac{x}{240}=\frac{100}{400}$ so $x = 60V$ meaning we can eliminate E, F, G and H.
Secondly, we can work out the input current as because the transformer is 100% efficient, we can use the equation: $V_pI_p=V_sI_s$ so 240V x I_p = 60V x 2.0A so I_p = 60 x 2/240 = 0.5A.
This eliminates C and D.
Output power can be calculated using P = IV where I and V are both at the secondary coil.
Hence P = 2 x 60 = 120W hence B is the answer.

2019 Section 3

To see the marking grid and mark bands that the BMAT examiners will use to mark your essays, please refer to the BMAT website.

'People are often motivated to deny the existence of problems if they disagree with the solutions to those problems.'

Explain what you think is meant by the statement.

This statement gets at the problem of disagreeing with something because dealing with it will have knock on effects that are undesirable to a person. An example of this is those who deny the existence of global warming as a problem. They may be motivated to disagree on the grounds that the solution to problems like global warming may include a carbon tax or major restructuring of lots of industries to make them sustainable - all of which creates huge chaos and costs money. If the individual disagrees with the solutions, then like the statement says, they may be motivated to deny the existence of a global warming problem in the first place.

Present a counterargument.

Almost every day people disagree with solutions to problems that they acknowledge exist and a clear example of this is the House of Commons. Some MPs would agree there is a lack of transport connecting the North of England to the South, but many would disagree with the HS2 rail project that has been planned to solve the problem. They may argue that it is not cost-effective, it causes environmental damage and runs very close to some people's homes which is unfair and undesirable.

To what extent do you agree with the statement?

You might like to argue that the statement is difficult to agree with given the ambiguity about the solutions to these problems. It implies that solutions do indeed exist, and it doesn't provide clarity on whether the person disagrees with all the solutions presented, or just some of them.
Alternatively you may align your views with this statement and appreciate the sentiment that it proposes which is that we ought to be more open-minded and not simply dismiss the existence of problems because we don't like the solutions as this will probably lead to the problem growing and causing more damage.

2019 Section 3

'In science, there are no universal truths, just views of the world that have yet to be shown to be false.' (*Brian Cox and Jeff Forshaw*)

Explain what you think is meant by the statement.

This statement means that we as humans cannot judge anything to be absolutely true but that our advancements to date stand as long as we haven't refuted them yet. In a sense, it is a sort of via negativa; we can say nothing positively about scientific truths, but we can show possibilities to be false. For example, when talking about enzymes and the induced fit hypothesis, we cannot claim this is a universal truth, we can only show that an alternative hypothesis such as the lock and key hypothesis isn't absolutely true; so we are narrowing the net of an infinite number of possibilities.

Argue that scientists need to accept some things as 'truths' to advance their understanding.

- If scientists were sceptical about all universal truths it would make lots of work and advancement incredibly difficult within the field. For example, if scientists didn't accept the truth of the Newtonian laws of physics as universal, how could they ever carry out reliable investigations into any form of motion if they weren't convinced that the motion could be explained by these laws?
- If scientists couldn't accept knowledge of atomic structure and reactivity as universal truths, then how could they manufacture drugs and be confident that those who take the drugs would see a benefit?
- To doubt all of these means a scientist limits the scope of what they can investigate and in our world of empirical data and checks and balances this isn't particularly useful for progression.

To what extent do you agree with the statement?

- You might like to express sympathy for the statement and take the view that as humans we really cannot judge whether something is a universal truth; hence there can be none for us. We are mortal beings that have our perception of the world and this perception could be faulty or incomplete so we cannot be arbiters of truth in this sense. An appreciation of this, you could argue, is integral to science because it shows an awareness of the inherent limitation of investigation.
- However, you may equally like to comment on the practicality of such a statement; while seeming noble and robust on the outside, how useful is it for our lives and for scientists themselves? It is all very well having an appreciation of the truth of the statement, but maybe you will argue that it needs to be overlooked in many situations to allow progress to be made to allow hypothesising that rests upon universal truths to take place and to allow investigation under the laws of the universe to take place.

Authors' tip: (*for q3*)

These sorts of questions give you the opportunity to show off your knowledge of recent medical advancements - make sure you include them in your answer, for example, here robotic surgery would be good.

'Teamwork is more important for surgical innovation than the skills of an individual surgeon.'

Explain the reasoning behind this statement.

Surgical innovation refers to advancement in surgical procedure or technology, whereas teamwork refers to the collaboration between different professionals (to aid surgery). The reasoning behind this statement is that collaboration and cooperation between different professionals, whether that be doctors, nurses, physicists, lab technicians etc, will have a greater impact on advancements in surgery than the abilities of an individual surgeon, potentially because surgical technique is already relatively refined, whereas there are always going to be advancements in technology.

Arguments for why teamwork is more important.

- Teamwork between for example engineers/physicists and medical professionals can lead to improved surgical technology, which can make surgeries safer, more efficient and cheaper. For example, keyhole surgery and the cameras used was developed through collaboration, which has allowed surgery to advance.
- Teamwork between different minded individuals can allow for quicker innovation, as ideas come from different people, who may look at a certain surgery/technique in a different way, which could indeed be beneficial.
- Collaboration between different surgeons (e.g. in MDT meetings), can lead to new surgeries being developed.

Argue that the skills of individual surgeons are more important for surgical innovation or progress.

- The surgeon is ultimately the individual performing the surgery, so improvements in his skills will overall lead to the greatest surgical innovation, for example if he/she develops a new technique.
- Surgery is an extremely delicate process, so individual skill may be far more important than teamwork between professionals, as it is ultimately the skill that will be improving the patient's life.
- In history, many surgical innovations were based on surgical skills. E.g. Robert F Spetzler developed the 'standstill surgical procedure', which has led to innovation in neurosurgery, especially treating brain aneurysms.
- Surgeons have the most responsibility so can be argued to be the most important in a surgery, so can be argued that his skills allow surgical innovation to progress the most.

To what extent do you agree with the statement?

Surgery is a complex matter, and has many different aspects, and therefore both teamwork and surgical skills of the surgeon are both important in allowing surgery to advance. However, in the modern world, it can be argued that teamwork between different fields and different professionals is becoming more important as technological advancements are what is driving current surgical innovation, for example robotic surgeries. Perhaps what may be more important than identifying the most important cause of surgical innovation, is ensuring that this surgical innovation is equitably shared across the world, and that surgical innovation focuses not only on improving quality of life, but on widening access to life-saving surgeries, for example in rural areas in the less developed world.

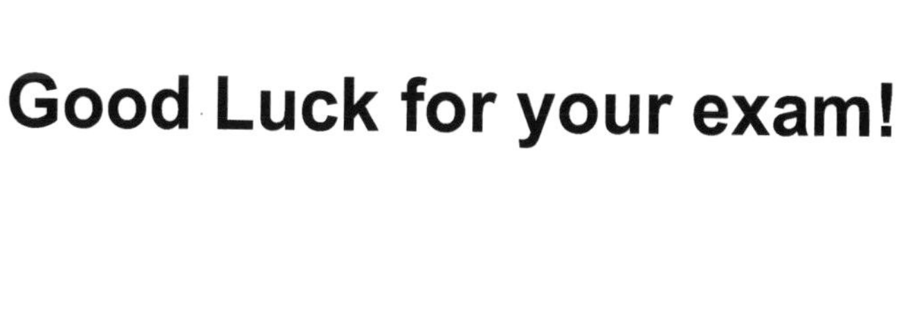
Good Luck for your exam!

For more information and advice about BMAT preparation please email:

bmatbook@gmail.com